Differential Diagnosis for Non-Medical Prescribers, Nurses and Pharmacists

A CASE-BASED APPROACH

Differential Diagnosis for Non-Medical Prescribers, Nurses and Pharmacists

A CASE-BASED APPROACH

PAUL RUTTER, PhD

Professor in Pharmacy Practice

School of Pharmacy and Biomedical Sciences

University of Portsmouth, Portsmouth, United Kingdom

ELSEVIER

Notices

Practitioners and researchers must always rely on their own experience and knowledge in evaluating and using any information, methods, compounds or experiments described herein. Because of rapid advances in the medical sciences, in particular, independent verification of diagnoses and drug dosages should be made. To the fullest extent of the law, no responsibility is assumed by Elsevier, authors, editors or contributors for any injury and/or damage to persons or property as a matter of products liability, negligence or otherwise, or from any use or operation of any methods, products, instructions, or ideas contained in the material herein.

ISBN: 978-0-443-11604-9

Printed in India
Last digit is the print number: 9 8 7 6 5 4 3 2 1

Content Strategist: Alexandra Mortimer
Content Project Manager: Abdus Salam Mazumder
Design: Brian Salisbury
Marketing Manager: Deborah Watkins

Working together
to grow libraries in
developing countries

www.elsevier.com • www.bookaid.org

Demand on healthcare professionals to deliver high quality patient care has never been greater. A multitude of factors impinge on healthcare delivery today, including an aging population, more sophisticated medicines, high patient expectations, health service infrastructure as well as adequate and appropriate staffing levels. In primary care, the medical practitioner's role is still central in providing this care, but shifting the workload from secondary to primary care is placing greater demands on their time, resulting in new models of service delivery.

This shift is leading to a break down of the traditional boundaries of care between doctors and other allied health professionals. In particular, certain activities once seen as medical practitioner responsibility, are now being routinely performed by nurses and pharmacists as their scope of practice expands.

The expansion of these roles has been supported by allowing non-medical practitioners to become prescribers. First recommended by Baroness Cumberlege in 1986, nurses (and latterly pharmacists and other non-medical practitioners) were allowed to prescribe from a limited formulary. However, in approximately 2006, independent prescribing rights were given, meaning a non-medical prescriber could, in theory, prescribe on a par with a doctor. Since that time the number of people training to hold such a qualification has markedly increased, especially in the last 10 years. For example, 25% (15,000) of pharmacists and 8% (60,000) of nurses were prescribers in 2023. Approximately one in three GP primary care practices and one in four hospitals and outpatient services now utilise non-medical prescribers.

In primary care, it is now commonplace for patients to be seen by a non-medical prescriber, rather than a doctor, for the treatment of both acute and long-term conditions. Research suggests that patients are broadly accepting of this shift in care, and the care received is safe and effective. The management of acute presentations in primary care is the focus of this book as many non-medical practitioners perform a triage role.

It is hoped that presenting conditions as cases will help foster clinical reasoning and support those training to be non-medical prescribers and those new in post to have greater confidence in making better decisions.

I would like to thank the people who took the time to read and sense check the cases – you know who you are!

Image courtesy for images used on the book cover:

Subconjunctival Haemorrhage. [From: Krachmer, J. H. & Paley, D. A. (2014). *Cornea Atlas* (3rd ed.). Saunders.]

Herpetic Gingivostomatitis. [From James, W. D. et al. (2016). *Andrews' diseases of the skin* (12th ed.). Philadelphia, Saunders.]

Impetigo Contagiosa. [From: Weston, W. L., Lane, A. T., & Morelli, J. G. (2007). *Color textbook of pediatric dermatology* (4th ed.). St. Louis, MO: Mosby.]

I would like to dedicate this book to my Dad. Sadly, he died Christmas 2023, just as I was finishing this book. Dad was always keen to know what I was doing, and he was amused to know that one of the cases was based on him.

HOW TO USE THE BOOK

The focus of this case study book is to utilise the principles of clinical reasoning as outlined in Chapter 1. The book covers 50 case presentations that are likely to be seen in primary care by nurses and pharmacists working either alongside or independently from a doctor. The structure of each case follows the clinical reasoning cycle given in Fig. 1.1:

- Presentation
- Problem representation
- Hypothesis generation
  - Likely diagnoses
  - Possible diagnoses
  - Critical diagnoses
- Continued information gathering
- Problem refinement
- Red flags
- Management
  - Self-care
  - Prescribing options
- Safety netting

A Type 2 reasoning approach has been adopted, as this book is targeted at undergraduates, relatively newly qualified practitioners and those new to clinical reasoning.

The question order and subsequent handling of this information to inform further questioning is based on the authors' own experiences (and with feedback from others) and therefore may differ in the approach taken by the reader. However, the way the information is presented tries to demonstrate Type 2 clinical reasoning, which will hopefully serve as a learning tool for others to improve their thinking. The cases have been written to encourage people to think about how to make a diagnosis – by asking the right question, at the right time, for the right reason. Elements of the consultation process (e.g., shared decision-making using tools such as 'ICE') are not specifically included.

After each case there is:

- An aide memoire

This serves to summarise the diagnoses that were considered for each case. In some cases, summary tables are presented. This information is designed to further knowledge, where appropriate, and help in the formation of illness scripts.

- Multiple choice questions (MCQs)

A minimum of five MCQs are given after each case relating to the problem and serve to test already acquired or new knowledge.

- Key points

These relate to the diagnosis made and cover three or four salient points in relation to that condition.

- Websites or further reading

This includes, for example, links to organisations (e.g., charities)

The 50 Cases Are Grouped Loosely Under Body Systems:		
Eyes, ears, nose and throat	Chapter 3:	12 cases
Gastrointestinal problems	Chapter 4:	7 cases
Skin	Chapter 5:	9 cases
Pain problems	Chapter 6:	9 cases
Respiratory problems	Chapter 7:	4 cases
Women's health issues	Chapter 8:	4 cases
General physical problems	Chapter 9:	5 cases

CONTENTS

Making a Diagnosis

THE USE OF CLINICAL REASONING

Making decisions is an everyday activity, whether it is at home or the workplace. They may range from straightforward and simple to difficult and complex. It is likely that everyone, to some extent, uses clinical reasoning, but not necessarily consciously or consistently. It is a learnt skill, and being more aware of its key elements should allow for better decisions to be made. The ability to effectively employ clinical reasoning is dependent on time and experience, and mastery of the process is often described as moving from 'novice' to 'expert' practice.

WHAT IS CLINICAL REASONING?

The ability of clinicians to take wise actions when faced with a problem is at the heart of clinical practice. Clinical reasoning is a process by which clinicians collect, process and interpret patient information and come to an understanding of a patient's problem or situation,
plan and implement interventions, evaluate outcomes, and reflect on and learn from the process.

Clinical reasoning is a complex cognitive process and is underpinned by the clinician having sound knowledge, good communication and consultation skills; employing patient-centred evidence-based practice; and facilitating shared decision making. These concepts are further discussed in Chapter 2.

Clinical reasoning is dynamic process where scientific knowledge, clinical experience and critical thinking, combined with existing and newly gathered information about the patient, is assessed against a backdrop of clinical uncertainty. This is not a linear process; rather it is more cyclical, as one step informs another (Fig. 1.1).

The cycle starts at initial contact with the patient where early information is given or sought, leading to formulation of the problem representation. At this point either a hypothesis is generated (and the reasoning process follows the right-hand side of Fig. 1.1) or a spot diagnosis is made (negating hypothesis generation) before both

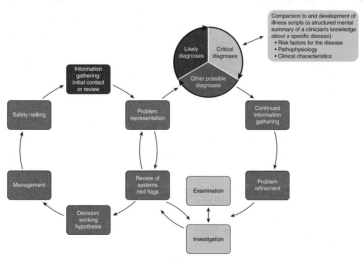

Fig. 1.1 Clinical Reasoning Cycle.

processes move to the left-hand side of the circle, where decisions are made, and treatment plans are put in place.

WHY USE CLINICAL REASONING?

Adverse patient outcomes are linked to poor clinical reasoning, such as misdiagnosis, inappropriate treatment and poor management of complications. A number of studies across different health disciplines have shown that healthcare professionals who have effective clinical reasoning skills have a positive impact on such patient outcomes. Within pharmacy education and practice, the use of mnemonics has been widely advocated for information gathering to generate a diagnosis. However, studies have shown this approach to offer limited clinical reasoning and to result in frequently arriving at the wrong diagnosis.

HOW EFFECTIVE IS CLINICAL REASONING?

Clinical reasoning is not perfect, and 10%–15% of patient consultations will result in diagnostic error either through a wrong, delayed or missed diagnosis, with the consequences being potentially harmful and costly. There are many factors that contribute to diagnostic error but they are usually related to healthcare process errors or individual human error, known as cognitive bias. There are a number of recognised cognitive bias types associated with clinical reasoning, especially when employing fast intuitive thinking. Common examples of this type of error include 'anchoring' – an over reliance on the first piece of information gained; search satisficing – when questioning stops because we have found something that fits instead of exploring alternatives; and confirmation bias – looking for information that supports your thinking rather than looking for evidence to refute it, when the latter is clearly present. Cognitive biases are subconscious, but strategies can be put in place to mitigate them; for example, deliberately 'slowing' down your thought process and adopting metacognition.

MODELS OF CLINICAL REASONING

Much has been written on the clinical reasoning process, and a number of models of reasoning have been described. The most commonly cited models in healthcare appear to be Type 1 and Type 2 thinking, often referred to as the dual process theory.

Type 1 thinking is usually used by clinicians who have prior experience dealing with a similar problem and have gained some level of expertise. Type 1 thinking is quick and intuitive and enables the clinician to make a person-centred diagnostic or treatment decision without needing to consult more widely. Shortcuts are used to aid this way of thinking and have been described as 'illness scripts', 'heuristics', and 'mindlines'.

Type 2 thinking is slow, analytical, controlled and deliberate – it is often utilised by 'novice' clinicians – i.e., those with limited exposure to the problem at hand. Using Type 2 thinking takes time and requires the clinician to research the problem so that they can make an informed decision.

The extent to which decision making is used can be described as a 'cognitive continuum' that runs from intuition (Type 1) at one end of the spectrum to analytical thinking (Type 2) at the other end. Usually, clinicians utilise intuition and experience to make decisions when there is a high volume of simple decisions to be made. At the other end of the spectrum, there may be complex decisions to be made, when the level of uncertainty is high and an analytical and evidence-based approach is needed. In other words, clinicians generally use Type 1 thinking, and only switch to Type 2 thinking when they override their Type 1 thinking. For example, when a person encounters a new clinical problem, they switch to using Type 2 reasoning.

HOW DO YOU DEVELOP YOUR CLINICAL REASONING SKILLS?

The foundations of clinical reasoning should be embedded within all healthcare curricula. However, this is currently not the case, and there is wide variation both within and across different professions, although it is the most developed in medical courses. For other professions, there is an acknowledgement that graduates often possess the prerequisite knowledge and procedural skills but are not 'work ready' as they lack clinical reasoning skills needed to respond to clinical situations. These 'novice' graduates therefore need to effectively learn clinical reasoning while 'on the job'. There are a number of strategies that can be employed to improve performance but require mentorship and/or coaching. For example:

Reflective Practice

Reflection allows for interpretation of experiences. In clinical reasoning, this involves evaluating all aspects of the clinical encounter – for example, yourself, the patient, the context, the environment you are operating in. This can occur directly after an encounter about what happened (reflection on action) or by thinking about previous encounters and identifying knowledge gaps in preparation for future encounters (reflection for action).

Think Aloud Technique

Here the person is encouraged to talk through their thoughts about a case. It allows the person to articulate their reasoning and explanations for the decisions they make in response to information they gain from the patient. This approach helps to build sound reasoning and become more aware of cognitive error.

Metacognition – Thinking About What You are Thinking

This involves self-monitoring and correcting your own learning processes. You should regularly ask questions such as: 'What do I already know?', 'Do I really know what I think I know?', 'How can I be sure of this?'.

MAKING A DIAGNOSIS
PROBLEM REPRESENTATION

The starting point in any consultation will be when the patient first presents or is identified for a review. This provides an opportunity to listen to the patient (as Osler's maxim states, "Listen to your patient, they are telling you the diagnosis") and acquire 'data' via exploratory information gathering of the patient's current health status. This is not limited to the information that the patient tells you and should be combined with cue acquisition – that is data about the person gained through observation (e.g., age, sex, ethnicity) and any clinical data (e.g., parameters that 'quantify' their management – this could be biochemical data, blood tests, etc.) available.

At this point, and often at the subconscious level, the practitioner will define the problem, known as problem representation. The problem representation is a one-sentence summary that highlights the defining features of a case. It comprises three critical components:

- **Clinical context** (Who is the patient? E.g., age, sex, risk factors from past, social, family, medication history)
- **Temporal pattern of illness** (Length and nature of symptom, e.g., acute vs. chronic, intermittent vs. constant or stable vs. progressive)
- **Key symptoms and examination findings** that relate to the presenting symptoms.

Construction of a problem representation helps practitioners crystallise their thoughts and helps them generate a hypothesis to test. As the practitioner gains more information from the patient, the problem representation will be refined and updated, and so is an iterative process.

To illustrate the properties of effective problem representations, consider the following case:

A father of a 5-year-old boy presents to the pharmacy on a Saturday morning. His son has a rash on his face that came on quickly over the last day or so. His son is at home as he is a bit off-colour, but the father has not taken his son's temperature.

This can be framed as:

A 5-year-old boy (*Who is the patient?*) presents with a 24-h history (*time course*) of acute onset facial rash with malaise (*clinical symptoms*).

HYPOTHESIS GENERATION

The problem representation activates clinician illness scripts, and through a comparison process, develops a prioritised differential diagnosis based on the degree of match between the patient's problem representation and previous illness scripts. At this point, a tentative differential diagnosis can be hypothesised and tested, but this prioritised list will also be shaped by 'Murtagh's process' – a diagnostic strategy that depends on learning the most common cause of the presenting problem and a shortlist of serious diagnoses which must be ruled out (most likely, possible and critical diagnoses, as seen in Fig. 1.1).

HYPOTHESIS TESTING AND REFINEMENT

Once a limited number of hypotheses have been formulated, they are used to guide subsequent data collection and integration. Each hypothesis can be used to predict what additional findings ought to be present if it were true, and then questions act as a guided search for these findings; hence, the method is hypothetico-deductive. Novices and experienced physicians alike attempt to generate hypotheses to explain clusters of findings. In short, hypothetico-deductive reasoning involves information from the patient that is gathered and used to construct a hypothesis, which is then tested; if this proves to be false, a further hypothesis is constructed.

There is no set order to which questions should be asked, but the responses given by the patient will influence thinking and consequently shape subsequent questions asked. It is therefore very likely that different practitioners will ask questions in a different order but ultimately arrive at the same conclusions. In summary, it is about asking the right question at the right time for the right reason.

As more information is gained, the hypotheses can be revised and reranked. It is likely that the clinician will work iteratively, refining problems, until a differential diagnosis is established. This is especially true if the clinician adopts a deductive clinical reasoning model. Where inductive reasoning is employed, 'short cuts' are often observed. This is seen extensively with expert practitioners drawing on memory from previous presentations. In effect, multiple previous cases are used as an overlay to help decision making to the case in front of the clinician, which incorporates an understanding of contributory risk factors, pathophysiology and clinical characteristics.

At the end of this process, the clinician should have a working diagnosis.

RED FLAGS

Red flags are troublesome or worrying symptoms that are suggestive of a patient who may be more acutely ill or who has more immediate and complex health needs. During the process of establishing a diagnosis it is likely that red flags will have been identified. However, taking a 'diagnostic pause' and further checking, where relevant, should be undertaken before considering management.

MANAGEMENT

Management plans should be made with the patient and take account of their ideas, concerns and expectations. This will involve measures that the patient can take themselves (self-care); prescriber interventions, including pharmacological or nonpharmacological; and instigation of further tests or referral to another healthcare professional.

Safety Netting

Clinical uncertainty will always exist, and we have to acknowledge that we cannot get things right all the time. Safety netting was formally introduced nearly 30 years ago by Roger Neighbour (see later consultation models). It has subsequently become an essential part of patient consultations and is widely recommended in national guidelines. This is despite a lack of consensus in terms of when it should be used or what information needs to be included. A 2019 review by Jones et al. set out to clarify this concept and concluded that safety netting is more than a mechanism to communicate uncertainty. Safety netting provides patient information on red-flag symptoms and a plan for timely reassessment of a patient's condition, and still relates closely to that proposed by Neighbour.

Effective safety netting should include three components:

- **What you think the problem is and what you expect to happen?** (Information on natural history of illness.) For example, 'I think the earache is likely to be caused by an infection and it should clear up in 2 or 3 days'.
- **How would the person know if you are wrong?** (Alert/advise on worrying symptoms.) For example, 'if the pain goes on longer than this or he develops a discharge from the affected ear'.
- **What they should do then?** (Information on follow-up investigations/referrals.) For example, 'Go and see your doctor'.

GLOSSARY OF TERMS

Clinical Prediction Rules

Utilisation of a well-defined and widely validated series of scoring systems to help increase diagnostic probability of a particular condition. For example, FEVERPain for streptococcal sore throat.

Expert and Novice Practitioner

The difference between novices and experts lies in the speed and accuracy of the hypotheses made, and the method and efficiency of weighing up evidence for and against the hypothesis.

Heuristics

Heuristics are mental shortcuts that allow people to solve problems and make judgements quickly and efficiently. These rule-of-thumb strategies shorten decision-making time and allow people to function without constantly stopping to think about their next course of action.

Illness Scripts

These are an abstract mental representation of an illness. They are used to compare and contrast a patient's clinical presentation (i.e., the patient's 'script') against the practitioners own mental models of a disease (i.e., our own illness scripts). They develop as a consequence of theoretical knowledge acquisition as well as accumulated experience. This means trainees or newly qualified practitioners may have had limited opportunities to build a repository of illness scripts. Through a comparison process, the clinician develops a prioritised differential diagnosis based on the degree of match between the patient's problem representation and previous illness scripts.

Mindlines

These are similar to the concept of illness scripts as they are learnt, internalised sequences of thought and behaviour but seem to be more reliant on professional interactions (e.g., a result of seeking a specialist's advice and discussion with others).

Murtagh's Process

This is a diagnostic strategy that depends on learning the most common cause of the presenting problem (the 'probability diagnosis') and a shortlist of serious diagnoses which must be ruled out. For example, viral cough is the commonest cough type, but malignancy, heart failure, etc. must routinely be ruled out, even if these diagnoses have not been triggered by the presentation.

Semantic Qualifiers

Semantic qualifiers are paired opposing descriptors that are used to compare and contrast diagnostic considerations, for example, sharp vs. dull, acute vs. chronic, tender vs. nontender. They help facilitate retrieval of stored information from illness scripts to aid diagnostic reasoning and reflect the meaning attached to the clinical data.

Spot Diagnosis

Recognition of a particular nonverbal pattern, usually visual (e.g., skin lesions) or auditory (cough). The spot diagnosis is almost instantaneous but relies on previous experience of the condition. It does not require any further questioning of the patient.

Self-labelling

The patient presents with a self-diagnosis, which may or may not be correct, and is often based on personal previous experience of similar signs or symptoms. This tends to influence the questioning strategy.

Pattern Recognition

Signs and symptoms are compared with those of previous patterns or cases, and a disease is recognised when the actual pattern fits. This is the refinement strategy and relies on memory of known patterns.

FURTHER READING

Anakin, M. G., Duffull, S. B., & Wright, D. F. B. (2021). Therapeutic decision-making in primary care pharmacy practice. *Research in Social & Administrative Pharmacy*, *17*(2), 326–331.

Andre, M., Borgquist, L., Foldevi, M., & Molstad, S. (2002). Asking for 'rules of thumb': A way to discover tacit knowledge in general practice. *Family Practice*, *19*(6), 617–622.

Bate, L., Hutchinson, A., Underhill, J., & Maskrey, N. (2012). How clinical decisions are made. *British Journal of Clinical Pharmacology*, *74*(4), 614–620.

Bowen, J. L. (2006). Educational strategies to promote clinical diagnostic reasoning. *New England Journal of Medicine*, *355*(21), 2217–2225.

Chernushkin, K., Loewen, P., de Lemos, J., Aulakh, A., Jung, J., & Dahri, K. (2012). Diagnostic reasoning by hospital pharmacists: Assessment of attitudes, knowledge and skills. *Canadian Journal of Hospital Pharmacy*, *65*(4), 258–264.

Gabbay, J., & le May, A. (2016). Mindlines: Making sense of evidence in practice. *British Journal of General Practice*, *66*(649), 402–403.

Jones, D., Dunn, L., Watt, I., & Macleod, U. (2019). Safety netting for primary care: Evidence from a literature review. *British Journal of General Practice, 69*(678), e70–e79.

O'Sullivan, E. D., & Schofield, S. J. (2018). Cognitive bias in clinical medicine. *Journal of the Royal College of Physicians of Edinburgh, 48*(3), 225–232.

Schmidt, H., & Rikers, R. (2007). How expertise develops in medicine: Knowledge encapsulation and illness script formation. *Medical Education, 41*(12), 1133–1139.

Sinopoulou, S., Gordon, M., & Rutter, P. (2019). A systematic review of community pharmacies' staff diagnostic assessment and performance in patient consultations. *Research in Social & Administrative Pharmacy, 15*(9), 1068–1079.

Wieringa, S., & Greenhalgh, T. (2015). 10 years of mindlines: A systematic review and commentary. *Implementation Science, 10*, 45.

Skills Needed to Facilitate Clinical Reasoning

Clinical reasoning is underpinned by having good subject knowledge and the ability to exercise:
- Good consultation and communication skills
- Evidence-based practice
- Shared decision making

CONSULTATION AND COMMUNICATION SKILLS

The medical consultation is the principal interaction between the patient and practitioner, enabling a two-way exchange of information and ideas that informs patient care. Unsurprisingly, many models have been developed to provide structure for these complex interactions (Table 2.1). An unstructured consultation can lead to less safe practice, a failure to recognise the real issues raised by the patient and an unclear shared management plan. Models allow us to have a better understanding of real-world systems, but no model is perfect and there is not a 'one size fits all', with different practitioners being drawn to different models.

A number of models have been developed that encourage a patient-centred, task-oriented and structured approach, for example, the Pendelton, Neighbour and Calgary–Cambridge models. These three models are widely taught in healthcare programmes.

Pendelton Model (1984)

This model was probably the first such model that was 'patient-centred', and specifically encourages the clinician to involve the patient in decision making and encourages the patient to take some ownership of their problem. The Pendelton model describes seven tasks that the doctor and patient should complete in the consultation as shown in Table 2.2.

Neighbour Model (1987)

The premise of the Neighbour model was to allow the clinician to consult more skilfully, efficiently and intuitively. It includes elements from the Pendleton model but introduced, for the first time, the concept of 'summarising, housekeeping and safety netting'. The model includes five elements to help uncover the patients' unspoken agenda (Table 2.3).

Calgary–Cambridge Model (1996)

This model builds on the connecting (rapport) element of the Neighbour model. It also incorporates effective communication (e.g., concepts of active listening and nonverbal behaviour. These are outside the scope of this introduction – see guided reading for further information) and considers the physical, psychological and social aspects of the consultation. It is broken down into four distinct sequential key steps:
- Initiating the session
- Gathering information (including physical examination, often listed as a fifth distinct step)
- Explanation and planning
- Closing the session

In addition to these steps there are two 'threads' that run through the consultation. These are:
- Providing consultation structure
- Building relationships

This model is now the most widely adopted model in healthcare courses, and therefore a detailed breakdown of each step is shown in Table 2.4.

Remote Consultations

Remote consultations can be conducted by telephone, video link or online. Consultation via telephone has been common practice for many years but because of the COVID-19 pandemic video and

TABLE 2.1 Commonly Encountered Medical Models of Consultation (Not Exhaustive)

Model Name	Pros	Cons
Traditional biomedical model	Concentrates on the diagnosis – this approach is still used when a patient is first admitted in to a hospital	Clinician centred Not concerned with what a patient thinks or the effect of the illness on the patient's life Time consuming and often covers areas of little relevance
Physical, psychological and social (1972)	First model to consider the patient's point of view	Simplistic regarding patient involvement
Health belief model (1975)	Introduced 'ICE' – Ideas, concerns and expectations of the patient Good model for the 'worried well' patient	Does not account for a person's attitudes or beliefs Does not account for environmental or economic factors that may prohibit or promote the recommended action
Six category intervention analysis (1976)	Provides 'options' in how the clinician can support the patient	Need to know which option to employ and when to switch to another option
Pendleton model (1984)	Involves the patient Encourages the patient to take responsibility	Less useful for acute (potentially serious) problems Can be time consuming
McWhinney's disease-illness model (1986)	Simple and practical Tries to meet both clinical and patient agenda	Can be time consuming
Neighbour model (1987)	Introduced safety netting Simple Encourages the patient to take responsibility	Can be more doctor centred than patient-centred
Calgary–Cambridge model (1996)	Comprehensive Structured but helps build rapport	Can be time consuming
Narrative based (2002)	Understanding of a patient's experience of their illness	Can be time consuming

TABLE 2.2 Pendleton Model of Consultation

1. Establish the patient's reason for attendance.	Determine the nature and history of the problem/s. Determine the cause of the problem. Explore their health beliefs. Establish the consequences of the problem/s.
2. Consider if there are other problems.	Consider factors that impact on the patient, for example, social issues.
3. Choose an appropriate management plan for each problem.	Work jointly with the patient.
4. Work together to achieve a shared understanding of each problem.	
5. Involve the patient in the management plan.	Encourage the patient to adopt an appropriate degree of responsibility for each problem.
6. Use time and resources efficiently.	This means both in the consultation and the longer term.
7. Establish and maintain a lasting relationship with the patient that helps to achieve other tasks.	Develop trust.

TABLE 2.3 Neighbour Model of Consultation

Connecting (rapport building)	• Establish a working relationship. • See things from the patient perspective.
Summarising (eliciting information)	• Why has the patient come? • Discover their ideas, concerns and expectations. • Summarise back to the patient. • Opportunity for the patient to correct the clinician before moving on with the consultation
Handover	• Clinician and patient formulate a management plan together. • Opportunity for checking understanding. • Patient takes responsibility for some aspects of the plan.
Safety netting	• Clinician and patient plan together to manage uncertainty. • Empower the patient to be aware of worrying signs or symptoms. • Know what to do and when to do it.
Housekeeping (for the clinician)	• Acknowledge and deal with emotions arising from the consultation prior to seeing the next patient.

TABLE 2.4 Calgary–Cambridge Model of Consultation

1. Initiating the Session

Establish initial rapport.	• Greet the patient and obtain the patient's name. • Introduce self and clarify role. • Demonstrate interest and respect.
Identify the reason(s) for the consultation.	• Identify the patient's problems. • Listen (actively) without interrupting or directing the patient's response. • Confirm list and screen for further problems. • Negotiate agenda taking both the patient's and physician's needs into account.

2. Gathering Information

Exploration of problems.	• Encourage the patient to tell the story in own words (clarifying reason for presenting now). • Use appropriate questioning. • Actively listen. • Facilitate the patient's responses verbally and nonverbally. • Pick up verbal and nonverbal cues. • Clarify patient's statements. • Periodically summarise to verify own understanding. • Use concise, easily understood jargon-free questions and comments. • Establish dates and sequence of events.
Additional skills for understanding the patient's perspective.	• Explore the patients' ideas, concerns, expectations. • Encourage the patient to express feelings.

3. Provide Structure

Make organisation overt.	• Summarise to confirm understanding. • Progress from one section to another using sign posting, transitional statements.
Attend to flow.	• Structure interview in logical sequence. • Attend to timing and keeping interview on task.

Continued

TABLE 2.4 **Calgary-Cambridge Model of Consultation—cont'd**	
4. Building the Relationship	
Use appropriate nonverbal behaviour.	• Use appropriate nonverbal behaviour. • Demonstrate appropriate confidence.
Develop rapport.	• Accept patient's beliefs. • Demonstrate empathy. • Provide support. • Deal sensitively with embarrassing and disturbing topics.
Involve the patient.	• Share thinking with patient. • Explain rationale for questions. • Explain process during physical exam.
5. Explanation and Planning	
Provide the correct amount and type of information.	• Chunks and checks: give information in assimilable chunks; check for understanding. • Assess the patient's starting point. • Ask the patient what other information would be helpful. • Give explanation at appropriate times.
Aid accurate recall and understanding.	• Organise explanation and judicious use of repetition and summarise to reinforce information. • Use concise, easily understood jargon-free statements. • Use visual methods of conveying information where appropriate. • Check patient's understanding of information.
Achieve a shared understanding: incorporating the patient's perspective.	• Relate explanations to patient's viewpoint. • Encourage the patient to contribute.
Planning: shared decision making.	• Share one's own thinking as appropriate. • Involve the patient by making suggestions not directives. • Encourage the patient to contribute their thoughts: ideas, suggestions and preferences. • Negotiate a mutually acceptable plan. • Offer choices: encourage the patient to make choices and decisions to the level that they wish. • Check with the patient: if plans are accepted; if concerns have been addressed.
6. Closing the Session	
Forward planning.	• Agree on next steps. • Safety nets.
Ensure appropriate point of closure.	• Summarise session briefly and clarify plan of care. • Final check that the patient agrees and is comfortable with plan.

online consultations are now almost universally available in general practice.

The General Medical Council has provided guidance to doctors on assessing if a remote consultation is appropriate and issued 10 principles for remote prescribing. Additionally, the Royal College of General Practitioners (RCGP) provides learning materials to support general practitioners (GPs) on remote consultation and triage, and bodies such as NHS Improvement provide templates on establishing remote 'total triage' models. In general, remote consultations are appropriate when:

• Clinical need or treatment is straightforward.
• There is no need for a physical examination.
• The patient has the capacity to decide about treatment.
• Safe systems are in place to prescribe.

Consultation Models vs. Remote Consultation

All models were developed for face-to-face consultations. One important critique of the Calgary–Cambridge and Neighbour models within a remote consultation is that the lack of face-to-face contact can make it hard to detect many of the cues described within the models. For example, visual cues (obviously absent in telephone calls) can be harder to see or pick up on a screen. Intonation of voice and pitch can also be more difficult to interpret and nonverbal behaviours harder to see or read. In addition, there are several cues that you need to be alert for on the telephone that are not included in these models, such as silence and hesitation. If these cues are missed, the rapport building and connecting stages of the consultation may be affected. This could impact subsequent stages. In spite of this, several sources (including the RCGP) have encouraged the use of the Neighbour model for remote consultations.

EVIDENCE-BASED PRACTICE

What is Evidence-Based Practice?

Evidence-based medicine (EBM) and evidence-based practice (EBP) are not new concepts. There are numerous definitions of EBM, but the most accepted comes from David Sackett and colleagues who described EBM as "...the conscientious, explicit, and judicious use of current best evidence in making decisions about the care of individual patients...integrating individual clinical expertise with the best available external clinical evidence from systematic research" (Sackett et al. 1996). This definition encapsulates the important aspects of practising in an evidence-based fashion. First, we need to be conscientious and explicit in the use of evidence, meaning that we need to seek out, and keep up to date with, the current evidence for the efficacy and safety of a medicine. Second, EBM involves integrating clinical knowledge with evidence, meaning that neither should dominate decision making. We should not make decisions based on our clinical experience alone, as our experiences may be biased. For example, we may get the impression that a treatment works because people return to tell us how 'wonderful' the treatment that we recommended was, without knowing how many people found the treatment useless and vowed never to use again. However, evidence from clinical trials should not be the sole basis for decision making either, as they may not be applicable to the patient you have before

you - incorporating both clinical experience and evidence is required. Some critics have accused EBP as being too 'standardised', with all clinicians practising the same way. However, this in fact ignores the important fundamental principle that each clinician must use their clinical experience, in addition to good external evidence, to reach a decision. Therefore, by definition, each decision-making process using EBP will be different. Finally, we should seek out the 'best' evidence, meaning that we need to understand which types of evidence are more robust, and which types of evidence are less reliable.

What is Good Evidence?

Practising in an evidence-based way means using the *best* available evidence. As a guide, a hierarchy of evidence has been developed. The grading is based on the level of potential bias in the study design, with those with the lowest potential for bias given the highest ranking. The abbreviated ranking, from highest to lowest is:

- Systematic reviews of randomised controlled trials (RCTs)
- Well-conducted RCTs
- Observational studies (e.g., cohort and case-control)
- Case series and case studies

Thus ideally, decisions should be based on systematic reviews followed by RCTs. It is important to note that 'expert opinion' is no longer considered a reliable source of evidence.

To have confidence in the findings from such data, studies need to be designed in a robust way that is subject to external scrutiny that assesses the 'quality' of the evidence. Thankfully, assessment tools have been developed (e.g., PRISMA - http://www.prisma-statement.org/) and are used to determine quality, allowing clinicians to trust evidence that is readily accessible to them through portals such as the Cochrane Library (https://www.cochranelibrary.com/).

Interpreting the Evidence

When examining the outcome of a study two things need to be considered: was the effect seen *statistically* significant, and was the effect seen *clinically* significant? To do this we need to first look at the metrics used to measure outcomes in studies. The outcomes that are measured in clinical trials can range from surrogate outcomes to patient-relevant outcomes. Surrogate outcomes are generally biomedical markers and examples include blood pressure, white blood cell counts and bone mineral density. An important feature of a surrogate outcome is that the patient generally cannot feel or report what the outcome is. At the other end of the spectrum we have patient-relevant outcomes. Arguably, these are the things that we ultimately want to change for a person and include outcomes such as improved quality of life, relief of pain and the ability to undertake normal daily activities. In between are what are called clinical outcomes. These are outcomes directly related to an underlying condition, such as fracture rates in osteoporosis and myocardial infarctions in cardiovascular disease. Examples of surrogate, clinical and patient-relevant outcomes can be found in Table 2.5.

The advantages of surrogate outcomes are that they are usually easy to measure and can be quantified with a reasonable amount of objectivity. By contrast, patient-relevant outcomes are the most subjective and are often difficult to measure reliably. However, interpreting changes in a surrogate outcome can be difficult unless we know what a change in a surrogate outcome does to a clinical or patient-relevant outcome. For example, what improvement in forced expiratory volume (FEV_1) is needed before a person can function normally? Most clinical outcomes are examples of dichotomous outcomes such as death, cure, achieving a 10% reduction in body weight and so on. These are commonly expressed by things such as the number needed to treat (NNT), relative risk (RR) or odds ratio (OR).

Statistical vs. Clinical Significance

Being statistically significant does not make the difference clinically significant. Statistical testing is dependent on the variability in the outcome, which is often related to the sample size used in the study. The larger the sample size, the more precise your results usually are and thus the greater the ability to detect even very small differences as being statistically significant. The question that has to be asked is 'Would the patient notice this difference?' or 'Am I going to notice a difference in my patients?'

Developing an Evidence-Based Personal Formulary

The concept of a 'personal formulary' and the selection of a personal formulary drug ('p-drug') is based on the World Health Organisation (WHO) Guide to Good Prescribing which is used to teach medical students to prescribe. Selecting a 'p-drug' involves a systematic, evidence-driven approach to selecting the best medicine to manage a particular condition.

The WHO approach to select between the possible therapies uses four criteria:
- Efficacy
- Safety
- Patient suitability
- Cost

The first thing you look at is comparative efficacy. If there is nothing to differentiate the treatments based on efficacy, we then consider safety. Again, if there are no significant differences in terms of safety, we would then consider patient suitability and so on. When considering patient suitability, we are looking at things such as ease of use, better adherence and so forth. The issue of cost is interesting; if you have two or more products that are considered equivalent in terms of efficacy, safety and patient acceptability, then it would seem reasonable to offer the patient the less expensive option. An example of this would be comparing imidazoles (e.g., clotrimazole) with terbinafine cream for tinea pedis. There is no appreciable difference in terms of efficacy and safety. However, imidazoles are usually applied several times a day for several weeks, whereas terbinafine is applied once a day for 1 week. If they were the same cost, you would clearly choose terbinafine. However, terbinafine is generally costlier and therefore it would seem reasonable

TABLE 2.5	Examples of Outcome Measures in Relation to Clinical Conditions		
Condition Outcome	**Surrogate Outcome**	**Clinical Outcome**	**Patient-Relevant**
Osteoporosis	Bone mineral density	Spinal fractures	Pain relief, ability to do normal daily activities
Asthma	FEV_1 or peak flow	Wheeze, use of rescue medication	Ability to play sport
Respiratory tract infection	Viral count/load	Sore throat, fever	Ability to go to work/school

FEV_1, Forced expiratory volume.

to offer both products to the patient, explaining the difference in dosing and cost and allowing the patient to choose which they would prefer.

SHARED DECISION MAKING (SDM)

There is a wealth of information supporting SDM contributing to positive patient outcomes and it is now embedded in UK law (e.g., Health and Social Care Act 2012). The National Institute for Health and Care Excellence (NICE) defines SDM as *"a collaborative process that involves a person and their healthcare professional working together to reach a joint decision about care"*.

This could be care the person needs straightaway or care in the future, for example, through advance care planning. It involves choosing tests and treatments based both on evidence and on the person's individual preferences, beliefs and values. It means making sure the person understands the risks, benefits and possible consequences of different options through discussion and information sharing. This joint process empowers people to make decisions about the care that is right for them at that time.

Despite this, recent (2020 and 2022) surveys show people want to be more involved than they currently are in making decisions about their own health and health care. NICE offers guidance to organisations and individual clinicians on how to embed SDM into everyday practice. NICE suggests that SDM should be considered:

Before a patient appointment
- Offer the person access to resources that encourage them to think about what matters to them, what they hope will happen as a result of the discussion and what questions they would like to ask.
- Ask if the person wants someone else to be with them during the consultation. If this is not possible or practicable, offer someone from the team to be their advocate/support.

During the appointment
- Encourage the person to participate and invite questions.
- Discuss the pros and cons of any treatment or intervention.
- Ensure 'ICE' (ideas, concerns and expectations) are covered.
- Make records, including what the patient says or wants to happen, and any letters to other professionals that need to be shared with the patient.

Following the appointment
- Provide appropriate resources to help the person understand what was discussed and agreed upon, and offer additional support where needed.
- Provides details of who to contact if they have further questions.

Shared Decision Making in Practice

There are a number of tools that can be used by patients and clinicians to facilitate and monitor SDM.

The Ask 3 Questions campaign is designed to encourage patients to ask questions and play a more active role in decisions about their treatment and care.

Q1 – What are my choices?

Q2 – What is good and bad about each choice?

Q3 – How do I get support to help me make a decision that is right for me?

Another option is the **It's OK to ASK campaign** which adopts the BRAN mnemonic.

Q1 – What are the **b**enefits of my treatment?

Q2 – What are the **r**isks of my treatment?

Q3 – Any **a**lternatives I can try?

Q4 - What if I do **n**othing?

The patient could also be asked to complete the SDM-Q-9 survey that looks at how well the clinician (states doctor on the survey) involved and explained things to the patient.

FURTHER READING

Denness, C. (2013). What are consultation models for? *InnovAiT*, *6*(9), 592–599.

General Medical Council (2024). Guidance – remote consultations. https://www.gmc-uk.org/ethical-guidance/ethical-hub/remote-consultations

Goodman, K. (2003). Foundations and history of evidence-based practice. In *Ethics and evidence-based medicine: Fallibility and responsibility in clinical science*. Cambridge: Cambridge University Press.

Harper, C., & Ajao, A. (2010). Pendleton's consultation model: Assessing a patient. *British Journal of Community Nursing*, *15*(1), 38–43.

Kurtz, S. M., & Silverman, J. D. (1996). The Calgary-Cambridge Referenced Observation Guides: An aid to defining the curriculum and organising teaching in communication training programmes. *Medical Education*, *30*, 83–89.

RCGP Learning (2024). Remote consultation and triaging. https://elearning.rcgp.org.uk/mod/page/view. php?id=10551

Sackett, D. L., Rosenberg, W. M., Gray, J. A., Haynes, R. B., & Richardson, W. S. (1996). Evidence based medicine: What it is and what it isn't. *BMJ*, *312*(7023), 71–73.

Schulz, K. F., Chalmers, I., Hayes, R. J., & Altman, D. G. (1995). Empirical evidence of bias: Dimensions of methodological quality associated with estimates of treatment effects in controlled trials. *JAMA*, *273*, 408–412.

WEBSITES

Care Quality Commission. Adult inpatient survey 2022.
https://www.cqc.org.uk/publications/surveys/adult-inpatient-survey

Centre for Evidence-Based Medicine
www.cebm.net
GP Patient Survey
https://www.gp-patient.co.uk/surveysandreports
SDM-Q-9: The 9-item Shared Decision Making Questionnaire
http://www.patient-als-partner.de/index.php?article_id=20&clang=2
Shared Decision Making. NICE guideline (NG197). June 2021
https://www.nice.org.uk/guidance/ng197/chapter/recommendations#shared-decision-making

Eyes, Ears, Nose and Throat

EYES

CASE 1: ACUTE RED EYE

PRESENTATION

Mrs P, a 42-year-old woman, woke up this morning with a bright right red eye. She also says that her eye is aching.

PROBLEM REPRESENTATION

A 42-year-old woman presents with acute sudden onset unilateral red eye.

HYPOTHESIS GENERATION (LIKELY, POSSIBLE AND CRITICAL DIAGNOSES)

The commonest forms of red eye seen in primary care are associated with some form of conjunctivitis and should be explored as a cause of Mrs P's symptoms. However, allergic conjunctivitis presents bilaterally and tends not to have such sudden onset and therefore can be discounted from our early thoughts. Another common cause of red eye is subconjunctival haemorrhage (SCH). This has unilateral presentation and is sudden in onset and should be considered as a likely cause alongside bacterial and viral conjunctivitis.

Likely Diagnoses

- Bacterial conjunctivitis
- SCH
- Viral conjunctivitis

Possible Diagnoses

- Allergic conjunctivitis
- Blepharitis
- Chlamydial conjunctivitis
- Dry eye syndrome

- Episcleritis
- Herpes simplex
- Scleritis

Critical Diagnoses

- Acute closed-angle glaucoma
- Anterior uveitis
- Corneal abrasion/foreign body injury
- Keratitis (corneal ulcer)

CONTINUED INFORMATION GATHERING

Signs and symptoms of red eye include eye discharge, redness, varying levels of eye discomfort and visual changes. Given the conditions we are initially considering, a better understanding of the distribution of redness, the aching feeling she describes and the presence of discharge need to be explored.

Mrs P tells you that she has not noticed any discharge and repeats that her eye is just aching; she denies having any form of true eye pain or discomfort in her eye. A visual inspection of her right eye reveals an obvious red patch in the centre of the sclera and no abnormal pupil responses (Fig. 3.1). Her left eye is unaffected. Based on this information and a unilateral presentation, it appears that both forms of infective conjunctivitis seem unlikely, as both tend to cause diffuse and generalised redness with associated discharge, watery discharge in viral conjunctivitis and mild to moderate mucopurulent discharge in bacterial conjunctivitis. In addition, Mrs P does not describe any discomfort, which should be present in both forms of conjunctivitis.

SCH therefore seems likely given it presents with little or no discomfort and has a bright red injection that is well demarcated on the sclera. Mrs P also only has unilateral involvement, which is typical in SCH, although both forms of conjunctivitis usually start unilaterally before

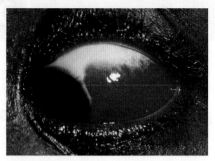

Fig. 3.1 Subconjunctival Haemorrhage. (Source: Krachmer, J. H. & Paley, D. A. (2014). *Cornea Atlas* (3rd ed.). Saunders.)

bilateral involvement and so cannot be considered discriminatory given the nature of Mrs P's presentation.

PROBLEM REFINEMENT

To help confirm your diagnosis and further rule out viral conjunctivitis, you could ask about recent symptoms of an upper respiratory tract infection (URTI) and check if close contacts have similar symptoms – which are likely if viral conjunctivitis was the cause.

Mrs P confirms that she has had no other symptoms, her eye was fine before going to bed, and it was red when she woke up. Her partner's eyes are fine. It seems that Mrs P is suffering from an SCH. Episcleritis, listed as a possible cause, also needs to be considered, as this

can present with unilateral eye redness. However, the suddenness of onset of Mrs P's symptoms points more towards haemorrhage (see Table 3.1).

> ⚡ **RED FLAGS**
>
> A reduction in normal vision, a cloudy/hazy cornea and the absence of pupillary response or irregularly shaped pupils all suggest a critical diagnosis. Inspection showed normal pupil responses. Mrs P also reported no true eye pain, which is usually associated with sinister pathology.

MANAGEMENT

Self-care Options

The condition does not require treatment. Artificial tears may be used if the patient experiences mild irritation. If she is a contact lens wearer, it would be advisable to not wear them.

Prescribing Options

None.

Safety Netting

You tell Mrs P that you think her red eye is caused by a burst blood vessel and it is nothing to worry about, but the redness can take 1–2 weeks to disappear. If the redness persists or she develops any other eye symptoms, she should come back so you can reassess her symptoms.

TABLE 3.1	Condition Summary of the Four Common Causes of Red Eye Seen In Primary Care			
	Bacterial Conjunctivitis (Fig. 3.2)	**Viral Conjunctivitis (Fig. 3.3)**	**Allergic Conjunctivitis (Fig. 3.4)**	**Subconjunctival Haemorrhage (Fig. 3.1)**
Eyes affected	Normally both; occasionally unilateral	Both, but one eye is often affected first	Both	One
Discharge	Often mucopurulent secretions with bilateral glued eyes upon awakening	Watery	Watery	None
Pain	Mild to moderate. Gritty discomfort often described as a 'foreign body' sensation	Gritty discomfort and associated mild itching	Itching (can be intense)	None
Distribution of redness	Generalised and diffuse	Generalised	Generalised but greatest in fornices	Localised or generalised
Associated symptoms	None commonly	Cough and cold symptoms	Rhinitis (may also have family history of atopy)	None

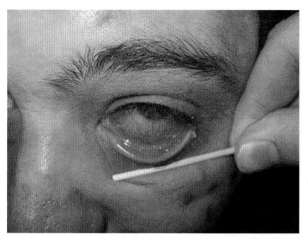

Fig. 3.2 Bacterial Conjunctivitis. Staphylococcal conjunctivitis of the left eye with mild erythema and inflammatory oedema of the eyelids. Purulent exudate can be seen at the lateral canthus. (Source: Durkin, S. R., Selva, D., Huilgol, S. C., Guy, S., & Leibovitch, I. (2006). Recurrent staphylococcal conjunctivitis associated with facial impetigo contagiosa. *American Journal of Ophthalmology*, 141(1), 189–190. https://doi.org/10.1016/j.ajo.2005.07.079)

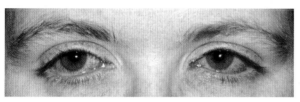

Fig. 3.3 Diffuse injection of the conjunctiva with a watery discharge is evident in this case of viral conjunctivitis. (Source: Palay, D. A., & Krachmer, J. H. (2005). *Primary care ophthalmology* (2nd ed.). Elsevier Mosby.)

AIDE MEMOIRE

Possible Diagnoses

Blepharitis

Typically, blepharitis is bilateral with symptoms ranging from irritation, itching and burning of the lid margins. Lid margins may appear red and raw, accompanied with excessive tearing and crusty debris or skin flakes around the eyelashes. In chronic cases, madarosis (missing lashes) and trichiasis (inturned lashes) can occur. This latter symptom can lead to further local irritation and result in conjunctivitis. The mean age of occurrence is 50 years.

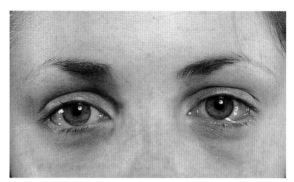

Fig. 3.4 Allergic Conjunctivitis With Swelling of the Bulbar Conjunctiva. (Source: Spalton, D., Hitchings, R., & Hunter, P. (2004). *Atlas of clinical ophthalmology* (3rd ed.). Mosby.)

Chlamydial Conjunctivitis

Usually bilateral with diffuse redness, gritty sensation and mucopurulent discharge. Chlamydial conjunctivitis should be suspected in young (15–35 years) sexually active patients. Most often, patients with chlamydial conjunctivitis will have an associated genital infection (of which they may be unaware). Bilateral red eye within the first month of birth is associated with maternal chlamydial infection. The baby will present with purulent or mucoid discharge and diffuse redness.

Dry Eye Syndrome

Symptoms are bilateral red itchy/burning/irritated eyes with a gritty or foreign body sensation. Eyes exhibit intermittent excessive watering. Vision and pupil reactions are normal. Dry eye disease is more common in women than in men and has an increased prevalence with age.

Episcleritis

Episcleritis is a localised area of inflammation involving superficial layers of episclera. It is generally seen as unilateral isolated patches of red injection. Mild (sometimes moderate) pain is usual, and patients often describe tenderness over the affected area but do not exhibit discharge, photophobia or reduced visual acuity.

Herpes Simplex

Associated with cold sores and genital herpes, but it can cause eye infections, usually affecting one eye. In addition to red eye symptoms, watery discharge, blurred vision, reduced visual acuity and eye pain can be experienced. Besides eye symptoms the person may exhibit

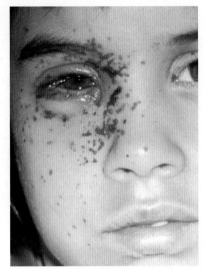

Fig. 3.5 Primary Herpes Simplex Infection of the Facial Skin. There are multiple vesicular lesions, some of which are crusted over. A blepharoconjunctivitis is present in the right eye. (Source: Krachmer, J. H., & Palay, D. A. (2006). *Cornea Atlas*. (2nd ed.). Mosby.)

crops of vesicles along the lid margin or periocular skin (Fig. 3.5). Recurrence is common and can cause corneal scarring as a complication.

Scleritis

Symptoms are similar to episcleritis, but onset tends to be more gradual. Pain is a much more prominent feature; pain increases with eye movements. Photophobia and reduced visual acuity may be present.

Critical Diagnoses

Acute Closed-angle Glaucoma

Onset can be rapid and characteristically occurs in the evening. Severe unilateral eye pain is associated with a headache on the same side as the painful eye. The eye appears red, watering and may be cloudy. Vision is blurred/decreased, and the patient might also notice haloes around lights. Vomiting is often experienced due to the rapid rise in intraocular pressure. Pupils are semidilated and fixed. It classically occurs in older, far-sighted patients.

Anterior Uveitis

Acute anterior uveitis can be unilateral or bilateral. Photophobia and pain are prominent features with the pain described as a dull ache (radiating into brow/temple). Redness is often localised to the limbal area (known as the ciliary flush). The affected pupil may be constricted

or irregular in shape and reduced visual acuity may be observed. The likely cause is an antigen–antibody reaction, which can occur as part of a systemic disease.

Corneal Abrasion/Foreign Body

They are generally a result of trauma to the surface of the eye and symptoms will depend on the cause and severity of injury. However, red watering eyes accompanied with photophobia, severe eye pain and possible loss of visual acuity can be seen.

Keratitis (Corneal Ulcer)

Pain, which can be very severe, is a prominent feature. The patient usually complains of photophobia, redness around the iris (limbal redness), a watery discharge and lid oedema. Physical examination shows a loss of visual acuity often accompanied with a small pupil.

▌ MCQs

1. A 32-year-old woman presents with a bright red eye that she describes as being sticky with a 'gunky' discharge. Her other eye appears to be normal. Which ONE of the following is the most likely diagnosis?
   (a) Allergic conjunctivitis
   (b) Bacterial conjunctivitis
   (c) Episcleritis
   (d) Keratitis
   (e) Viral conjunctivitis

2. A 28-year-old man complains of a red and sore left eye. He describes the pain as discomfort. Visual acuity is normal. Which ONE of the conditions is the most likely cause of the red eye?
   (a) Allergic conjunctivitis
   (b) Episcleritis
   (c) Keratitis
   (d) Scleritis
   (e) Viral conjunctivitis

3. A 51-year-old woman presents with generalised redness in her left eye. Which ONE of the symptom clusters most likely warrants referral to an optician?
   (a) Moderate pain with slight discharge and vision unaffected
   (b) Slight pain with little discharge and blurred vision
   (c) Slight pain with little discharge and vision unaffected
   (d) Slight pain with mucopurulent discharge and vision unaffected
   (e) Slight to moderate eye discomfort but no discharge with vision unaffected

4. Which ONE of the following conditions is most closely associated with the symptoms of redness in the fornices?
   (a) Allergic conjunctivitis
   (b) Bacterial conjunctivitis
   (c) Episcleritis
   (d) Scleritis
   (e) Viral conjunctivitis
5. A middle-aged woman presents with a red left eye. The redness appeared quite quickly, and she has no other symptoms. Based on this information which ONE of the following is the most likely diagnosis?
   (a) Allergic conjunctivitis
   (b) Bacterial conjunctivitis
   (c) Episcleritis
   (d) Keratitis
   (e) SCH

Answers

1. b; 2. e; 3. a; 4. a; 5. e

KEY POINTS: SUBCONJUNCTIVAL HAEMORRHAGE

- Caused when a blood vessel breaks and bleeds into the subconjunctival space
- Unilateral painless area of localised well-demarcated redness
- Symptoms should resolve in approximately 2 weeks
- No treatment required

WEBSITES

Eyecare Trust
http://www.eyecaretrust.org.uk/index.php
International Glaucoma Association
http://www.glaucoma-association.com/
The Royal College of Ophthalmologists
https://www.rcophth.ac.uk
American College of Optometrist Clinical Guidelines
https://www.college-optometrists.org/guidance/clinical-management-guidelines.html

CASE 2: ACUTE RED EYE

PRESENTATION

Mr C, a 40-year-old man, who is unknown to you, asks for some eye drops to help with a sore right red eye. He has had the symptoms for 2 days and describes the soreness as a general discomfort.

PROBLEM REPRESENTATION

A 40-year-old man presents with a 2-day history of unilateral eye redness causing discomfort.

HYPOTHESIS GENERATION (LIKELY, POSSIBLE AND CRITICAL DIAGNOSES)

From the presenting symptoms it appears that Mr C is probably suffering from either viral or bacterial conjunctivitis.

Likely Diagnoses

- Bacterial conjunctivitis
- Viral conjunctivitis

Possible Diagnoses

- Allergic conjunctivitis
- Blepharitis
- Chlamydial conjunctivitis
- Dry eye syndrome
- Episcleritis
- Herpes simplex
- Scleritis
- SCH

Critical Diagnoses

- Acute closed-angle glaucoma
- Anterior uveitis
- Corneal abrasion/foreign body
- Keratitis (corneal ulcer)

CONTINUED INFORMATION GATHERING

On presentation we know he has had the symptoms for 2 days and is experiencing some level of discomfort. We need to establish the nature and severity of this discomfort. Both forms of conjunctivitis can cause irritation/discomfort but would not be severe enough to be debilitating. Mr C reports that his eye is sore and aching and is 'bothering him' and that his eye keeps watering.

On inspection his eye is diffusely red. His left eye appears normal. At this point his symptoms seem a better fit for viral conjunctivitis (watery discharge) than a bacterial cause (mucopurulent discharge).

PROBLEM REFINEMENT

To further explore if his symptoms are viral in origin, it would be worth asking about associated symptoms. Often patients with viral conjunctivitis will exhibit upper respiratory tract symptoms. However, Mr C reports no such recent symptoms. This casts some doubt on your thinking. Viral conjunctivitis causes follicles on the palpebral conjunctiva and so eversion of the upper lid can be performed. The findings for Mr C are negative. Your differential diagnosis of viral conjunctivitis is now more uncertain. At this point we need to consider other possible diagnoses of his red eye.

Allergic and chlamydial conjunctivitis (bilateral presentation), SCH (painless), blepharitis (lid margins, longer duration and wrong age group) and dry eye syndrome (wrong age group) do not seem to be the cause of his symptoms.

We therefore need to further consider episcleritis, scleritis, uveitis and herpes simplex as possible causes. To help differentiate, testing visual acuity can be helpful as this will usually be reduced in uveitis, scleritis and herpes simplex but not in episcleritis. In addition, the pupil seen in uveitis is likely to be smaller and irregular compared with that of the unaffected eye, but this is not seen in episcleritis, scleritis or herpes simplex. You perform these two tests and find Mr C's vision to be slightly decreased, and his right pupil seems smaller compared with his left. Episcleritis can now be discounted (normal acuity and pupils) and scleritis and herpes simplex would show normal pupil reflexes and therefore seem unlikely as the cause of his symptoms.

Signs and symptoms now point most to a diagnosis of uveitis.

Other symptoms of uveitis include eyebrow ache and mild photophobia. Enquiry as to whether Mr C has had such symptoms reveals he has noticed the pain across his forehead as well as eye discomfort. This seems to support your differential diagnosis.

> ⚡ **RED FLAGS**
>
> Those causing true and severe eye pain (glaucoma, corneal abrasion and keratitis) can be eliminated from our thinking as Mr C does not report such symptoms.

MANAGEMENT

Uveitis will be outside the remit of most practitioners. Mr C requires urgent referral to an ophthalmologist for further assessment.

Self-care Options

If Mr C wears contact lenses, he should be advised to stop wearing them prior to attending an ophthalmologist.

Prescribing Options

Specific treatment will depend on the underlying pathology. Treatment consists of pupil-dilating agents, analgesics and corticosteroids. Where an infective cause is responsible, topical antimicrobial agents should be used.

Safety Netting

Early and frequent follow-up should be instigated to assess response to treatment and monitor for complications, for example, deterioration in vision.

AIDE MEMOIRE

Table 3.2 summarises those eye conditions where pain is a prominent feature. For descriptions of other causes of red eye please see Case 1: Acute Red Eye.

TABLE 3.2	**Summary of Eye Conditions Where Pain Is Prominent**						
	Discharge	Visual Disturbance	Pupil Shape/ Reaction	Visual Acuity	Eyes Affected	Redness	Severity of Pain
Uveitis (Fig. 3.6)	No	Photophobia	Abnormal	Reduced	one	Often pronounced around iris	Moderate
Keratitis (Fig. 3.7)	Watery	Photophobia	Abnormal	Reduced	one or both	Often pronounced around iris	Severe
Scleritis (Fig. 3.8)	Unusual	No	Normal	Can be reduced	one	Segmental	Moderate
Corneal abrasion (Fig. 3.9)	Watery	Photophobia	Normal	Can be reduced	one	Generalised	Severe
Glaucoma (Fig. 3.10)	Watery	Blurred	Abnormal	Reduced	one	Haloes	Severe

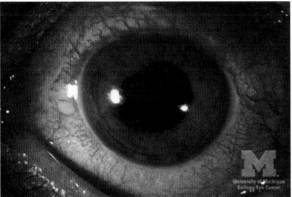

Fig. 3.6 Anterior Uveitis. With permission from Jonathan Trobe, MD, W.K. Kellogg Eye Center.

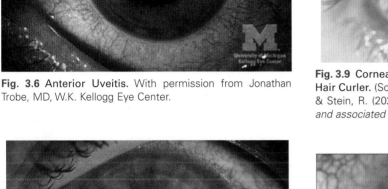

Fig. 3.7 Acanthamoeba Keratitis in a 12-Year-Old. Initial diagnosis was herpes keratitis, which delayed the initiation of the correct treatment for several weeks. (Source: Lyons, C. J., & Lambert, S. R. (2023). *Taylor and Hoyt's pediatric ophthalmology and strabismus* (6th ed.). Elsevier.)

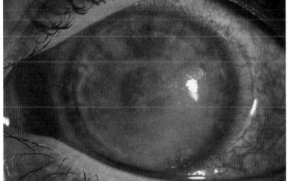

Fig. 3.8 Scleritis. (Kanski J. J. (2006) *Clinical diagnosis in ophthalmology* (1st ed.). St Louis, Mosby.)

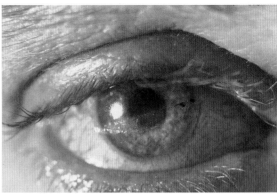

Fig. 3.9 Corneal Abrasion as a Result of Thermal Burn From Hair Curler. (Source: Stein, H. A., Stein, R. M., Freeman, M. I., & Stein, R. (2023). *The ophthalmic assistant: A text for allied and associated ophthalmic personnel* (11th ed.). Elsevier.)

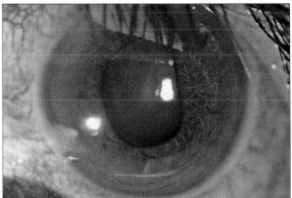

Fig. 3.10 Acute Closed-Angle Glaucoma. (Source: Y. Myron & J. S. Duker (2023). *Ophthalmology* (6th ed.). Elsevier.)

▌ MCQs

1. A young woman asks for help with her sore left eye. On examination you notice an area of injected conjunctiva in the nasal canthus (corner of the eye where the upper and lower eyelids meet). Which ONE of the following conditions is the most likely diagnosis?
   - (a) Acute angle glaucoma
   - (b) Allergic conjunctivitis
   - (c) Episcleritis
   - (d) Keratitis
   - (e) Uveitis

2. A 27-year-old woman presents with a sore left eye. She describes experiencing a watery discharge and generalised scleral redness. You check for visual acuity and find it to be normal. Which ONE of the following conditions is the most likely diagnosis?
   (a) Allergic conjunctivitis
   (b) Bacterial conjunctivitis
   (c) Blepharitis
   (d) Episcleritis
   (e) Viral conjunctivitis

3. A woman presents with watery, itchy and irritating eyes. Upon examination you notice that both eyes are very inflamed. Which ONE of the following conditions best explain her symptoms?
   (a) Allergic conjunctivitis
   (b) Bacterial conjunctivitis
   (c) Blepharitis
   (d) Stye
   (e) Viral conjunctivitis

4. A female patient asks for your advice. She says her right eye is 'achy' for the last 3 days and looks red. She also says her vision is normal and is generally fit and healthy. Which ONE of the following conditions is the most likely diagnosis?
   (a) Episcleritis
   (b) Keratitis
   (c) Scleritis
   (d) Uveitis
   (e) Viral conjunctivitis

5. A 27-year-old woman presents with bilateral red eye of 3 days duration. She also complains of slight discharge. Visual examination reveals nothing untoward. Your differential diagnosis is conjunctivitis. Which ONE of the following symptoms helps to differentiate allergic conjunctivitis from bacterial and viral conjunctivitis?
   (a) Discharge is mucopurulent.
   (b) Redness is distributed throughout the conjunctiva.
   (c) She also has nasal congestion.
   (d) She complains of itching eyes.
   (e) Symptoms were sudden in onset.

Answers

1. c; 2. e; 3. a; 4. d; 5. d

KEY POINTS: UVEITIS

- Commonly caused by infection, autoimmune disease or trauma
- Key symptoms of pain, ciliary flush and photophobia
- Symptoms settle within a few days with treatment, but inflammation may take several weeks to disappear.
- Treatment with corticosteroids for inflammation and, if infective in origin, an appropriate antibacterial

WEBSITES

Uveitis Information Group
http://www.uveitis.net/

CASE 3: ACUTE RED EYE

PRESENTATION

Ms K, a 41-year-old woman, presents with left eye redness and pain. The symptoms came on suddenly. She is otherwise fit and healthy but was diagnosed with arthritis about 9 months ago for which she takes regular ibuprofen.

PROBLEM REPRESENTATION

A 41-year-old woman presents with sudden onset unilateral painful red eye.

HYPOTHESIS GENERATION (LIKELY, POSSIBLE AND CRITICAL DIAGNOSES)

Epidemiologically, conjunctivitis is the commonest cause of red eye. However, all forms of conjunctivitis do not cause eye pain, but various levels of itching and discomfort. It appears from this presentation that we are dealing with a more unusual cause of red eye, potentially something with sinister pathology. Based on the information at presentation, we need to first consider those conditions where eye pain is a clinical feature.

Likely Diagnoses

- Acute closed-angle glaucoma
- Anterior uveitis
- Corneal abrasion/foreign body
- Episcleritis

CHAPTER 3 Eyes, Ears, Nose and Throat   23

- Keratitis (corneal ulcer)
- Scleritis

Possible Diagnoses

- Allergic conjunctivitis
- Bacterial conjunctivitis
- Blepharitis
- Chlamydial conjunctivitis
- Dry eye syndrome
- Herpes simplex
- SCH
- Viral conjunctivitis

Critical Diagnoses

- Acute closed-angle glaucoma
- Anterior uveitis
- Corneal abrasion/foreign body
- Keratitis (corneal ulcer)

CONTINUED INFORMATION GATHERING

Exploration of the level of eye pain Ms K is experiencing is important as most causes of true eye pain have sinister pathology. They also tend to affect vision, and assessments of visual acuity and pupil responses need to be performed.

Questioning reveals that Ms K describes the pain as annoying and is not so bad that it is stopping her from doing her daily activities. Ms K's symptoms suggest her pain as low to moderate. Examination shows localised sectoral redness of the left eye (Fig. 3.11). Visual acuity and pupil reactions are normal.

Negative findings towards visual acuity and pupil response are useful as glaucoma, keratitis, uveitis (and possibly corneal abrasion and scleritis) would show abnormal findings. In addition, the level of pain is also a useful indicator as to the cause. Moderate to severe pain is experienced in scleritis, glaucoma, keratitis and corneal abrasion.

A combination of normal findings and low/moderate pain levels indicates episcleritis to be the most likely diagnosis.

PROBLEM REFINEMENT

To test this hypothesis, you ask about the presence of discharge and associated symptoms. She reports neither discharge nor other symptoms. It appears Ms K has unilateral sectoral redness associated with some pain

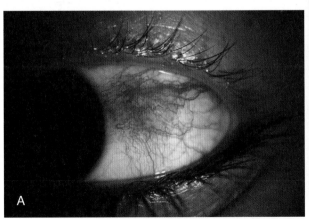 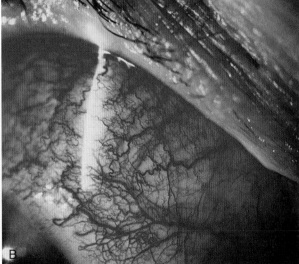

Fig. 3.11 Simple Episcleritis. (A) Sectoral. (B) Diffuse. (Source: Krachmer, J. H., Mannis, M. J., & Holland, E. J. (2005). *Cornea*. Mosby Elsevier; B, *Kanski, J. J., & Bowling, B. (2016). Kanski's clinical ophthalmology: A systemic approach* (8th ed.). Elsevier.)

but no discharge or other symptoms. This presentation seems consistent with episcleritis.

Epidemiological data further support this differential diagnosis as roughly two-thirds of cases occur in women with a peak incidence in their fourth decade. We also know that Ms K was diagnosed with rheumatoid arthritis 9 months ago; this positive medical history further strengthens a diagnosis of episcleritis, as approximately a third of patients have an associated autoimmune disorder.

> ⚡ **RED FLAGS**
>
> Visual inspection and pain assessments have already been performed and the likelihood of Ms K's symptoms being caused by a critical diagnosis is low.

MANAGEMENT

Self-care Options

A cold compress may be applied to provide symptomatic relief of any pain.

Prescribing Options

Although the condition is usually self-limiting, artificial tears can be given to reduce discomfort.

Safety Netting

You tell Ms K you believe the redness is caused by something called episcleritis. This is a self-limiting condition and will go away on its own in 7–10 days. You recommend artificial tears to help with the eye discomfort which Ms K accepts. You ask her to return if her symptoms have not cleared up after 14 days.

AIDE MEMOIRE

Please see Case 1: Acute Red Eye and Case 2: Acute Red Eye for descriptions of red eye conditions.

■ MCQs

1. A patient presents with circumcorneal hyperaemia. Which ONE of the following is the most likely diagnosis?
   (a) Allergic conjunctivitis
   (b) Anterior uveitis
   (c) Episcleritis
   (d) Inflamed pinguecula
   (e) Viral conjunctivitis

2. A female patient complains of having an achy red right eye for the last 4 days. She has no other symptoms apart from a dislike of bright lights. Which ONE of the following is the most likely diagnosis?
   (a) Acute closed-angle glaucoma
   (b) Anterior uveitis
   (c) Episcleritis
   (d) Keratitis
   (e) Scleritis

3. A middle-aged man presents with a history of a redness in his right eye for the last 24 h. Which ONE of the following symptoms should alert you to potential sinister pathology?
   (a) Discomfort in the eye
   (b) Excessive tearing
   (c) Mucopurulent discharge
   (d) Redness located in the fornice
   (e) Reduction in visual acuity

4. A 22-year-old man with a previous history of eczema presents to you complaining of a painful red right eye. The eye is generally red, but the cornea is bright and the pupil small. Which ONE of the following is the most likely diagnosis?
   (a) Acute angle glaucoma
   (b) Allergic conjunctivitis
   (c) Corneal abrasion
   (d) Keratitis
   (e) Scleritis

5. A 54-year-old man presents with a red right eye. He has had the symptoms for a week or so. He is complaining of photophobia. He takes methotrexate for rheumatoid arthritis. Which ONE of the following is the most likely diagnosis?
   (a) Episcleritis
   (b) Glaucoma
   (c) Keratitis
   (d) Scleritis
   (e) Uveitis

Answers
1. b; 2. b; e; 4. d; 5. e

> **KEY POINTS: EPISCLERITIS**
> - Often of unknown cause
> - Key symptoms are unilateral segmental redness associated with aching.
> - Symptoms should improve within 10 days.
> - No treatment is usually needed in mild cases.

CASE 4: EYE IRRITATION

PRESENTATION

Miss L, a 37-year-old female patient, presents to your morning clinic. She describes a history of irritation in both eyes for the last 3–4 months. Her predominant symptoms are intermittent itching and watery eyes. She bought over-the-counter chloramphenicol on two previous occasions. These seemed to have helped for a short period of time before her symptoms returned. She denies any problems with her vision. On initial inspection her eyes look generally healthy, but the eyelid margins appear to be inflamed.

PROBLEM REPRESENTATION

A 37-year-old woman presents with a 4-month history of bilateral eye soreness involving the lid margins.

HYPOTHESIS GENERATION (LIKELY, POSSIBLE AND CRITICAL DIAGNOSES)

Common causes of eyelid dysfunction include blepharitis, hordeola (styes), dermatitis and chalazion. In this case hordeola and chalazion seem unlikely. The chronic nature rule outs hordeola, and the bilateral nature of her symptoms rules out chalazion. In addition, there are a number of asymptomatic conditions affecting the eyelids and surrounding skin, and therefore can also be discounted; these include hydrocystoma and xanthelasma.

Likely Diagnoses

- Blepharitis
- Dermatitis (atopic, contact, seborrhoeic)

Possible Diagnoses

- Acne rosacea
- Blocked tear duct/inflammation of the lacrimal sac
- Chalazion
- Ectropion
- Entropion
- Hordeola
- Molluscum contagiosum

Critical Diagnoses

- Actinic keratosis
- Periorbital/orbital cellulitis
- Malignancy
  - Basal cell carcinoma
  - Squamous cell carcinoma

CONTINUED INFORMATION GATHERING

On the basis of trying to differentiate between blepharitis and dermatitis it is necessary to get a fuller history of her symptoms and inspect both the anterior and posterior lid margins. Miss L has complained of intermittent itching and watery eyes, and initial visual inspection revealed inflamed eyelid margins. These symptoms are consistent with blepharitis. Examination usually also reveals eyelash loss or misdirection accompanied with debris within the lashes. Varying degrees of conjunctival redness may also be present.

You inspect Miss L's eyes and note some lash loss in both eyes, slight conjunctival redness and normal findings for visual acuity and pupil responses (Fig. 3.12). There also appears to be no obvious redness of the eyelids or surrounding skin.

These findings are further consistent with a differential diagnosis of blepharitis.

PROBLEM REFINEMENT

At this point dermatitis, in its various forms, has not been fully excluded. Cosmetics are an obvious cause of contact dermatitis. You ask Miss L about what products she uses and if the symptoms are experienced at such times. Miss L cannot think of any time where her makeup or facial products have caused her symptoms to flare up.

Seborrhoeic and atopic dermatitis can cause blepharitis-like symptoms, but rash is seen elsewhere (in adults), such as the face, scalp or trunk in the seborrheic

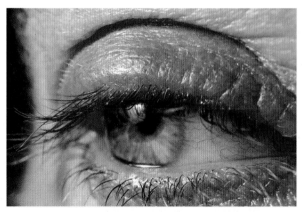

Fig. 3.12 Blepharitis. (Source: Islam, S. (2023). *Infectious diseases: Smart study guide for medical students, residents, and clinical providers.* Elsevier.)

form and hands in atopic dermatitis. This seems to rule out dermatitis and also acne rosacea as the cause.

Other possible causes can be excluded based on age and findings. For example, ectropion and entropion are associated with older age. Lacrimal duct/sac issues are most common in the young as is molluscum contagiosum.

It appears that dermatitis is not the cause of her symptoms and blepharitis is your differential diagnosis.

> ⚡ **RED FLAGS**
>
> Malignant causes are seen in people older than Miss L, and visual inspection did not reveal any lesions or growths. Finally, no swelling or redness of orbital tissues were noted thus ruling out periorbital and orbital cellulitis.

MANAGEMENT

Self-care Options

The mainstay of treatment for blepharitis is improved lid hygiene and warm compresses. You advise Miss L to wet a cloth or cotton bud with a diluted mixture of baby shampoo (1:10) in warm water and gently clean her eyelids. You recommend her to do this twice a day initially and reduce to once a day if symptoms improve. Warm compresses can also be applied to closed eyelids for up to 15 min twice a day.

Prescribing Options

If lid hygiene measures are ineffective, you could give topical antibiotics, although previous use of chloramphenicol failed to resolve symptoms.

Safety Netting

You tell Miss L that you think she has blepharitis and that it is a chronic problem that is associated with flare-ups and remission and that treatment is not curative. Symptom improvement may take several weeks, and you advise Miss L to return after 4 weeks to see if her symptoms have improved.

AIDE MEMOIRE

Likely Diagnoses

Blepharitis

Typically, blepharitis is bilateral with symptoms ranging from irritation, itching and burning of the lid margins.

Lid margins may appear red and raw, accompanied with excessive tearing and crusty debris or skin flakes around the eyelashes. In chronic cases, madarosis (missing lashes) and trichiasis (inturned lashes) can occur. This latter symptom can lead to further local irritation and result in conjunctivitis. Symptoms also tend to be worse in the mornings, and patients might complain of eyelids being stuck together. Symptoms are often intermittent, with exacerbations and remissions occurring over long periods. The mean age of occurrence is 50 years.

Dermatitis

Contact dermatitis can be caused by many products—especially cosmetics—which can be sensitising and result in itching and flaking skin that mimics blepharitis. Additionally, systemic atopy or atopic dermatitis can manifest on the eyelid causing erythema, scaling and itch. In the adult form of seborrhoeic dermatitis, it can also affect the eyelids causing local redness, swelling, itching and skin flaking (Fig. 3.13). It is unusual for only lid involvement to occur in both forms, and other sites are usually affected.

Possible Diagnoses
Acne Rosacea

Rosacea is a characterised by facial skin findings including erythema, telangiectasia, papules and pustules that

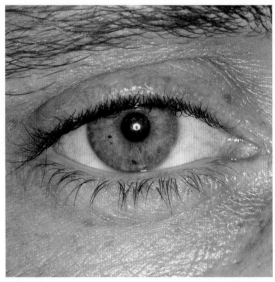

Fig. 3.13 Patient With Characteristic Involvement of Seborrheic Dermatitis on the Eyelid Margin. (Source: *The Fitzsimons Army Medical Center Collection.* Aurora, CO.)

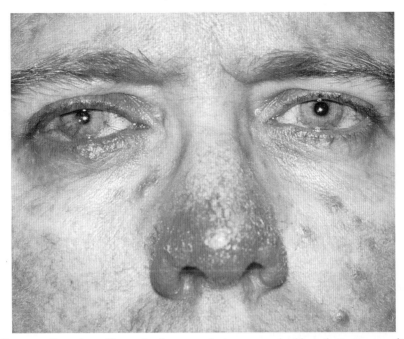

Fig. 3.14 **Rosacea.** Occurring with greater frequency in women, as in this patient, rosacea often involves erythema, telangiectasia and acne as common skin findings. (Source: Krachmer, J. H., & Palay, D. A. (2006). *Cornea atlas* (2nd ed.). Mosby.)

mimic acne vulgaris, although many patients also suffer from marginal blepharitis (Fig. 3.14).

Blocked Tear Duct/Inflammation of the Lacrimal Sac

Dacryocystitis is infection of the tear (lacrimal) sac, and dacryostenosis is narrowing/blockage of the tear (naso-lacrimal) duct. Dacryostenosis can be present from birth (congenital) or develop after birth (acquired). Either type can lead to tearing or an infection of the tear sac. In infants the blockage usually disappears without treatment by the age of 6–9 months. Acquired dacryo-stenosis is often a result of age-related narrowing of the duct. It can also result from scarring after an injury or surgery or from disorders that cause inflammation.

In acute dacryocystitis, the area around the tear sac is painful, red and swollen. The area around the eye may become red and watery and may ooze pus. Because drainage is affected, there is excessive tearing from the eye. If it becomes chronic, the tear sac may bulge, and conjunctivitis can be present.

Entropion and Ectropion

Both problems are associated with older age groups. Entropion is the inward turning of the eyelid margin

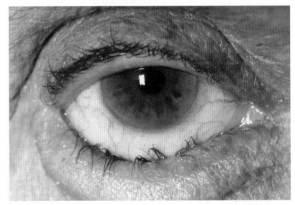

Fig. 3.15 **Involutional Entropion of the Lower Lid With Trichiasis.** (Source: Palay, D. A., & Krachmer, J. H. (2005). *Primary care ophthalmology* (2nd ed.). Philadelphia: Elsevier Mosby.)

(Fig. 3.15), and ectropion is the outward turning of the eyelid margin (Fig. 3.16). They cause similar symptoms, affecting the lower lid and causing irritation, redness and tearing. Entropion can also cause a white mucoid discharge.

Chalazion

A chalazion is a noninfectious mass that results from the obstruction of the meibomian gland. The upper

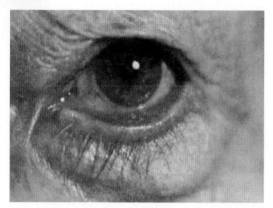

Fig. 3.16 Ectropion of the Lower Lid. (Source: *Zenith, Medical Assistant: Integumentary, Sensory Systems, Patient Care and Communication Module A,* (2nd ed.) 2016, Elsevier.)

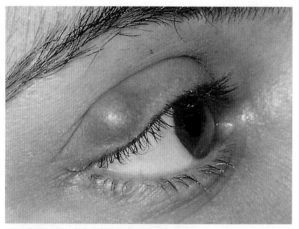

Fig. 3.17 Chalazion (Right Upper Eyelid). (Source: Newell, F. W. (1992). *Ophthalmology: Principles and concepts* (7th ed.). CV Mosby.)

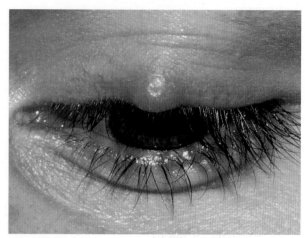

Fig. 3.18 Hordeolum (stye). This is an acute inflammation of the lid margin. An internal hordeolum originates in the meibomian glands, and an external hordeolum originates in Moll's glands, Zeis' glands, or lash follicles. This external hordeolum is on the upper eyelid. (Source: Krachmer, J. H., & Palay, D. A. (2006). Cornea Atlas. (2nd ed.). Mosby.)

Molluscum Contagiosum

Typically seen in preschool children and frequently involves the face, but rarely includes the eyelids, but can lead to conjunctivitis due to viral particle shedding. The trunk and extremities are more often affected. Lesions appear in crops and appear as pink pearl-like spots usually less than 0.5 cm in diameter. All lesions have a central punctum which is a diagnostic feature.

Critical Diagnoses
Actinic Keratosis

Actinic keratosis is a premalignant condition observed in older people and found on sun-damaged skin – hence the face is a common site. Appearance is variable and can occur as single or multiple lesions. Typically, lesions are 1 to 2 cm in size, flat, flaky, white and scaly. They can feel rough to the touch and are likened to the touch of sandpaper. Itching can also be experienced.

Periorbital/Orbital Cellulitis

Periorbital and orbital cellulitis are infections of the soft tissues of the orbit. Distinguishing between them can be difficult as both can present with sudden onset of eyelid redness, swelling and fever. However, orbital cellulitis tends to cause more severe symptoms and is also associated with painful and restricted eye movement, eye bulging and decreased visual acuity.

eyelid is most affected. It may develop from a hordeolum and tends to be present for weeks. Initially tenderness and erythema can be present before evolving into a nontender lump (Fig. 3.17). Associated blepharitis is frequently present. It is most often seen in people aged between 30 and 50 years.

Hordeola (Stye)

Hordeola present as acute painful tender well-defined swelling on the eyelid margin (Fig. 3.18). They can be either internal infections (of the meibomian gland) or external (glands of Zeiss or Moll). They tend to look like a pus-filled lump or pimple at the edge of the eyelid. The patient may also complain of eye discomfort and excessive tearing.

Malignancy

Basal cell carcinoma (90%) and squamous cell carcinoma (5%–10%) account for most malignancies of the eyelid.

Basal Cell Carcinoma

Basal cell carcinoma usually appears on the lower lid. The lesion is firm and pearly with an elevated border. Telangiectasia may overlie the lesion and show central ulceration, which fails to heal. The lesion may bleed or itch but is rarely painful. If located along the lid margin, eyelashes may be missing in the region of the lesion.

Squamous Cell Carcinoma

Lesions present similarly to basal cell carcinomas but occur frequently on the upper lid. They appear erythematous, raised with a rough surface and centrally ulcerated (Fig. 3.19). They can cause pain. Squamous cell carcinoma is quicker growing and more aggressive than basal cell carcinoma.

■ MCQs

1. A 56-year-old Asian man has a sore right eye. He says that his eye is watering and irritated. The symptoms have been present for quite some time. Eye examination is normal. Based on this information which ONE of the following is the most likely diagnosis?
   (a) Blepharitis
   (b) Conjunctivitis
   (c) Dry eye syndrome
   (d) Entropion
   (e) Stye

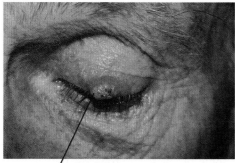

Squamous cell carcinoma

Fig. 3.19 Squamous cell carcinoma of the left upper eyelid, demonstrating erythematous lesion with central scaly plaque. (Source: Kaiser, P. K., & Friedman, N. J. (2014). *The Massachusetts eye and ear infirmary illustrated manual of ophthalmology* (4th ed.). Saunders.)

2. A mother of a 10-year-old boy asks you to look at her son's sore left eye. On examination you notice that his upper eyelid is slightly swollen and tender to touch. Which ONE of the following is the most likely diagnosis?
   (a) Bacterial conjunctivitis
   (b) Blepharitis
   (c) Chalazion
   (d) Hydrocystoma
   (e) Stye

3. An 88-year-old man asks to speak with you. Both eyes are irritated and sore. The symptoms have been present for quite some time. Eye examination reveals a degree of generalised scleral redness with no abnormal lid findings, visual acuity or pupil reflex. Based on this information which ONE of the following is the most likely diagnosis?
   (a) Blepharitis
   (b) Dry eye syndrome
   (c) Conjunctivitis
   (d) Ectropion
   (e) Entropion

4. A 41-year-old man asks for some eye drops to help with his irritated eyes. He reports having sore eyes for the last 2 months. Both eyes are mildly red, and you notice some crusting on the eyelids. Which ONE of the following is the most likely diagnosis?
   (a) Bacterial conjunctivitis
   (b) Blepharitis
   (c) Pterygium
   (d) Sjögren's syndrome
   (e) Viral conjunctivitis

5. Mrs K, a 61-year-old woman, presents with eyes that are sore, feel itchy and watery. The symptoms have been present for quite some time. On examination her eyes are not red and lid margins are normal. Based on this information which ONE of the following is the most likely diagnosis?
   (a) Blepharitis
   (b) Conjunctivitis
   (c) Dry eye syndrome
   (d) Entropion
   (e) Stye

Answers

1. c; 2. e; 3. b; 4. b; 5. c

KEY POINTS: BLEPHARITIS

- A disorder characterised by either infection or gland dysfunction
- Key symptoms are bilateral burning, itching and red eyelid margins.
- Chronic in nature
- Treatment may involve antibacterials if unresponsive to lid hygiene measures.

CASE 5: EYE SORENESS

PRESENTATION

A middle-aged woman who is unknown to you presents with sore eyes that she describes as burning, which are worse on waking, but she complains of eye irritation during the day. She has had the symptoms for a few weeks but not sought help until today. She takes no medicines from the doctor for any medical problems.

PROBLEM REPRESENTATION

A middle-aged woman presents with bilateral eye soreness and irritation of relatively long duration.

HYPOTHESIS GENERATION (LIKELY, POSSIBLE AND CRITICAL DIAGNOSES)

The woman's symptoms are suggestive of lid pathology and/or dry eye disease. Both are common presentations and should be initially considered.

Likely Diagnoses
- Blepharitis
- Dry eye disease

Possible Diagnoses
- Conjunctivitis
- Ectropion
- Environmental factors
- Eyelid abnormality or dysfunction leading to exposure (exposure keratopathy)
- Medicine-induced dry eye (n/a in this case)
- Rosacea
- Systemic diseases
  - Sjögren's syndrome
  - Rheumatoid arthritis

- Lupus
- Thyroid disease
- Nocturnal lagophthalmos
- Ocular pemphigoid

Critical Diagnoses
- Bell's palsy
- Corneal abnormalities

CONTINUED INFORMATION GATHERING

Further exploration of her symptoms is needed, which includes assessing the frequency and severity of discomfort, if her eyes are watering, and location of any redness.

Questioning reveals that she experiences the symptoms on an almost daily basis with early morning symptoms being the most bothersome, where she feels the need to apply a warm flannel to her eyes to ease the discomfort. During the day her eyes frequently water and now she routinely carries a handkerchief with her to dab away the tears. She denies her eyes being stuck together in the morning, and a visual inspection of her eyes shows little to no scleral redness and lid margins are marginally inflamed with no obvious signs of debris.

Her symptoms seem to overlap between dry eye syndrome and blepharitis; excessive tearing is suggestive of dry eye syndrome, and symptoms being worse in the morning fits with blepharitis, although limited redness of the lid margins is not consistent with blepharitis.

PROBLEM REFINEMENT

As dry eye has a number of systemic causes, it is worth asking the patient about any other symptoms that she is experiencing even though she has reported having no medical conditions. For example, Sjögren's syndrome commonly causes dry mouth as well as dry eyes; skin rashes can suggest rosacea or lupus; joint pain might indicate rheumatoid arthritis; and fatigue could be suggestive of thyroid or lupus.

Our patient does not report any other symptoms except some recent sleep problems, but she attributes that to being busy at work and thinking about work-related problems when she goes to bed. She works as a university administrator, and you ask about changes to the work environment to rule out occupational exposure. She tells you nothing has changed.

Dry eye syndrome still seems likely, but the fact that her symptoms are worse in the morning and that she has some sleep disturbances could suggest hyperthyroidism – early morning eye soreness might be associated with eyelid retraction leading to incomplete closure of the eyelids when asleep, and insomnia is a commonly reported symptom.

Based on a suspicion that her symptoms might be due to hyperthyroidism, it is important to check visual acuity and pupil responses as these can be reduced. Additionally, it would be worth asking again about other symptoms but being more specific to those associated with hyperthyroidism, for example, palpitations, fatigue, tremor, anxiety, weight loss, heat intolerance and sweating.

Findings show normal acuity, pupil reflexes and no visual changes or facial skin problems. She does repeat she is tired but again puts that down to her poor sleeping patterns.

Normal findings, whilst not helpful in hyperthyroidism, do allow conjunctivitis, ectropion, rosacea, nocturnal lagophthalmos and ocular pemphigoid to be ruled out.

Some uncertainty exists about the diagnosis, but hyperthyroidism at this point cannot be dismissed.

⚡ RED FLAGS

Visual inspection showed no signs of ectropion or facial skin problems (e.g., rosacea) nor facial paralysis (e.g., Bell's palsy).

MANAGEMENT

Self-care Options

An ocular lubricant could be given to help reduce symptoms in the short term.

Prescribing Options

None. Thyroid function tests should be performed and involve checking serum thyroid stimulating hormone (TSH) levels in the first instance.

Safety Netting

You tell the woman that you are uncertain as to the cause of her symptoms although there are a number of conditions which can cause the problem, and by doing some tests it might be possible to work out what is

causing the dry eyes. If hyperthyroidism is confirmed, treatment should be instigated on consultation with a specialist and follow-up appointments arranged in 3–4 weeks to assess symptoms.

If results are negative, the patient needs to be reassessed.

AIDE MEMOIRE

Likely Diagnoses
Blepharitis

Typically, blepharitis is bilateral with symptoms ranging from irritation, itching and burning of the lid margins. Lid margins may appear red and raw, accompanied with excessive tearing and crusty debris or skin flakes around the eyelashes. In chronic cases, madarosis (missing lashes) and trichiasis (inturned lashes) can occur. This latter symptom can lead to further local irritation and result in conjunctivitis. Symptoms also tend to be worse in the mornings and patients might complain of eyelids being stuck together. Symptoms are often intermittent, with exacerbations and remissions occurring over long periods. The mean age of occurrence is 50 years.

Dry Eye Disease

Dry eye disease is also known as dry eye syndrome or keratoconjunctivitis sicca. It is a chronic condition characterised by reduction in the quality and/or quantity of tears and manifests with a range of symptoms, which include dry, tired and irritated eyes accompanied by epiphora, varying degrees of pain/discomfort and redness of eyelids or conjunctiva with intermittent blurry vision. Dry eye disease is more common in women than in men and has an increased prevalence with age. Causes can be anatomical or systemic. A number of validated questionnaires are available (e.g., Dry Eye Questionnaire (DEQ-5)) that may be useful in assessing dry eye symptoms.

Possible Diagnoses
Conjunctivitis

All forms of conjunctivitis cause a degree of eye discomfort and redness. Infective causes are acute and sudden in onset with watery or mucopurulent discharge. Allergic conjunctivitis will cause itching eyes and be present whilst exposed to the allergen and so can last weeks or months. It is also associated with sneezing and watery nasal discharge. Conjunctivitis tends not to cause lid irritation.

Ectropion

Ectropion is the outward turning of the lower eyelid margin that overexposes the conjunctiva to the atmosphere, leading to eye dryness. Other symptoms include irritation, redness and tearing. It is associated with older age groups.

Environmental Factors

Exposure to irritants such as chemical fumes, cigarette smoke, pollution or low humidity can all cause dry eyes. Symptoms can be exacerbated by wind or heat.

Eyelid Abnormality or Dysfunction Leading to Exposure (Exposure Keratopathy)

Exposure keratopathy occurs when the eyelids do not close fully leading to inadequate protection. Symptoms include dry and irritated eyes, eye redness and blurred vision. Underlying systemic disease may be responsible, for example, thyroid disorders (see below).

Medicine-induced Dry Eye

A number of medicines can exacerbate or produce side effects of dry eyes as a result of decreased tear production. These include systemic medications such as antihistamines, antihypertensives, anxiolytics/benzodiazepines, diuretics, systemic hormones, nonsteroidal antiinflammatory drugs (NSAIDs), androgen antagonists, cardiac arrhythmic drugs and selective serotonin reuptake inhibitors.

Rosacea

Typically presenting with facial skin findings, commonly persistent central facial redness, telangiectasia and inflammatory pustules and papules. In three-quarters of women, eye involvement is also apparent that mimics blepharitis/dry eye syndrome. Eye symptoms include eyelid redness, eye irritation/discomfort/dryness and blurred vision. It is most common in women aged between 30 and 50 years.

Systemic Diseases

Sjögren's syndrome. An autoimmune disease and usually appears in middle- to older-aged adults. Salivary and lacrimal glands are commonly affected, and therefore dry mouth and dry eyes are usually experienced. Symptoms closely mimic dry eye syndrome, although symptoms tend to be more severe. Some people experience tiredness and muscle and joint pain.

Rheumatoid arthritis. A chronic inflammatory disease that primarily affects the joints, but also affects other parts of the body including the eyes. The most common symptom is dryness.

Lupus. Systemic lupus erythematosus is an autoimmune disease, causing widespread inflammation and tissue damage. Patients may therefore experience a variety of symptoms, but common symptoms include fatigue, headaches, skin rash (e.g., butterfly-shaped rash on the cheeks), fever and pain or swelling in the joints. Dry eye is found in about one-third of all patients.

Thyroid disease. Eye symptoms are very common in thyroid disease and include dry eyes, watery eyes and red eyes. In addition, in hyperthyroidism, bulging eyes, double vision, difficulty closing the eyes and reduction in visual acuity can be experienced. Other classic symptoms of thyroid disease include weight changes, heat intolerances, fatigue and anxiety.

Nocturnal Lagophthalmos

Nocturnal lagophthalmos is the inability to close the eyelids during sleep. Symptoms are most obvious on waking and tend to gradually improve during the day. Patients experience soreness/dryness in one or both eyes, often associated with watering. Blurred vision and eye redness may also be present.

Ocular Pemphigoid

This is a rare autoimmune disease that damages the conjunctiva. It usually affects both eyes. Early symptoms are conjunctivitis that can become persistent. Dryness of the eye and trichiasis are common. Scarring of the conjunctiva occurs but is difficult to detect with the naked eye.

Critical Diagnoses
Corneal Abnormalities

There are several common conditions that affect the cornea ranging from small abrasions, foreign bodies and allergies. Most conditions will cause true eye pain (e.g., keratitis, corneal abrasion) and/or affect vision. Other symptoms can mimic dry eye, such as watering and irritation.

Bell's Palsy

Bell's palsy is characterised by unilateral facial paralysis, often with sudden onset. A complication of Bell's palsy is that the patient might be unable to close one eye or blink, leading to decreased tear film, excessive tearing and paradoxically dry eye.

MCQs

1. You speak with an elderly woman about her sore eyes. You diagnose dry eyes that have probably been caused through her medicines. Which ONE of the following medicines is known to cause dry eye?
   (a) Atenolol
   (b) Isosorbide mononitrate
   (c) Nifedipine
   (d) Ramipril
   (e) Valsartan
2. Which ONE of the following is not a common sign of thyroid ophthalmopathy?
   (a) Conjunctival injection (redness)
   (b) Double vision
   (c) Dry eyes and irritation
   (d) Enophthalmos
   (e) Eyelid retraction
3. Dry eyes can be a symptom of lupus. From the following, which ONE of the common symptoms would you associate lupus with?
   (a) Blurred vision
   (b) Fatigue and weight change
   (c) Joint pain
   (d) Joint pain and dry mouth
   (e) Joint pain and fatigue
4. Ocular lubricants are often prescribed to ease dry eye symptoms. Which ONE of the following lubricants has the advantage of infrequent application?
   (a) Carbomer
   (b) Carmellose sodium
   (c) Hypromellose
   (d) Sodium hyaluronate
   (e) Polyvinyl alcohol
5. When performing thyroid function tests, which ONE of the values suggests that a person has hypothyroidism?
   (a) High TSH and high T4
   (b) High TSH and low T4
   (c) Low TSH and low T4
   (d) Low TSH and high T4
   (e) None of the above

Answers

1. a; 2. d; 3. e; 4. a; 5. b

KEY POINTS: DRY EYE SYNDROME

- Caused by an imbalance between either poor or inadequate tear production and tear drainage
- Key symptoms are feelings of dryness, grittiness or soreness in both eyes, which worsen through the day.
- The condition is chronic.
- Treat with artificial tears and ointments if advice alone is insufficient.

WEBSITES

The British Sjögren's Syndrome Association
https://www.bssa.uk.net/
Sjögren's foundation
https://sjogrens.org/

EARS

CASE 6: EARACHE

PRESENTATION

Mrs Y, the mother of a 4-year-old boy, asks if you can give her son some painkillers stronger than paracetamol for his earache. He has been complaining of right ear pain for the last 24 h and is not eating properly. Paracetamol seems to ease the pain, but he is still complaining of pain.

PROBLEM REPRESENTATION

A 4-year-old boy presents with a 1-day history of acute unilateral earache and poor appetite.

HYPOTHESIS GENERATION (LIKELY, POSSIBLE AND CRITICAL DIAGNOSES)

Ear pain (otalgia) is classed as either primary (originating from the external, middle or inner ear) or secondary (originates outside the ear (i.e., referred)). In children primary otalgia is most common, typically otitis media or otitis externa, and as such form our initial hypotheses to test.

Likely Diagnoses

- Otitis media (acute)
- Otitis externa

Possible Diagnoses

- Dental infection/abscess
- Eustachian tube dysfunction/barotrauma
- Foreign body
- Temporomandibular joint disorders (unusual in children)

Critical Diagnosis

- Mastoiditis

CONTINUED INFORMATION GATHERING

Otitis media and otitis externa can present with similar symptoms – both show rapid onset that causes ear pain, which can be persistent; decreased hearing is also observed, although this tends to be more common in otitis media. Further information about the pain and any associated symptoms should be sought.

You find out that pain is the predominant symptom. He has not described any loss of hearing and his mother seems to think that his hearing is normal. This description seems to fit both otitis media and externa, although given that he may have constitutional symptoms (not eating) thinking of otitis media can be favoured.

PROBLEM REFINEMENT

At this point an ear examination should be performed. Manipulation of the tragus and/or pinna would usually cause tenderness or pain if otitis externa was the cause, and inflammation of the ear canal is common. Visualisation of a distinctly red, yellow or cloudy bulging tympanic membrane, with or without loss of landmarks, is observed in otitis media.

Examination reveals a red ear canal and a slightly red nonbulging tympanic membrane; manipulation of the outer ear caused some but not excessive discomfort.

These signs and symptoms now point more towards a differential diagnosis of otitis externa. To help support

this hypothesis asking the child's mother about any ear discharge and possible precipitating factors should help rule in/rule out otitis externa.

In otitis externa, otorrhoea is common and symptoms are usually caused by local trauma to the ear canal by items used in an attempt to clean the ears, for example, cotton buds, hairgrips, etc., which is then predisposed to infection from water which enters during swimming, hair washing, showering, etc. His mother tells you that prior to the earache he seemed fit and healthy, she has not been cleaning his ears with cotton buds and she has not noticed any ear discharge, but her son has started swimming lessons recently. Otitis media seems less likely now due to no ear discharge and the absence of any respiratory symptoms prior to the earache.

You check that none of the possible causes could be responsible. Her son's symptoms seem to poorly fit: dental infection (fever and local mouth pain), barotrauma (no history pressure changes), foreign body (no discharge) and temporomandibular joint disorders (no local jaw pain).

Given his symptoms and the recent history of swimming you are relatively confident of a diagnosis of otitis externa rather than otitis media.

> ⚡ **RED FLAGS**
>
> Physical examination has ruled out mastoiditis as he did not have any pain, redness and swelling behind the ear.

MANAGEMENT

Self-care Options

Mrs Y should be advised that her son should avoid swimming for at least a week, and care should be taken when he is showering or bathing to keep water out of the ear. His ear pain could be managed by switching to ibuprofen. If this does not help, alternating use of both paracetamol and ibuprofen could be tried.

Prescribing Options

You could recommend acetic acid (Earcalm Spray) as current UK guidelines advocate its use for mild cases.

Safety Netting

You tell Mrs Y that as you suspect her son has an ear infection, his symptoms should improve within 72 h;

however, if the pain persists or she notices discharge, she needs to bring her son back to reassess his symptoms. At that point ear drops containing an antibiotic and corticosteroid could be considered. Choice of drug will depend on clinical judgement, consideration of patient adherence regarding dosing and local antibiotic prescribing guidelines.

AIDE MEMOIRE

Likely Diagnoses
Otitis Media (Acute)

Acute otitis media (AOM) is most common in children of up to the age of 4 years. Symptoms develop rapidly. Young children often hold or rub their ear or have nonspecific symptoms such as fever, crying, poor feeding and restlessness. In older children, ear pain/earache is the predominant feature and tends to be throbbing. An examination of the ear should reveal a red/yellow and bulging tympanic membrane with a loss of normal landmarks. Otitis media often follows URTI. A complication of AOM is conductive hearing loss.

Otitis Externa

Patients experience itching of the ear canal, ear pain and tenderness on manipulation of the pinna or tragus, and their ear canal is oedematous and can be filled with infectious debris. Ear discharge is often seen. Conductive hearing loss may occur if swelling and debris occlude the canal.

Possible Diagnoses
Dental Infection/Abscess

The main symptom is sudden onset pain in the affected tooth, which can be intense and throbbing. Other symptoms include tooth sensitivity to heat and cold, unpleasant taste in the mouth, fever and malaise. The pain can radiate to the ear.

Eustachian Tube Dysfunction/Barotrauma

Ear barotrauma is discomfort in the ear due to pressure differences between the inside and outside of the eardrum. It is usually observed with altitude changes such as flying, although it can be experienced when suffering from URTIs. Ear discomfort/pain and a sensation of ear fullness (often described as being underwater or ears with cotton wool) are the commonest symptoms. Other symptoms that may be experienced are tinnitus, dizziness and popping or clicking noises.

Foreign Body

It most often occurs in toddlers. A foreign object in the ear can cause pain, hearing loss and over time, infection where redness, swelling and discharge may be present.

Temporomandibular Joint Disorders

Temporomandibular disorder (TMD) is most common among people between the ages of 20 and 40 years. Symptoms include pain or tenderness in the face, jaw joint area, neck and shoulders and in or around the ear. Pain worsens on chewing, speaking or opening the mouth. Clicking or grating sounds in the jaw joint can be heard when the mouth is opened and closed. Patients with TMD also report headaches and otological symptoms such as otalgia, tinnitus, vertigo, ear fullness and hearing loss.

Critical Diagnosis
Mastoiditis

The person generally presents as systemically unwell with fever. Ear pain, mastoid tenderness and swelling are seen. A history of a recent episode of AOM is common.

▌ MCQs

1. An 8-year-old girl complains of constant pain in her left ear. You inspect the outer ear and see that it is red, inflamed and hot to the touch, with a small amount of visible crust. Her father also noticed a sticky yellow discharge this morning. Which ONE of the following is the most likely diagnosis?
   (a) AOM
   (b) Chronic otitis media
   (c) Excessive ear wax
   (d) Glue ear (otitis media with effusion)
   (e) Otitis externa

2. A 30-year-old man presents to you complaining of constant pain in his left ear. Upon examination you see that his tympanic membrane appears red and inflamed. Which ONE of the following is the most likely diagnosis?
   (a) Eustachian tube dysfunction
   (b) Glue ear (otitis media with effusion)
   (c) Otitis externa
   (d) Otitis media
   (e) Perforated eardrum

3. A 19-year-old Caucasian woman with 2-day history of left-sided earache presents to your walk-in clinic. Pain has worsened over the last 24 h and she says there has been some 'rubbish' coming out of her ear. She denies feeling feverish and has not noticed any loss of hearing. Which ONE of the following is the most likely diagnosis?
   - (a) Acute otitis externa
   - (b) AOM
   - (c) Chronic otitis externa
   - (d) Chronic otitis media
   - (e) Mastoiditis

4. On examination of the ear you observe a pearly white lesion on the tympanic membrane. The patient has had some hearing loss and a recently perforated tympanic membrane. Which ONE of the following is the most likely diagnosis?
   - (a) Cerumen impaction
   - (b) Cholesteatoma
   - (c) Glue ear
   - (d) Mastoiditis
   - (e) None of the above

5. You take the history of an adult male patient. He tells you that he has ear pain, tinnitus and a sensation of fullness in his left ear. He also tells you he has recently returned from a holiday. Which ONE of the following is the most likely diagnosis?
   - (a) Barotrauma
   - (b) Cervical lymphadenitis
   - (c) Glue ear
   - (d) Temporomandibular joint disorder
   - (e) Trauma

Answers

1. e; 2. d; 3. a; 4. b; 5. a

KEY POINTS: OTITIS EXTERNA

- Most cases are caused by a bacterial infection but can be due to fungal infection, irritation, trauma and allergy.
- Key symptoms are itch, ear pain, discharge and pinna tenderness.
- Symptoms should resolve within 10 days.
- Mild cases – acetic acid drops; moderate to severe cases – topical antibiotics with or without corticosteroids.

WEBSITES

Otitis media (acute): antimicrobial prescribing NG91
https://www.nice.org.uk/guidance/ng91

CASE 7: DIZZINESS

PRESENTATION

A 76-year-old man (Mr T) presents complaining of recent episodes of dizziness. Yesterday was probably the worst as he kept getting short-lived dizziness throughout the day and felt sick, although he did not vomit. He tells you he has felt unsteady on his feet and is worried that he is going to fall. You check his medical history, and it shows he has long-standing cardiovascular disease and chronic obstructive pulmonary disease (COPD). He has also been recently diagnosed with benign prostrate hyperplasia (BPH).

PROBLEM REPRESENTATION

Recent onset of intermittent and unpredictable dizziness in an elderly man with comorbidities.

HYPOTHESIS GENERATION (LIKELY, POSSIBLE AND CRITICAL DIAGNOSES)

The term dizziness describes sensations of feeling faint, unsteady/off balance or woozy. When dizziness creates a false sense that your surroundings are spinning or moving, then it is defined as vertigo. Dizziness is a common symptom and can be caused by diverse aetiologies including vestibular, cardiovascular, neurological and psychogenic causes. It may be part of a symptom cluster but not the presenting symptom, for example, acute otitis externa or anxiety. In this case dizziness is a predominant symptom, and we need to consider:

Likely Diagnoses

- Benign positional paroxysmal vertigo (BPPV)
- Diabetes (hypoglycaemia)
- Labyrinthitis
- Ménière's disease
- Postural (orthostatic) hypotension
- Vestibular neuronitis

Possible Diagnoses

- Cardiovascular causes
- Migraine
- Persistent postural–perceptual dizziness (PPPD)
- Otosclerosis
- Perilymphatic fistula
- Superior semicircular canal dehiscence

Critical Diagnoses

- Acoustic neuroma
- Cholesteatoma
- CO poisoning
- Multiple sclerosis (MS)
- Vertebrobasilar insufficiency

CONTINUED INFORMATION GATHERING

Knowing more about the dizziness episodes Mr T has been experiencing is needed, for example, when and how do they start, how long do they last and what does he mean by the use of the word dizziness.

Mr T tells you that he has had about five or six episodes in the last month or so. They never last very long and seem to be very unpredictable, which worries him. He cannot really think that they occur more at any time of day, but they do not seem to happen when he is sitting down or in bed. He says he feels very wobbly when they happen, and it is disconcerting. He says that the nausea has only happened the last time he went dizzy.

This description of unpredictable short-lived dizziness, which is usually not associated with nausea, seems to point away from the two most common causes of dizziness, BPPV and vestibular neuronitis, as both are associated with nausea and vomiting. BPPV is also associated with head movement. The shortness of each episode also points away from labyrinthitis, Ménière's disease and vestibular neuronitis.

Based on the most likely causes, it seems we may be dealing with episodes of hypoglycaemia or postural hypotension.

PROBLEM REFINEMENT

Mr T has not reported other symptoms apart from a one-off episode of nausea. You specifically ask him if he has had any tiredness, feels hungry or feels shaky. He reports no such symptoms. This seems to rule out hypoglycaemia. We know he has comorbidities and therefore will be taking many medicines. Medicine side effects are usually associated with the introduction of new medicines or dosage modifications. You ask him about this. He says the only thing that has recently changed is that he now takes something for his waterworks. We know BPH is often treated using alpha-blockers, which can cause postural hypotension. This therefore could be the cause of his symptoms. You ask, specifically, if the

dizziness is noticed when getting up and down, for example, out of bed or from a chair. He tells you that, although he had not thought of that, it does seem to fit when he gets dizzy.

Checks on his medical history are needed to see what he was given. You see he was given alfuzosin. You are now relatively confident it is medication-related hypotension.

> ### ⚡ RED FLAGS
>
> You ask if his hearing has worsened over the time of his dizzy spells. He says his hearing is about the same. No reduction in hearing suggests that acoustic neuroma and cholesteatoma are not the cause of his symptoms. He seems alert and reports no neurological deficits, suggesting that CO poisoning, MS or vertebrobasilar insufficiency can be discounted.

MANAGEMENT

Self-care Options

Mr T could try drinking more fluids but should restrict his caffeine intake. He should take his time when standing and make sure he has support in case he feels dizzy. If he does feel dizzy, he should sit down.

Prescribing Options

Consideration should be given to stopping alfuzosin. If this is stopped, finasteride may be tried instead.

Safety Netting

You tell Mr T you think it is his new medicine that is causing his dizziness. If Mr T wanted, he could stop taking this medicine and try a different one instead. If he did this, then you would want to see him in a week's time.

AIDE MEMOIRE

Likely Diagnoses
Benign Positional Paroxysmal Vertigo

This is the most common cause of vertigo and is caused by dislodged canaliths in the semicircular canals of the inner ear. It tends to occur in people older than 50 years and is more common in women. Episodic vertigo and nausea are experienced when the head is in certain positions (e.g., lying on one side or face up in bed). Episodes tend to be short-lived – typically less than 1 min, but people can feel off balance for several hours after symptoms have gone.

Hypoglycaemia

Low blood sugar is a common problem primarily associated with diabetes. Various signs and symptoms can be experienced, with dizziness and light-headedness being common. Others include sweating, feeling tired and hungry, shakiness, difficulty concentrating, tingling lips and irregular or fast heartbeat.

Labyrinthitis

Labyrinthitis is an inner ear infection. The most common symptoms are dizziness, hearing loss and vertigo. These symptoms can range from mild to severe. Other symptoms may include tinnitus, nausea, aural fullness (pressure in the ear), ear pain and visual disturbances.

Ménière's Disease

Ménière's disease causes vertigo and unilateral hearing loss. It is more common among people aged between 20 and 60 years. Vertigo associated with Ménière's disease is often severe enough to necessitate bed rest and can cause nausea, vomiting and loss of balance. It can occur suddenly, is not provoked by changes in position and, unlike BPPV, lasts much longer, anywhere from 30 min to several hours. Other symptoms include sudden slips or falls, tinnitus and headache.

Postural (Orthostatic) Hypotension

Postural hypotension is a symptom rather than a condition but is associated with Parkinson's disease, certain medication and increasing age, especially those aged more than 60 years. An abnormal drop in blood pressure when changing from lying/sitting to a standing position gives rise to light-headedness or dizziness and can lead to falls. Classic postural hypotension occurs within 3 min of standing, although delayed symptoms beyond 3 min are sometimes seen. It can be experienced at any time of the day. Many medicines are implicated, including antihypertensives and nitrates, although polypharmacy (more than five medicines) is probably more of a contributory factor to causes of hypotension and dizziness.

Vestibular Neuronitis

Vestibular neuronitis is the second most common cause of vertigo. It most commonly affects persons aged 30–50 years. Symptoms are acute in onset and generally severe, although they tend to subside over a few days. Nausea and vomiting are common but auditory symptoms (e.g., hearing loss) are not present. Balance can be affected. A prior viral illness is often experienced. Nystagmus (rhythmical, repetitive and involuntary movement of the eyes) is present.

Possible Diagnoses
Cardiovascular Causes

Dizziness, light-headedness or syncope can be experienced by people who have underlying cardiovascular problems, for example, arrhythmia, aortic stenosis and sick sinus syndrome. However, common to cardiac pathology, patients should exhibit other symptoms including irregular pulse, palpitations, chest discomfort, shortness of breath and fatigue. These may be exacerbated by activity.

Migraine

Episodic vertigo and dizziness in a patient with a history of migraine headaches suggests vestibular migraine. Patients will experience 'typical' migraine symptoms such as intense headache, nausea or vomiting.

Persistent Postural–Perceptual Dizziness

Characterised by persistent sensations of rocking or swaying unsteadiness and/or dizziness without vertigo lasting 3 months or more. Most patients have daily symptoms, although the severity will fluctuate. Symptoms are related to body posture and are more severe when walking or standing compared with sitting or lying down. A previous vestibular disorder is often a triggering event for PPPD.

Otosclerosis

The most frequently reported symptom of otosclerosis is gradual hearing loss, which usually starts in one ear and then moves to the other. Many people with otosclerosis first notice that they are unable to hear low-pitched sounds or cannot hear a whisper. Some people may also experience dizziness, balance problems and tinnitus. It typically affects middle-aged White women. There is usually a positive family history.

Perilymphatic Fistula

This is a rare condition. It causes acute onset unilateral sudden hearing loss, tinnitus, vertigo and unsteadiness.

There is usually a history of barotrauma head or ear trauma.

Superior Semicircular Canal Dehiscence

This is a rare condition characterised by vertigo and the apparent motion of objects that are known to be stationary in response to loud noises. Symptoms can be triggered by heavy lifting, straining or coughing. Other symptoms include fullness in the ear and autophony (which is 'hearing oneself', in which sounds from inside the body, such as breathing, heartbeat and blood flow, can be heard).

Critical Diagnosis

Acoustic Neuroma

A benign tumour which can cause hearing loss, vertigo and unsteadiness by compressing the cochlear nerve. Tinnitus may also be present. Symptoms tend to develop gradually usually affecting one ear. They occur most frequently in adults aged 30–60 years.

Cholesteatoma

Cholesteatoma is a destructive and expanding growth in the middle ear and/or mastoid process. They are characterised by persistent or recurrent malodorous purulent discharge and fullness. Conductive hearing loss is present in 90% of patients. Dizziness and vertigo are possible but are uncommon.

Carbon Monoxide Poisoning

Dizziness is a common symptom of CO poisoning, along with headache, weakness, vomiting, chest pain, shortness of breath and confusion.

Multiple Sclerosis

MS presents with wide-ranging neurological signs and symptoms and includes vertigo. The most common initial presentation is unilateral visual loss, muscle weakness and paraesthesia. Onset is usually before the age of 50 years.

Vertebrobasilar Insufficiency

The blood supply to the brainstem, cerebellum and inner ear is derived from the vertebrobasilar system. Any major branch occlusion (through atherosclerosis) can cause vertigo and is the most common symptom and is also often the initial symptom. Dizziness/fainting is also frequently reported. Diagnosis usually relies on a history of symptoms such as loss of vision, diplopia, confusion, numbness or tingling, slurred speech and loss of coordination. Risk factors for cerebrovascular disease are those associated with atherosclerosis, such as smoking, hypertension, older age, hyperlipidaemia and family history.

■ MCQs

1. A 37-year-old woman presents with severe vertigo which started whilst she was taking a course of antibiotics for a urinary tract infection. Which ONE of the following antibiotics is most likely to be the cause of her symptoms?
   (a) Amoxicillin
   (b) Cephalexin
   (c) Ciprofloxacin
   (d) Nitrofurantoin
   (e) Tetracycline

2. A 75-year-old woman was admitted following a fall. During an assessment of her fall, she complained of balance problems and dizziness whenever she looked upwards, for example, to hang laundry on her washing line outside. Her past medical history reveals she has hypertension, for which she was taking amlodipine 10 mg daily. On examination her gait and balance and neurological examination were normal and there were no injuries. Which ONE of the following is the most likely diagnosis?
   (a) BPPV
   (b) Cervical spondylosis
   (c) Ménière's disease
   (d) Otosclerosis
   (e) Vertebrobasilar insufficiency

3. Almost all patients with vertigo feel worse with:
   (a) Being in the supine position
   (b) Exposure to visual stimuli
   (c) Head movement
   (d) Physical exertion
   (e) Valsaver movement

4. Labyrinthitis can present with a range of symptoms. Which ONE of the following is least likely?
   (a) Aural fullness
   (b) Nausea
   (c) Severe headache
   (d) Severe vertigo
   (e) Tinnitus

5. Which ONE of the following is false regarding vestibular neuronitis?
   (a) A viral inflammatory aetiology is thought to precipitate vestibular neuronitis
   (b) It is the second most common cause of vertigo
   (c) Men and women are equally affected
   (d) The sudden onset of severe symptoms can raise concerns of a central aetiology
   (e) Vestibular and cochlear components of the eighth cranial nerve are both affected

Answers

1. c; 2. a; 3. c; 4. c; 5. e

KEY POINTS: POSTURAL (ORTHOSTATIC) HYPOTENSION

- Postural hypotension is a drop in blood pressure ($\geq 20\,mm\,Hg$ systolic and/or $\geq 10\,mm\,Hg$ diastolic) that occurs within 3 min of standing.
- Key symptoms are light-headedness and dizziness.
- The goal of treatment is to alleviate symptoms and lower the risk of falls.

WEBSITES

Ménière's Society
https://www.menieres.org.uk/

CASE 8: HEARING LOSS

PRESENTATION

Mr F, a 66-year-old man, presents to you complaining of hearing loss. He says he has been struggling to catch what people say when he is having conversations, and it has been noticeable for a few months now. This seems to be worse when he is with a group of people.

PROBLEM REPRESENTATION

A 66-year-old man with a history of gradual hearing loss.

HYPOTHESIS GENERATION (LIKELY, POSSIBLE AND CRITICAL DIAGNOSES)

Hearing loss can be categorised as conductive, sensorineural or both. Conductive hearing loss occurs when sound conduction is impeded through the external ear, the middle ear or both. Sensorineural hearing loss occurs when there is a problem within the cochlea or the neural pathway to the auditory cortex. Many people with sensorineural hearing loss report that they struggle to understand speech, especially in the presence of background noise.

For Mr F, based on his symptoms and age, the likely conditions to consider initially are:

Likely Diagnoses

- Ageing (presbycusis)
- Impacted earwax
- Noise exposure
- Otosclerosis
- Tympanic membrane perforation (trauma)

Possible Diagnoses

- Exostoses and osteomas
- Foreign bodies
- Head trauma
- Infection
- Medication
- Ménière's disease
- Otitis externa
- Otitis media
- Otitis media with effusion
- Perilymphatic fistula

Critical Diagnoses

- Tumours
  - Acoustic neuroma
  - Cholesteatoma
  - Glomus tumours

CONTINUED INFORMATION GATHERING

Age-related hearing loss seems likely, but more information is needed about his symptoms. Is the hearing loss unilateral or bilateral? Are there particular frequencies at which hearing loss occurs? He tells you that both ears are affected and high-pitched sounds are difficult to hear – he says that some noises that his grandchildren can hear he cannot, and he likes birds but some of their songs he can now just not hear. The loss of high-frequency sounds does not fit with otosclerosis, in which there is a loss of low frequency sounds. The gradual onset of symptoms rules out sudden noise exposure but not chronic exposure. Enquiry to his job history or if he frequently attended music concerts would enable noise exposure to be eliminated. He tells you he is a retired teacher and only occasionally used to go to concerts. Chronic noise exposure does not seem to be the cause.

Bilateral gradual loss of high-frequency sounds is consistent with age-related hearing loss and is now your differential diagnosis.

PROBLEM REFINEMENT

A physical examination should be normal if it is age-related hearing loss. Signs of redness, discharge or changes to the tympanic membrane would exclude impacted earwax, tympanic membrane perforation, otitis media, otitis externa and foreign bodies.

You also ask if he has experienced any other symptoms. He says he has only noticed the hearing loss. No symptoms of tinnitus or dizziness also seem to rule out conditions such as exostoses, trauma, Ménière's disease or perilymphatic fistula. Finally, you take a medication history to rule out ototoxicity. You ask if he takes anything from the doctor and he tells you he is diabetic and asthmatic. He takes metformin and inhalers. Based on this, medicines can be ruled out as a cause.

> ⚡ **RED FLAGS**
>
> Tumours can be discounted as they are unilateral.

MANAGEMENT

Self-care Options
Not applicable.

Prescribing Options
Arrangements should be made for an audiological assessment for the need of hearing aids.

Safety Netting
You tell Mr F that you believe his hearing difficulties are due to him getting older and that he probably would benefit from hearing aids, and you will make an onward referral for hearing tests.

AIDE MEMOIRE

Likely Diagnoses
Age-related Hearing Loss (Presbycusis)
Hearing loss is progressive and occurs in older patients. High-frequency hearing and speech discrimination ability are most affected. Because this type of loss occurs over time, people may not easily notice deterioration.

Impacted Earwax
The key features of earwax impaction are a history of gradual hearing loss (most common symptom) and variable degrees of ear discomfort. Itching, tinnitus and dizziness occur infrequently.

Noise Exposure
Occupational, recreational or accidental exposure to sounds greater than 85 decibels can produce hearing loss accompanied by tinnitus. It occurs more commonly in people working in environments with chronic exposure to loud noises and having insufficient ear protection or from a one-off loud noise such as an explosion or gunfire. Patients typically report that the symptoms are worse in noisy or crowded environments.

Otosclerosis
Otosclerosis refers to abnormal bone growth affecting the small bones of the ear. It typically starts in one ear and then moves to the other. Hearing loss occurs gradually. Many people with otosclerosis first notice that they are unable to hear low-pitched sounds or cannot hear a whisper. Some people may also experience dizziness, tinnitus and balance problems. It typically affects middle-aged White women. There is usually a positive family history.

Tympanic Membrane Perforation (Trauma)
The main causes of tympanic membrane perforations are chronic otitis media and trauma. Traumatic perforations of the tympanic membrane can occur because of water accidents, barotrauma, explosions, penetrating injury or temporal bone fractures.

Possible Diagnoses
Exostoses and Osteomas
These are rare benign bony growths of the external auditory canal that lead to occlusion and conductive hearing loss. Patients may also experience a sense of ear

fullness, tinnitus or otorrhoea. Exostoses are multiple and bilateral and are found adjacent to the tympanic membrane. Patients with exostoses often report a history of cold-water swimming. Osteomas are single and unilateral and are found at the bony–cartilaginous junction and are generally asymptomatic and only discovered on examination.

Foreign Bodies

Foreign bodies (in adults can be things such as insects) in the external auditory canal can cause unilateral conductive hearing loss but discharge is generally a more prominent feature.

Head Trauma

Damage to the inner ear can be caused by a blow to the head. Concussions are linked to hearing loss and tinnitus.

Infections

Complications of certain viral infections such as measles, meningitis and mumps can cause sensorineural hearing loss.

Medications

Ototoxicity specifically affects the cochlea or auditory nerve and sometimes the vestibular system. Medications include aminoglycoside antibiotics (e.g., gentamicin), loop diuretics (e.g., bumetanide and furosemide), nonsteroidal antiinflammatory drugs (NSAIDs), aspirin, antimalarials (e.g., quinine and chloroquine) and cytotoxic drugs (e.g., cisplatin and bleomycin). Symptoms are bilateral and the effect can either be reversible and temporary or irreversible and permanent.

Ménière's Disease

This can occur at any age but is more common in people aged between 40 and 60 years. It can cause severe dizziness (vertigo), unilateral fluctuating hearing loss with a feeling of pressure in the ear and tinnitus. Initially, the hearing loss is in low frequencies, but higher frequencies are affected as the disease progresses. Some people with Ménière's disease have vertigo so extreme that they lose their balance and fall.

Otitis Externa

Otitis externa is an infection of the skin of the external auditory canal. Patients experience itching of the ear canal, ear pain and tenderness on manipulation of the pinna or tragus, and their ear canal is oedematous that can be filled with infectious debris. Ear discharge is often seen. Conductive hearing loss may occur if swelling and debris occlude the canal.

Otitis Media

AOM is most common in children up to the age of 4 years. Symptoms develop rapidly. Young children often hold or rub their ear or have nonspecific symptoms such as fever, crying, poor feeding and restlessness. In older children ear pain/earache is the predominant feature and tends to be throbbing. An examination of the ear should reveal a red/yellow and bulging tympanic membrane with a loss of normal landmarks. A complication of AOM is conductive hearing loss.

Otitis Media With Effusion

Children may go on to have persistent otitis media after bouts of AOM. This is either known as chronic suppurative otitis media or otitis media with effusion (glue ear). It is characterised with ear discharge (through perforation in the tympanic membrane), lasting more than 2 weeks that is not associated with pain or fever. Glue ear is symptomless, apart from impaired hearing, but can have a negative impact on a child's language and educational development if unresolved.

Perilymphatic Fistula

This is a rare condition. It causes acute onset unilateral sudden hearing loss, tinnitus, vertigo and unsteadiness. There is usually a history of barotrauma head or ear trauma.

Critical Diagnoses
Tumours

Acoustic neuroma. A benign tumour which can cause hearing loss, vertigo and unsteadiness by compressing the cochlear nerve. Symptoms tend to develop gradually usually affecting one ear. They occur most frequently in adults aged 30–60 years.

Cholesteatoma. Cholesteatoma is a destructive and expanding growth in the middle ear and/or mastoid process. They are characterised by persistent or recurrent malodorous purulent discharge and fullness. Conductive hearing loss is present in 90% of patients.

Glomus tumours. These are a rare cause of conductive hearing loss. Characteristically, patients are women aged 40–50 years who report pulsatile tinnitus and hearing loss.

MCQs

1. Regarding cholesteatoma, which ONE of the following is true?
   (a) It consists of squamous epithelium.
   (b) It is mainly treated medically.
   (c) It is a malignant tumour.
   (d) It may metastasise to distant sites.
   (e) It should be left untreated.
2. Which ONE of the following conditions most commonly observed in children causes bilateral conductive deafness?
   (a) AOM
   (b) Cholesteatoma
   (c) Chronic suppurative otitis media
   (d) Otitis media with effusion
   (e) Otosclerosis
3. A number of medicines are known to cause ototoxicity. Which ONE of the following does not cause ototoxicity?
   (a) Aspirin
   (b) Cisplatin
   (c) Furosemide
   (d) Gentamicin
   (e) Paracetamol

4. Which ONE of the following conditions is least associated with progressive deafness?
   (a) Otitis media with effusion
   (b) Otosclerosis
   (c) Medicine-induced deafness
   (d) Ménière's disease
   (e) Presbycusis
5. An adult patient presents with unilateral deafness and tinnitus. Based on these symptoms, which ONE of the following is the most likely diagnosis?
   (a) Exostoses
   (b) Foreign body
   (c) Ménière's disease
   (d) Otosclerosis
   (e) Presbycusis

Answers

1. a; 2. d; 3. e; 4. c; 5. c

KEY POINTS: AGE-RELATED HEARING LOSS

- Causes are multifactorial and include physiological degeneration plus the accumulated effects of noise exposure, medical disorders and hereditary susceptibility.
- Key symptoms are gradual hearing loss in both ears.
- Prognosis is of progressively deteriorating hearing.
- Hearing aids are generally required.

WEBSITES

Tinnitus UK
http://www.tinnitus.org.uk

NOSE

CASE 9: UPPER RESPIRATORY TRACT

PRESENTATION

Mrs L, a 25-year-old woman, says she has had cold-like symptoms for the last 10 days. Her nose is still blocked up, and she has been continually nose blowing. She also says she is experiencing some pain across her nose and face.

PROBLEM REPRESENTATION

A 25-year-old woman presents with a 10-day history of worsening URTI symptoms mainly affecting the nose.

HYPOTHESIS GENERATION (LIKELY, POSSIBLE AND CRITICAL DIAGNOSES)

Nasal congestion can be a symptom of many conditions. However, based on her age, we can draw up a relatively short list of those that should be initially considered, as things such as adenoiditis, nasal foreign body (both seen in children) and malignancy (older age groups) can be discounted from early thinking. Therefore, for Mrs L, we should initially consider the following conditions:

Likely Diagnoses
- Allergic rhinitis
- Common cold
- Sinusitis

Possible Diagnoses
- Adenoiditis
- Deviated nasal septum
- Facial pain
  - Cluster headache
  - Dental
  - Giant cell arteritis (GCA)
  - Migraine
  - Neuropathic pain – for example, trigeminal neuralgia
  - TMDs
- Nasal foreign body
- Nasal polyp
- Turbinate hypertrophy

Critical Diagnosis (Sinonasal Tumour)
- Malignancy

CONTINUED INFORMATION GATHERING

Mrs L's symptoms appear to be typical of URTI, with nasal congestion as the predominant symptom. At this point it would be useful to know about what, if any, other symptoms she has experienced over the last 10 days and details about her current nasal and facial symptoms.

She tells you that she started off with a sore throat, which lasted a few days but has then been replaced with her blocked-up nose, which is now making her face ache. On nose blowing, she says the discharge is yellowish green. She said she was sneezing quite a bit at the start but that seems to have settled down. At present she has no cough and does not report having a temperature.

Her previous and present symptoms seem to suggest that she has a common cold, although she now has facial pain and symptoms seem to have lasted longer than a

typical cold – symptoms peak after 2–3 days and last about 1 week.

Allergic rhinitis seems unlikely as discharge is mucopurulent, sneezing is not prominent, and she has facial pain. To further rule out allergic rhinitis, one would expect a negative history of atopy. Mrs L confirms that this is the case.

PROBLEM REFINEMENT

Duration of symptoms and now presence of facial pain point towards Mrs L developing sinusitis. However, a number of conditions do cause facial pain, but her symptoms of mucopurulent discharge and location of pain do not match any of those presentations.

In sinusitis, many patients experience local tenderness and an increase in pain when bending over or lying down. You ask if this is the case and Mrs L says her cheek area is sore to touch but she has not noticed an increase in pain when she bends down. This supports a differential diagnosis of common cold that has developed into sinusitis.

⚡ RED FLAGS
You confirm with her that nasal blockage affects both nostrils, allowing you to rule out conditions in which unilateral nasal blockage or discharge is prominent, for example, deviated nasal septum, turbinate hypertrophy and malignancy.

MANAGEMENT
Self-care Options
Very limited evidence exists for the effectiveness of simple analgesia, saline nose drops or decongestants (National Institute for Health and Care Excellence (NICE) Guidance 79). However, based on clinical experience, NICE recommends use of simple analgesia to manage pain and nasal saline or nasal decongestants for congestion. Prior to recommendation of any of the above interventions, a check on Mrs L's medical history would be appropriate. You find out she has no underlying medical conditions and takes the contraceptive pill. You decide to recommend paracetamol to help with facial pain.

Prescribing Options
Beyond self-care measures, no intervention is required.

Safety Netting

You tell Mrs L you think her symptoms are caused by a cold, but you suspect she may have developed sinusitis, and if her symptoms worsen (develop fever and severe local pain) or persist beyond 2–3 weeks, then you need to review her symptoms to see if she has developed bacterial sinusitis.

AIDE MEMOIRE

Likely Diagnoses
Allergic Rhinitis

Symptoms are usually restricted to bilateral nasal symptoms of sneezing, itching and nasal congestion/discharge. Associated conjunctivitis and cough can be present. Suspect where there is a history of allergy or atopy; mucopurulent discharge or loss of smell are unlikely.

Common Cold

Initial symptoms are sore throat of sudden onset that then rapidly resolves, followed by profuse nasal discharge, congestion and sneezing. Cough commonly follows. In addition, headache, mild to moderate fever and general malaise may be present. Symptoms tend to improve within 3–5 days.

Sinusitis

Sinusitis is defined as inflammation of the paranasal sinuses caused by predominantly viral pathogens (e.g., common colds) but can be followed by a bacterial infection. It can affect any age group, although it is more common in adults. Symptoms that are highly suggestive of sinusitis are nasal obstruction and discharge and severe facial pain. Other symptoms include frontal headache, fever, loss of smell and tenderness over the cheekbones. The pain tends to be bilateral but often has a unilateral predominance. The pain can also increase on lying down or bending over.

Possible Diagnoses
Adenoiditis

Seen in children, the main symptoms of adenoiditis are difficulty in breathing through the nose. This can lead to dry mouth and disturbed sleep. However, adenoiditis can be difficult to differentiate from sinusitis in children.

Deviated Septum

A septal deviation occurs when the line of cartilage between the nostrils is not straight. When a deviated septum is severe, it can block one side of the nose and reduce airflow, causing difficulty in breathing. The exposure of a deviated septum to the drying effect of airflow through the nose may sometimes contribute to crusting or bleeding. Patients might report noisy breathing during sleep.

Facial Pain

A number of conditions cause substantial pain in and around the face that may also present with URTI-like symptoms.

Cluster headache. Presents with short-lasting (15 min to 3 h) severe unilateral orbital or temporal pain that causes the patient to be restless (e.g., pacing the floor) due to pain severity. Associated nasal congestion, conjunctivitis/eye watering, drooping and swelling of one eyelid and facial flushing and sweating may be observed. Attacks often start at night. Typically, people experience bouts of attacks (clusters) that last a week to months, followed by lengthy periods of remission. It is more common in men.

Dental pain. The main symptom is sudden onset pain in the affected tooth, which can be intense and throbbing. Other symptoms include pain on biting the tooth, tooth sensitivity to heat and cold, unpleasant taste in the mouth, fever and malaise. Associated swelling in the jaw, trismus (inability to open the mouth) or lymphadenopathy may indicate a spreading infection.

Giant cell arteritis. Unilateral temporal headache is the predominant symptom in most patients. Scalp tenderness (classically pain on combing hair), visual changes and jaw pain are common symptoms. Less common symptoms include fever and URTI symptoms.

Migraine. Unilateral moderate to severe throbbing pain associated with nausea and/or photophobia and phonophobia with or without preceding aura is typical.

Neuropathic pain. For example, trigeminal and glossopharyngeal

Characterised by episodic severe, unilateral, short-lived lancing/shooting pain that follows the branches of each nerve; for trigeminal neuralgia, this is the lower jaw and cheek, and in glossopharyngeal neuralgia, pain is experienced at the back of tongue, tonsils and neck.

Other nonpain-related symptoms experienced by some people include nasal congestion/discharge, facial sweating and conjunctivitis.

TMD. Temporomandibular disorder is most common among people aged between 20 and 40 years, especially women. Symptoms include pain or tenderness in the face, jaw joint area, neck and shoulders and in or around the ear. Pain worsens on chewing, speaking or opening the mouth (where restricted jaw movements are often seen). Clicking noises are heard during mandibular movements. Patients with TMD also report headaches and otological symptoms.

Nasal Foreign Body

Children under 5 years are most affected. Typically, it causes a unilateral mucopurulent foul-smelling discharge. Pain is usually absent but can cause headaches.

Nasal Polyps

Polyps most common in people aged between 20 and 40 years. When small, they can be asymptomatic, but as they grow, they cause blocked or runny nose, loss of smell, nosebleeds, postnasal drip and sinus pain. They are usually bilateral.

Turbinate Hypertrophy

Symptoms are very similar to those of a common cold that does not go away. Symptoms include prolonged nasal congestion, mild facial pain and more difficulty in nose breathing, which can cause snoring and mouth dryness on awakening. Sense of smell can also be affected. Symptoms are similar to septal deviation.

Critical Diagnosis

Sinonasal Tumours

These are rare forms of cancers. They are more common in people aged more than 50 years. Suspicion should be raised in those with persistent unilateral symptoms of nasal obstruction, nasal congestion and discharge, frequent nose bleeds and facial swelling.

▌ MCQs

1. Acute sinusitis can become chronic. Which ONE of the following imaging techniques is the most appropriate to help with the diagnosis of chronic sinusitis?
   (a) CT
   (b) MRI
   (c) Positron-emission tomography
   (d) Ultrasound
   (e) X-ray

2. Which ONE of the following is the most definitive method to detect the presence of nasal polyps?
   (a) CT scan of the sinus
   (b) MRI of the sinus
   (c) Nasal endoscopy
   (d) Rhinoscopy
   (e) X-ray of the sinus

3. Acute sinusitis in adults is relatively common. Which ONE of the following is the estimated prevalence of acute sinusitis?
   (a) <2%
   (b) <5%
   (c) 5%–15%
   (d) 15%–25%
   (e) >30%

4. Chronic sinusitis is defined as symptoms that last for more than 12 weeks. In which ONE of the following groups is it more common?
   (a) In those with asthma
   (b) In those with COPD
   (c) In men
   (d) People with history of allergies
   (e) With increasing age

5. Sinusitis can present with a range of symptoms. Which ONE of the following is NOT a common symptom of a sinusitis?
   (a) Coughing
   (b) Loss of smell
   (c) Pain/pressure in the face
   (d) Sore throat
   (e) Stuffy or runny nose

Answers

1. a; 2. c; 3. c; 4. c; 5. d

> **KEY POINTS: ACUTE SINUSITIS**
> - Acute sinusitis of viral origin causes 98/100 cases.
> - Cardinal symptoms are purulent nasal discharge/congestion and facial pain.
> - Symptoms should improve within 10 days.
> - Treatment with analgesia, saline irrigation or nasal decongestants can be tried.

WEBSITES

NHS Inform
https://www.nhsinform.scot/illnesses-and-conditions/ears-nose-and-throat/sinusitis
Self Care Forum
https://www.selfcareforum.org/wp-content/uploads/2022/11/12-Sinusitis-2022.pdf

CASE 10: EPISTAXIS

PRESENTATION

Mrs J presents with her 5-year-old son. She reports that he has been getting frequent nosebleeds over the last 2–3 months. He is otherwise fit and healthy. She is concerned that he seems to be experiencing these almost weekly and wants to know what can be done.

PROBLEM REPRESENTATION

A 5-year-old boy presents with a 3-month history of recurrent nosebleeds.

HYPOTHESIS GENERATION (LIKELY, POSSIBLE AND CRITICAL DIAGNOSES)

Nosebleeds are common. Up to 60% of people will experience a nosebleed at least once, although they affect children and the elderly more frequently. Most people do not seek medical help. Usually they are spontaneous (primary bleeds) with no obvious cause but can be secondary bleeds, attributed to local or systemic aetiology, as well as drug-induced bleeding.

Local (and Likely) Diagnoses

- Complication of local infections
- Environmental – temperature and humidity changes
- Epistaxis digitorum (nose picking)
- Foreign body
- Medicine-induced
- Rhinitis
- Trauma

Local (and Possible) Diagnoses

- Deviated nasal septum
- Polyp

Local (and Critical) Diagnosis

- Tumour

Systemic (and Possible) Diagnosis

- Hypertension

Systemic (and Critical) Diagnoses

- Alcoholism/liver disease
- Granulomatosis with polyangiitis
- Inherited bleeding disorders

CONTINUED INFORMATION GATHERING

Nosebleeds, in an otherwise healthy child, are usually caused or aggravated by minor trauma, for example, nose picking, crusting from nasal inflammation, or nasal foreign bodies, and should form your initial hypotheses to test.

Further information needs to be sought from the child's mother about the onset, duration, frequency and severity of nosebleed. Questioning reveals that the nosebleeds tend to occur randomly, last for a few minutes each time and bleeding is usually bilateral.

From this description it appears that most, if not all, local likely causes can be excluded from our thinking. Nose picking has not been described and the random nature of events suggests it is not trauma. Foreign bodies present with unilateral and not bilateral symptoms. The child is fit and healthy eliminating medicine-induced nose bleed as a cause.

You ask if he experiences any other symptoms around the time of the nosebleeds, such as a cold. His mother says she has noticed nothing unusual apart from the nosebleeds. Rhinitis seems unlikely given he does not have nasal congestion or other symptoms associated with rhinitis.

PROBLEM REFINEMENT

Idiopathic nose bleeding therefore seems to be the cause of the nosebleeds, but nasal inflammation, possibly precipitated via environmental factors has not been fully excluded. At this point we can also exclude nasal polyps and deviated nasal septum as both would present with nasal congestion/obstruction often accompanied with facial pain (more so in polyps). Additionally, deviated nasal septum would present unilaterally.

⚡ RED FLAGS

At this stage idiopathic nose bleeding seems likely but systemic causes should be ruled out, although only inherited causes need to be considered in a 5-year-old child. Inherited causes, whilst rare, would present with more frequent and severe nose bleeding than in this case. In addition, the absence of a history of bruising also does not support these as the cause.

It appears that Mrs J's son has no symptoms that warrant concern at the present time.

MANAGEMENT

Nosebleeds are usually benign, self-limiting and spontaneous, with many children 'growing out' of the problem.

Self-care Options

As the child has not got an active nosebleed, advice on how to manage further episodes would be appropriate. Nose pinching is likely to resolve bleeding. Sustained nasal compression to the lower third of the nose (direct pressure at the tip of the nose) for 5 min or longer should be performed. If this fails to resolve bleeding, Mrs J should be told to seek medical attention.

Beyond controlling any future nosebleeds, her son should avoid activities that could traumatise the nose further, for example, sports.

Prescribing Options

If on future occasions compression fails to control the bleeding, either nasal cautery or nasal packing could be considered.

In most cases, on examination, the source of bleeding is clearly visible, and the bleeding point is cauterised with a silver nitrate stick. If the bleeding point cannot be seen, then nasal packing is recommended.

Safety Netting

In this case no further action is need.

AIDE MEMOIRE

Likely Diagnoses (Local)

Complication of Local Infections (e.g., Common Cold)

Symptoms of sore throat, nasal congestion/rhinorrhea, general malaise, fever and cough are typical presenting symptoms.

Environmental

Temperature and humidity changes can result in mucosal drying and epithelial damage making nose bleeds more likely. Other factors implicated include exposure to chemicals and cigarette smoke.

Epistaxis Digitorum (Nose Picking)

Most commonly seen in toddlers.

Foreign Body

Foreign body in the nose is associated with young children and produces unilateral mucopurulent foul-smelling nasal discharge although this discharge can become blood stained or lead to nose bleeds.

Medicines

Corticosteroids, NSAIDs, anticoagulant and antiplatelet medications increase the risk of nosebleeds as does illicit drug use (e.g., cocaine).

Rhinitis

Symptoms of nasal discharge, itching and sneezing predominate. Associated symptoms of conjunctivitis, cough and itching oral palate are also common.

Trauma

External nasal trauma results from a force to the nose. Typically, this may be from a fall, sports injury or motor vehicle accident.

Possible Diagnoses (Local)

Deviated Septum

When a deviated septum is severe, it can block one side of the nose and reduce airflow, causing difficulty breathing. The exposure of a deviated septum to the drying effect of airflow through the nose may sometimes contribute to crusting or bleeding. Patients might report noisy breathing during sleep.

Polyps

Polyps affect 1%–4% of the general population, with peak incidence in individuals aged between 20 and 40 years. Usually bilateral and when small they can be asymptomatic but as they grow, they cause blocked or runny nose, loss of smell, nosebleeds, postnasal drip and sinus pain.

Critical Diagnosis (Local)

Tumour

Tumours, either benign (e.g., angiofibroma) or cancerous, cause nasal obstruction, rhinorrhoea, facial pain, hearing loss, persistent lymphadenopathy and/or evidence of cranial neuropathy (e.g., facial numbness or double vision). Most cancers are more common in people aged more than 50 years.

Possible Diagnosis (Systemic)
Hypertension
The association between hypertension and nosebleed is inconsistent in the medical literature and there is a lack of evidence to establish a causal relationship.

Critical Diagnoses (Systemic)
Alcoholism/Liver Disease
Regular alcohol consumption reduces platelet aggregation and prolongs the bleeding time; these effects, coupled with haemodynamic changes such as vasodilatation and changes in blood pressure, may be important in causing some cases of arterial nose bleeds in adults. Liver disease can lead to clotting factor deficiencies leading to increased likelihood of nosebleeds.

Granulomatosis With Polyangiitis
Signs and symptoms of granulomatosis with polyangiitis are wide ranging but the first warning signs usually involve the sinuses, throat or lungs. The condition often worsens rapidly, affecting blood vessels and the organs they supply, leading to symptoms such as sinus infections, nosebleeds, coughing, shortness of breath or wheezing, fever, fatigue and joint pain.

Inherited Blood Disorders
For patients with known inherited bleeding disorders, such as von Willebrand disease or haemophilia, as well as for patients with abnormal nasal vasculature, for example, hereditary haemorrhagic telangiectasia (HHT), nosebleeds are a recognised problem. Such conditions are usually identified in children/adolescents. Patients will bruise easily and show slow healing times for cuts. In HHT patients, lacy red vessels or tiny red spots are seen, particularly on the lips, face, fingertips, tongue and inside surfaces of the mouth.

▌ M C Q s

1. From the following, which ONE is the most effective medical treatment of nasal polyps?
   (a) NSAIDs
   (b) Systemic antihistamines
   (c) Topical antihistamines
   (d) Topical decongestants
   (e) Topical steroids

2. A 4-year-old child presents with bleeding from right side of his nose. He also gets purulent discharge from the same side. From the following, which ONE is the most likely diagnosis?
   (a) Foreign body
   (b) Local trauma
   (c) Polyps
   (d) Septal deviation
   (e) Tumour

3. From the following, which ONE is the most common cause of epistaxis?
   (a) Angiofibroma
   (b) Blood disorders
   (c) Blunt trauma
   (d) Hypertension
   (e) Idiopathic

4. Nasal obstruction can be unilateral or bilateral. Which ONE of the following is usually a bilateral presentation?
   (a) Adenocarcinoma
   (b) Angiofibroma
   (c) Deviated nasal septum
   (d) Foreign body
   (e) Polyp

5. From the following conditions, which ONE of the following is the most likely cause of nosebleed?
   (a) Angiofibroma
   (b) Dry nasal passages
   (c) Hypertension
   (d) NSAID use
   (e) Polyps

Answers
1. e; 2. a; 3. e; 4. e; 5. e

KEY POINTS: EPISTAXIS
- Rupture of a blood vessel within the nasal mucosa but usually no identifiable cause
- Key symptom is bilateral bleeding.
- Local pressure usually controls most acute bleeds

WEBSITES
ENT UK
https://www.entuk.org/default.aspx

CASE 11: NASAL CONGESTION

PRESENTATION

A 29-year-old Caucasian woman presents to you on a Saturday morning in March. She asks for your advice about her blocked nose. She has been suffering for a week or so and describes generalised bilateral congestion with occasional bouts of sneezing. She appears to be otherwise fit and healthy.

PROBLEM REPRESENTATION

A 29-year-old woman presents with a 7-day history of acute bilateral nasal congestion.

HYPOTHESIS GENERATION (LIKELY, POSSIBLE AND CRITICAL DIAGNOSES)

Nasal congestion is a common and predominant symptom of various forms of rhinitis, especially those associated with URTI (infective rhinitis) and allergies.

Likely Diagnoses

- Intermittent allergic rhinitis (hay fever)
- Infective rhinitis
- Persistent allergic rhinitis

Possible Diagnoses

- Nonallergic rhinitis
  - Endocrine in origin
  - Medicines
- Structural
  - Deviated nasal septum
  - Nasal polyps
  - Foreign body (unlikely in this case)
  - Adenoidal hypertrophy

Critical Diagnosis

- Tumours

CONTINUED INFORMATION GATHERING

Her symptoms match all three of the most likely causes and requires focusing on the presence of other symptoms, trigger factors and personal and family histories of atopy.

On questioning the patient tells you her main symptom is the blocked nose. She has not really experienced any excessive sneezing and has not been coughing. She cannot remember having similar symptoms like this in previous years and nobody in the family has asthma or eczema. She also has no pets, as pets are not allowed where she lives.

Her symptoms do not match that of hay fever (nasal itch, sneeze and ocular irritation are common) or infective rhinitis (cough and sore throat are prominent) but do fit with persistent allergic rhinitis (where congestion is more prominent and sneezing, cough and ocular irritation are unusual). She does not have a positive family history of the atopic triad of hay fever, asthma or eczema meaning hay fever is now unlikely.

It appears that her symptoms point away from a diagnosis of hay fever and infective rhinitis. Symptoms most closely resemble persistent allergic rhinitis despite its recent onset (ARIA defines this as symptoms present for more than 4 days a week for 4 consecutive weeks).

PROBLEM REFINEMENT

We now need to eliminate other possible conditions as the cause. You establish a medication history and find out she takes the pill and is very confident that she is not pregnant. The contraceptive pill can affect hormonal levels and is known to cause rhinitis, so we need to establish how long she has been on the pill. She tells you she has been on the same pill for 3 years. This seems to exclude rhinitis as a possible cause.

Her symptoms are bilateral suggesting that structural problems can be discounted, for example, deviated nasal septum, foreign body and tumours. Moreover, her symptom profile does not fit that of adenoidal hypertrophy (snoring, sleep problems, sore throat) or nasal polyps (loss of smell, snoring, nose bleeds).

The only condition yet to be considered is nonallergic rhinitis. This presents in a similar fashion to persistent allergic rhinitis and the two conditions can be difficult to tell apart. Asking about other triggers such as worsening symptoms after exposure to changes in temperature or humidity points towards nonallergic rhinitis.

She says she has not noticed any changes in her symptoms when going from hot to cold places.

Based on the information gained it appears that she could be at the initial stage of persistent allergic rhinitis.

> ⚡ **RED FLAGS**
>
> Her age and bilateral symptoms imply that a tumour is very unlikely.

MANAGEMENT

Self-care Options

Instigating measures to reduce house dust mite may lead to an improvement in symptoms. You can tell her that washing bedlinen and mattress covers at high temperatures once a week may be helpful. In the longer term, she might want to consider replacing carpets with wooden floors.

Prescribing Options

It appears her symptoms are relatively mild as she has not spoken about her symptoms affecting her day-to-day routine, and on that basis, an intranasal antihistamine used when needed is recommended as first-line treatment. If she does not want to use a nasal spray, an oral antihistamine could be provided. Choice will be driven by patient preference as all are effective and have broadly the same side effect profile.

Safety Netting

You tell the patient that you are not certain of the cause of her symptoms but it does appear to be allergy related and symptoms will be experienced whilst exposed to the allergen. You say this might be due to house dust mite, and hence, the patient should try to mitigate these around the house. If her symptoms fail to respond to antihistamines over the next 2 weeks, she should come back and an intranasal corticosteroid could be tried.

AIDE MEMOIRE

Likely Diagnoses
Intermittent Allergic Rhinitis (Hay Fever)

Classically associated with bilateral nasal itching, sneezing, congestion and rhinorrhoea. Associated symptoms include bilateral conjunctivitis and postnasal drip. Often there is a personal or family history of atopy. Allergen exposure dictates when symptoms are experienced, for example, tree pollens in early spring, grass pollen in the summer and fungal spores in late summer/autumn.

Infective Rhinitis (Common Cold)

The first symptoms noted are usually a sore or irritated throat with associated sneezing, followed closely by profuse nasal discharge and congestion. The sore throat usually resolves quickly, and by the second and third day of illness, nasal symptoms predominate. A cough can develop in approximately 30% of people typically after nasal symptoms have cleared. Systemic symptoms are uncommon, but people can experience headache, mild to moderate fever and general malaise.

Persistent Allergic Rhinitis

This can present with a similar symptom complex to hay fever. However, symptoms are generally experienced all the time. House dust mite and animal dander are two common allergens.

Possible Diagnoses
Nonallergic Rhinitis

Nonallergic rhinitis is thought to be due to either an overactive parasympathetic nervous system response, or hypoactive sympathetic nervous system response to irritants such as dry air, pollutants, or strong odours. Symptoms are similar to allergic rhinitis yet an allergy test will be negative. Itching and sneezing are less common, and patients might experience worsening nasal symptoms in response to climatic factors such as a sudden change in temperature.

Endocrine in origin. A hormonal cause should be considered where symptoms coincide with starting contraceptives, hormone replacement therapy or pregnancy. In pregnancy, it usually starts after the second month of the pregnancy and resolves spontaneously after childbirth. Hypothyroidism can also cause rhinitis.

Medicines. Rebound congestion is well recognised with local decongestant use. Systemic medicines associated with congestion/rhinorrhoea include alpha-blockers (common), Angiotensin converting enzyme inhibitors (uncommon), beta-blockers (rare).

Structural

Deviated nasal septum. When a deviated septum is severe, it can block one side of the nose and reduce airflow causing difficulty breathing. The exposure of a deviated septum to the drying effect of airflow through the nose may sometimes contribute to crusting or bleeding. Patients might report noisy breathing during sleep.

Nasal polyps. Polyps affect 1%–4% of the general population with peak incidence in individuals aged between 20 and 40 years. Usually bilateral and when small they can be asymptomatic but as they grow, they cause blocked or runny nose, loss of smell, nosebleeds, postnasal drip and sinus pain.

Foreign body. Foreign body in the nose is associated with young children and produces unilateral mucopurulent foul-smelling nasal discharge although this discharge can become blood stained or lead to nose bleeds.

Adenoidal hypertrophy. Characterised by rhinorrhoea, difficulty breathing through the nose, chronic cough, postnasal drip and snoring. If the nasal obstruction is significant, the patient can suffer from sinusitis.

Critical Diagnosis
Tumours

Tumours, either benign (e.g., angiofibroma) or cancerous, cause unilateral nasal obstruction, rhinorrhoea (can be bloody), nose bleeds, facial pain, hearing loss, persistent lymphadenopathy, and/or evidence of cranial neuropathy (e.g., facial numbness or double vision). Most cancers are more common in people aged more than 50 years.

MCQs

1. A man with a blocked nose, facial pain and a reduced sense of smell. Upon further questioning he adds that he suffers from hay fever and was playing football in a field with his friends yesterday. Which ONE of the following is the most likely diagnosis?
   (a) Allergic rhinitis
   (b) Common cold
   (c) Influenza
   (d) Postnasal drip
   (e) Sinusitis
2. A woman enters the pharmacy complaining of hay fever which is affecting her eyes. Which ONE of the following symptom clusters best describes allergic conjunctivitis?
   (a) Bilateral redness with mucopurulent discharge
   (b) Bilateral redness with watery discharge
   (c) Bilateral redness with watery discharge and pain described as discomfort
   (d) Unilateral redness in the fornices
   (e) Unilateral redness with watery discharge
3. A 52-year-old patient presents with symptoms of nasal congestion, slight sore throat, cough and headache. You decide to make a referral to the doctor because the diagnosis suggests:
   (a) Adenoidal hypertrophy
   (b) Infective rhinitis
   (c) Influenza
   (d) Nasal polyps
   (e) Sinusitis
4. A 24-year-old male patient asks to buy fexofenadine (Allevia) to treat his hay fever. You find out he is taking an antibiotic for sinusitis, but he cannot remember the name of the antibiotic. Which ONE of the following antibiotics should be avoided when taking fexofenadine?
   (a) Amoxicillin
   (b) Cefalexin
   (c) Doxycycline
   (d) Erythromycin
   (e) Flucloxacillin
5. A young mother of two wants to buy an antihistamine for her hay fever. You find out she is currently breast feeding her youngest child. According to manufacturer SmPC data, which ONE of the following antihistamines is most appropriate?
   (a) Cetirizine
   (b) Chlorphenamine
   (c) Fexofenadine
   (d) Loratadine
   (e) None of the above

Answers
1. e; 2. b; 3. b; 4. d; 5. e

KEY POINTS: PERSISTENT ALLERGIC RHINITIS

- Typically caused by animal dander and house dust mite
- Key symptom is nasal congestion.
- Allergen avoidance/eradication (where possible) and intranasal antihistamines are first-line treatment. Systemic antihistamines and nasal steroids are second-line treatment or used if symptoms are severe.

WEBSITES

Allergy UK
https://www.allergyuk.org/
British Society for Allergy and Clinical Immunology
https://www.bsaci.org/about-bsaci/who-are-bsaci/
European Forum for Research and Education in Allergy and Airway Diseases - ARIA
https://www.euforea.eu/aria

THROAT

CASE 12: SORE THROAT

PRESENTATION

Mrs B, approximately 30 years old, asks for your advice on a sore throat she has. Her symptoms started about 3 days ago, but she has not yet taken anything to help. You find out she takes no medication from the doctor.

PROBLEM REPRESENTATION

A 30-year-old woman presents with a 3-day history of acute sore throat.

HYPOTHESIS GENERATION (LIKELY, POSSIBLE AND CRITICAL DIAGNOSES)

Viral infection accounts for 70%–90% of all sore throat cases. The remaining cases will be mostly bacterial infection; the most common being infection with Group A beta-haemolytic *Streptococcus*. However, there are a number of other conditions where sore throat is one of the major presenting symptoms, and we need to consider if infection does not appear to be the cause.

Likely Diagnosis
- Infection (either viral or bacterial)

Possible Diagnoses
- COVID-19
- Glandular fever (adolescents)
- Herpangina (children)
- Herpetic pharyngitis (children)
- Influenza
- Irritation/trauma
- Medicines

Possible Diagnoses (Where Sore Throat is a Symptom but Not a Major Presenting Symptom)
- Allergic rhinitis
- Behcet's syndrome
- Dyspepsia
- Human immunodeficiency virus (HIV)
- Sexually transmitted diseases (STDs)

- Stevens–Johnson syndrome (SJS)
- Thrush
- Vaccine preventable diseases

Critical Diagnosis
- Malignancy

CONTINUED INFORMATION GATHERING

The default diagnosis will be a viral sore throat but an assessment to confirm viral infection needs to be conducted. Differentiating between a viral and bacterial cause is not easy, and the National Institute for Health and Care Excellence (NICE) recommends two clinical prediction rules (CPRs), FeverPAIN and Centor, to guide decision making.

FeverPAIN score range is from 1 to 5 and Centor score range is from 1 to 4. The likelihood of a bacterial cause increases with the increase in the score. For example, a score of 1 (on either criteria) gives only approximately 17% chance of it being bacterial. A score of 4 or 5 respectively increases the probability to 56%–65%.

Common to both criteria are:
- Presence of tonsillar exudate
- Presence of fever
- Absence of cough

FeverPAIN criteria also considers onset (within 3 days) and severity of tonsillar inflammation, whereas Centor looks at anterior cervical lymphadenopathy.

Applying the FeverPAIN criteria to Mrs B's initial presentation, we know about onset (3 days), which meets the criteria. In relation to the other four criteria, you find out that she does not have a cough and is not showing any signs of systemic illness (e.g., fever). A visual inspection reveals soreness of the throat and tonsil area with some exudate, but inflammation does not look severe.

Mrs B's symptoms therefore score 3/5 (attended within 3 days, no cough and has tonsillar exudate), which is associated with a 34%–40% likelihood of isolating *Streptococcus*.

It seems the default position of viral sore throat is still the most likely diagnosis.

PROBLEM REFINEMENT

Although we are relatively confident of our diagnosis, it is worth checking that Mrs B has no symptoms that would cause us to rethink. Checks on any other symptoms being experienced or triggers causing sore throat should be conducted. For Glandular fever (and influenza) we would expect signs of malaise; influenza also produces debilitating symptoms; COVID-19 other symptoms would be more obvious, such as new continuous cough and a loss or change to sense of smell or taste and herpetic pharyngitis would show mouth ulceration. For irritation/trauma, one would expect Mrs B to recall an event causing the sore throat.

Mrs B reports no other symptoms and cannot think of anything that might have caused the sore throat.

You are now confident of your diagnosis of viral sore throat.

> **RED FLAGS**
>
> Malignancy can be ruled out based on Mrs B's age and lack of other symptoms such as dysphagia and hoarseness.

MANAGEMENT

Self-care Options

Simple analgesia can be tried, for example, paracetamol/ibuprofen or local application of lozenges containing flurbiprofen. Other nonmedicated lozenges that either contain lidocaine to help with pain or demulcents to help lubricate the throat could be offered.

Prescribing Options

None required beyond self-care measures.

Safety Netting

You tell Mrs B that her sore throat is likely because of a viral infection and should clear in the next 5 days, and symptoms should be managed through pain relief and lozenges. However, if her symptoms worsen or fail to clear up, she needs to be reassessed to see if she has developed a secondary bacterial infection.

AIDE MEMOIRE

Likely Diagnoses
Viral or Bacterial Infection

Characterised by rapid onset of symptoms and pharyngeal inflammation (with or without exudate). Sore throat can be an isolated symptom or as part of a cluster of symptoms that include rhinorrhoea, cough, malaise, fever, pharyngeal inflammation, tonsillar exudate, headache and hoarseness.

Possible Diagnoses (Where Sore Throat is One of the Major Presenting Symptoms)
COVID-19

COVID-19 presents with a wide range of symptoms, but the most common presentations include a new continuous dry cough, high temperature or a loss or change to sense of smell or taste. Other symptoms that can be experienced include shortness of breath, tiredness, sore throat, nasal congestion, gastrointestinal disturbances and loss of appetite.

Glandular Fever

Generally seen in young adults. Malaise, fatigue and headache are often seen before sore throat (often severe), fever and lymphadenopathy. A maculopapular rash on the trunk is seen in about 10% of people.

Herpangina

Herpangina is seen mainly in children up to 10 years of age. Clinically it presents as an acute febrile illness with a sore throat and ulcers at the back of the mouth. Red spots appear within hours (up to 1 day later) in the mouth and throat. The lesions are raised into small vesicles, which form a tiny yellowish ulcer with a red rim. The ulcers are generally 1–2 mm in diameter. The ulcers take 5–10 days to heal. Nausea and abdominal symptoms can also be seen.

Herpetic Pharyngitis

Primary herpetic gingivostomatitis is usually seen in childhood/young adults and presents with fever, sore throat and potential associated widespread superficial ulcers of the oral mucosa.

Influenza

The onset of influenza is sudden – within a few hours – and typical symptoms include cold-like symptoms, fever, a nonproductive cough, and generalised symptoms such as shivering, chills, malaise, marked aching of limbs, insomnia, fatigue, and loss of appetite. Influenza is therefore normally debilitating. Flu is typically seen between December and March.

Irritation/Trauma

Direct trauma (e.g., heat) and exposure to irritants (e.g., smoking) can cause sore throat.

Medicines

A small number of medicines are associated with sore throat as they can induce neutropenia, agranulocytosis or thrombocytopenia. These include penicillamine (common), sulfasalazine (uncommon), carbimazole (rare), clozapine (rare) and captopril (very rare). In addition, all cytotoxic medicines may cause these problems.

Thrush

Candida albicans may cause pharyngitis in immunosuppressed individuals, people who use inhaled corticosteroids or those undergoing chemotherapy or irradiation.

Possible Diagnoses (Where Sore Throat is a Symptom but Not a Major Presenting Symptom)
Allergic Rhinitis

Classically associated with bilateral nasal itching, sneezing, congestion and rhinorrhoea. Associated symptoms include bilateral conjunctivitis and postnasal drip, and occasionally sore throat. Often there is a personal or family history of atopy. Allergen exposure dictates when symptoms occur.

Behcet's Syndrome

This is a multisystem disorder characterised by recurrent inflammatory skin lesions, eye problems (e.g., uveitis) and oral and genital ulcers. Eye symptoms and genital lesions are more prominent than skin and oral lesions. Oral ulcers can appear anywhere in the oral cavity and tend to be large (1–3 cm) and cause pain affecting the pharynx.

Dyspepsia/Gastrooesophageal Reflux Disease

Typical symptoms are of upper abdominal discomfort, heartburn and acid reflux. Atypical symptoms can be experienced and include cough, hoarseness and sore throat.

Human Immunodeficiency Virus

Early signs and symptoms of primary HIV infection are similar to that of flu, such as fever, headache, fatigue, myalgia and sore throat. In some people a nonitchy maculopapular rash is seen.

Sexually Transmitted Diseases

STDs that cause sore throat symptoms are most commonly due to oral sex. However, in causes such as chlamydia and gonorrhoea, oropharyngeal infection is usually asymptomatic.

Stevens–Johnson Syndrome

SJS is a rare, acute, serious and potentially fatal skin reaction in which there are sheet-like skin lesions and mucosal loss. However, before skin symptoms start, many people feel generally unwell with symptoms including headache, joint pain, fever, cough, sore mouth and sore throat. Recent infection and new medication usually precipitate SJS.

Vaccine Preventable Diseases

In nonvaccinated individuals, prodromal symptoms of measles and German measles show cold-like symptoms including sore throat.

Critical Diagnosis
Malignancy

Tumours of the throat, tongue or larynx can cause a sore throat. Other signs or symptoms may include hoarseness, difficulty swallowing, noisy breathing, neck mass, and blood in saliva or phlegm.

■ MCQs

1. In which ONE of the following patient groups should flurbiprofen lozenges be avoided?
   (a) Asthmatics
   (b) Hypertensive patients
   (c) Patients with mild hepatic impairment
   (d) Patients with moderate renal impairment
   (e) Patients with peptic ulcers
2. Sore throat can be caused by many different types of infection. Which ONE of the following is the least common cause of sore throat?
   (a) Adenovirus
   (b) Epstein–Barr virus
   (c) *Haemophilus influenza* type b
   (d) Influenza type A virus
   (e) *Streptococcus*
3. A mother and her 3-year-old girl present to the pharmacy. The mother explains the child has had a temperature and sore throat but no cough or runny nose. Upon examination you note she has swollen lymph nodes and white pustules on the tonsils. Which ONE of the following conditions is the most likely diagnosis?
   (a) Bacterial sore throat
   (b) Leukoplakia
   (c) Oral thrush
   (d) Pertussis
   (e) Viral cough

4. A 24-year-old man presents with sore throat, which he has had for 4 or 5 days with associated symptoms of malaise and fever. On examination, you note cervical adenopathy and tonsillar exudate. Which ONE of the following is the most likely cause of this patient's symptoms?
   (a) Group A beta-haemolytic *Streptococcus*
   (b) Group D *Streptococcus*
   (c) Epstein–Barr infection
   (d) Herpangina
   (e) Herpes simplex type 1

5. A 52-year-old man presents with symptoms of nasal congestion, sore throat, headache and loss of smell. You decide to make a referral to a doctor as the differential diagnosis most strongly suggests which ONE of the following?
   (a) Glandular fever
   (b) Influenza
   (c) Postnasal drip
   (d) Rhinitis
   (e) Sinusitis

Answers

1. e; 2. c; 3. a; 4. c; 5. e

KEY POINTS: VIRAL SORE THROAT

- Rhinoviruses are most common cause (accounting for 30%–50% of all cases); other causes include coronaviruses, parainfluenza virus, respiratory syncytial virus and adenovirus.
- Key symptom of sore throat associated with tonsillar involvement
- Symptoms should resolve within 7 days.
- No treatment is needed other than symptomatic treatment of pain.

WEBSITES

Scoring criteria - Sore throat (acute): antimicrobial prescribing NICE guideline [NG84]
https://www.nice.org.uk/guidance/ng84/chapter/terms-used-in-the-guideline
Diagnostic accuracy of FeverPAIN and Centor criteria for bacterial throat infection in adults with sore throat: a secondary analysis of a randomised controlled trial
https://bjgpopen.org/content/5/6/BJGPO.2021.0122

4

Gastrointestinal Problems

CASE 13: ABDOMINAL PAIN IN A CHILD

PRESENTATION

Mrs R brings in her 7-year-old daughter, 'E', this morning. She tells you E has been complaining of a tummy ache since yesterday evening. Her mother says she is off-colour and generally a bit lethargic.

PROBLEM REPRESENTATION

A 7-year-old girl presents with a 12–24-h history of abdominal pain associated with possible systemic upset.

HYPOTHESIS GENERATION (LIKELY, POSSIBLE AND CRITICAL DIAGNOSES)

The age of the child is a key factor in evaluating the cause and is a useful starting point in which to formulate a differential diagnosis. Table 4.1 lists causes of abdominal pain in other child age groups, but for our patient, e.g., children aged between 5 and 12 years, we need to consider:

Likely Diagnoses

- Appendicitis
- Constipation
- Gastroenteritis

Possible Diagnoses

- Henoch-Schönlein purpura
- Functional abdominal pain
- Pharyngitis
- Pneumonia
- Sickle cell disease complications (vasculo-occlusive crisis)
- Urinary tract infection (UTI)

Critical Diagnosis

- Abdominal trauma

CONTINUED INFORMATION GATHERING

We know Miss E has pain of recent onset but we need to know more about the onset, nature, severity and location of the pain.

Her mother tells you her symptoms have gradually worsened over the last 24 h. She points to an area below and to the left of the umbilicus as the origin of the pain. The best description of the nature of the pain from the mother is cramp-like, as when her daughter gets the pain, she seems to rub her belly a lot. With regards to severity, it appears relatively mild as her mother does not describe the pain as causing too much distress or crying.

This symptom cluster seems a poor fit for appendicitis. Appendicitis seems unlikely due to wrong location and intermittent pain which seems not too severe. Her symptoms do show characteristics of both constipation and gastroenteritis, although location is not consistent for either problem.

To determine if either are the cause you ask if Miss E has had any vomiting or diarrhoea. Mrs R states her daughter has not had any vomiting or diarrhoea. This seems to rule out gastroenteritis.

At this point constipation is left as the remaining likely cause of her symptoms but Mrs R denies any changes in her daughter's bowel habit.

PROBLEM REFINEMENT

It seems that one of the possible causes is responsible for her symptoms. From those listed, only functional abdominal pain and UTI seem plausible given her symptoms. Functional abdominal pain is recurrent and UTI

TABLE 4.1 Abdominal Causes in Other Paediatric Age Groups

	<5 Years Old	>12 Years Old
Likely	• Constipation • Gastroenteritis	• Appendicitis • Constipation • Gastroenteritis
Possible	• Infantile colic • Mesenteric adenitis • Meckel's diverticulum • Poisoning • Pyloric stenosis • Urinary tract infection	• Cholecystitis/ Cholelithiasis • Dysmenorrhoea • Inflammatory bowel disease • Mittelschmerz • Pelvic inflammatory disease
Critical	• Abdominal trauma • Hirschsprung's disease • Incarcerated hernia • Volvulus • Intussusception	• Abdominal trauma • Appendicitis • Ectopic pregnancy • Ovarian torsion • Testicular torsion

acute so knowing about the previous history of Miss E's symptoms will help in deciding which condition should be explored further. Mrs R says her daughter has very infrequently had a tummy ache and when she has had these symptoms previously, they have tended to go quickly. It seems UTI may be the cause given she has abdominal pain and is 'off-colour', but you would normally expect other symptoms to be present. You therefore now ask a general question about any other problems Mrs R has noticed. Mrs R states that her daughter has been going to the toilet for wees frequently.

It appears the differential diagnosis is a lower UTI.

⚡ RED FLAGS

The lack of other symptoms such as rash (purpura), upper respiratory symptoms (pharyngitis), breathing difficulties (pneumonia) and pain away from the abdomen (sickle cell) seem to rule out other possible causes. No recent injury has been reported that seems to rule out trauma.

MANAGEMENT

Self-care Options

You tell Mrs R that she needs to keep her daughter well hydrated, even though this may make her go the toilet more often. You could suggest she takes simple analgesia to treat the abdominal pain if deemed necessary.

Prescribing Options

You prescribe a 3-day course of trimethoprim at 100 mg bd.

Safety Netting

You tell Mrs R that you think her daughter has a bladder infection and her symptoms will start to get better over the next 48–72 h. However, if her symptoms worsen, she needs to be seen again to check that the infection has not gotten worse (e.g., upper UTI).

AIDE MEMOIRE (FOR CONDITIONS SEEN IN THE 5–12-YEAR-OLD AGE GROUP)

Likely Diagnosis

Appendicitis

For appendicitis, right lower quadrant (RLQ) pain has the highest positive predictive value, although migration from periumbilical to RLQ and fever also suggest appendicitis. The pain of appendicitis is described as colicky or cramp-like but after a few hours becomes constant. Movement tends to aggravate the pain and nausea/vomiting might also be present.

Constipation

Constipation is a symptom of many abdominal conditions. In addition to a reduced bowel movement, associated lower abdominal discomfort/pain is often present.

Gastroenteritis

Symptoms of diffuse cramping pain that follows or coincides with diarrhoea and nausea/vomiting are seen. General malaise, headache and abdominal bloating may also be present. Depending on the causative agent, diarrhoea may also be bloody (bacterial rather than viral cause). Dehydration is possible due to the loss of fluid through diarrhoea.

Table 4.2 summarises these three likely diagnoses.

TABLE 4.2 Condition Summary of Signs/Symptoms of the Likely Causes of Abdominal Pain in 5–12-Year-Old Children

	Sudden Onset	Nature of Pain	Severity	Location	Associated Symptoms
Appendicitis	Yes	Cramp-like/colicky that becomes constant	Moderate to severe	Right lower quadrant (RLQ)	Fever; nausea/vomiting
Constipation	No	Cramp-like	Mild to moderate	Diffuse but often RLQ	Unusual
Gastroenteritis	Yes	Cramp-like/colicky	Mild to moderate	Diffuse	Vomiting/diarrhoea (possibly bloody); fever; malaise

Possible Diagnoses
Henoch-Schönlein Purpura

Purpura occurs in all patients and is the presenting complaint in 75% of cases. Other symptoms include arthritis/arthralgia, nephritis and abdominal pain. It most commonly affects children aged 2–8 years.

Functional Abdominal Pain

This can have an organic cause (e.g., dyspepsia, irritable bowel syndrome (IBS)) but is also associated with psychological issues involving stress/anxiety or depression. It is associated with unexplained episodes of recurrent abdominal pain. Other symptoms such as vomiting, constipation, diarrhoea and headaches may be experienced.

Pharyngitis

Typically, pharyngitis presents with rapid onset of symptoms and pharyngeal inflammation (with or without exudate), swollen uvula and tender, enlarged anterior cervical lymph nodes. Sore throat can be an isolated symptom or as part of a cluster of symptoms that include rhinorrhoea, cough, malaise, fever, headache and hoarseness. Occasionally abdominal pain may also be present.

Pneumonia

The symptoms vary depending on the age of the child and causative agent. In general, the key symptoms are fever and rapid/difficult breathing. However, if the lower part of the lungs is affected near the abdomen, then the child might have fever, abdominal pain or vomiting.

Sickle Cell Disease Complications (Vasculo-occlusive Crisis)

Almost all cases of sickle cell disease are diagnosed as part of the UK national newborn screening programme. However, symptoms of crisis manifest as increasing pain over a period of days that can affect any part of the body, including the abdomen, although the back, chest and extremities are more commonly affected. It can be triggered by stress, dehydration, cold temperatures and infection.

Urinary Tract Infection (UTI)

It can be difficult to tell if a child has a UTI, as the symptoms can be vague. UTIs in children often present with generalised symptoms. In those under 3 months of age, poor feeding, irritability, vomiting and fever are seen. Other less common symptoms include abdominal pain. In older children, symptoms are clearer with UTI, e.g., frequency, dysuria, changes to urine, but fever and abdominal pain/loin tenderness are also commonly observed.

Critical Diagnosis
Abdominal Trauma

Injury in children is more severe than adults due to a thinner abdominal wall, a more pliable rib cage providing less protection and a relatively large liver and spleen in proportion to the abdominal cavity. Symptoms include abdominal pain, tenderness at the injury site, abdominal distension, blood in the urine and referred pain, for example, shoulder pain.

MCQs

1. A child presents with abdominal pain and fever. From the following, which ONE is most likely to be the cause of the symptoms?
   (a) Abdominal trauma
   (b) Appendicitis
   (c) Functional abdominal pain
   (d) Gastroenteritis
   (e) Henoch-Schönlein purpura

2. A child presents with abdominal pain and nausea/vomiting. From the following, which ONE is the most likely cause of the symptoms?
   (a) Abdominal trauma
   (b) Constipation
   (c) Functional abdominal pain
   (d) Gastroenteritis
   (e) Henoch-Schönlein purpura

3. Left lower quadrant pain is most closely associated with which ONE of the following conditions?
   (a) Appendicitis
   (b) Gastroenteritis
   (c) Infantile colic
   (d) Irritable bowel syndrome
   (e) Testicular torsion

4. Which ONE of the following conditions presents with pain that is not described as cramp/colicky-like?
   (a) Appendicitis
   (b) Constipation
   (c) Gastroenteritis
   (d) Mesenteric adenitis
   (e) Mittelschmerz (ovulation pain)

5. Which ONE of the following is most likely to present with severe abdominal pain?
   (a) Abdominal trauma
   (b) Constipation
   (c) Functional abdominal pain
   (d) Gastroenteritis
   (e) Henoch-Schönlein purpura

Answers
1. b; 2. d; 3. d; 4. d; 5. a

> ### KEY POINTS: LOWER URINARY TRACT INFECTION IN A CHILD
> - *Escherichia coli* is the predominant pathogen.
> - Key symptoms are frequency, dysuria, abdominal pain and fever.
> - Symptoms come on quickly and resolve within 48 h of appropriate antibiotic treatment.

WEBSITES

British Society of Gastroenterology
https://www.bsg.org.uk/

CASE 14: DIARRHOEA

> ### PRESENTATION
> Mr F, a 34-year-old man, tells you that he has been suffering from occasional diarrhoea for the last 4 months. He has not seen anybody so far to discuss it as it seems to come and go, but between episodes he is fine and his bowel movements are normal.

PROBLEM REPRESENTATION

A 34-year-old man presents with a 4-month history of altered bowel habit.

HYPOTHESIS GENERATION (LIKELY, POSSIBLE AND CRITICAL DIAGNOSES)

Before thinking about the likely causes for Mr F, it is necessary to establish what he means by diarrhoea, as diarrhoea is medically defined as an increase in the frequency of passage of soft or watery stools relative to the usual bowel habit for that individual. Once confirmed, we can see that the person has a long-standing history of the problem, thus ruling out acute causes (defined as diarrhoea lasting less than 14 days) such as infection (viral, bacterial or parasitic). Additionally, because of his age it also means the following conditions are very unlikely and can be discounted from our early thinking:
- Colorectal cancer (over 50s – highest in very elderly)
- Faecal impaction (elderly)
- Hyperthyroidism (increases with age and more common in women)
- Lactose intolerance (infants)

Given his presenting symptoms we should be considering:

Likely Diagnoses
- Anxiety
- Coeliac disease
- Excess alcohol
- Inflammatory bowel disease (IBD)
- IBS

Possible Diagnoses

- Diabetes
- Medicines
- Traveller's diarrhoea

Critical Diagnoses

- Addison's disease
- Colorectal carcinoma

CONTINUED INFORMATION GATHERING

Knowing more about when his symptoms occur will be helpful in ruling in/ruling out anxiety and excess alcohol, as the incidence of diarrhoeal episodes should coincide with acute alcohol intake and bouts of anxiety. Mr F says whilst he does drink, he rarely drinks to excess and has not experienced any hangovers over the last few months. He also says that he very rarely feels stressed and does not suffer from any sort of panic type attacks. This seems to rule out these as the cause of his symptoms.

PROBLEM REFINEMENT

IBS, IBD and coeliac disease show overlapping symptom profiles and to differentiate between these conditions we need to know more about the diarrhoea, if he experiences other symptoms and if anything aggravates, precipitates or ameliorates his symptoms.

Mr F tells you that he experiences bloating and lower abdominal discomfort during episodes of diarrhoea. He reports not seeing any blood in the diarrhoea and generally feels fit and healthy, both in between and during episodes of diarrhoea. He has not noticed anything that seems to worsen or help his symptoms. He says he has not been abroad for over a year.

This description best fits with IBS. In coeliac disease, fatigue and weight loss are common and in IBD, bloody diarrhoea, urgency and non-gastrointestinal (GI) symptoms such as fatigue and joint pain can be seen. Before deciding on management, it would be prudent to take a drug history, as it is well known that many medicines can cause diarrhoea. Mr F occasionally takes ibuprofen – known to cause diarrhoea. Causality between symptoms and taking ibuprofen needs to be established. Mr F believes that his symptoms do not coincide with him taking ibuprofen and he has had no problems previously taking the medicine which predates his current symptoms.

You arrive at a differential diagnosis of IBS.

⚡ RED FLAGS

We know Mr F has not reported symptoms of weight loss or fatigue (associated with colorectal cancer and Addison's disease) nor blood in the stool/rectal bleeding, which is associated with colorectal cancer. He also shows no signs associated with classical diabetes presentation such as polyuria or polydipsia.

MANAGEMENT

Self-care Options

Mr F should be given general advice on nutrition, for example, keeping adequately hydrated, eating regular meals and adjusting fibre intake. Mr F could buy loperamide to manage the diarrhoeal episodes.

Prescribing Options

Antispasmodics are generally first line in managing abdominal pain/spasms, for example, mebeverine, alverine or peppermint oil. Second-line treatment options include the use of low-dose tricyclic antidepressants such as amitriptyline at a dose of 5–10 mg at night, increasing the dose to a maximum of 30 mg. However, given his symptoms the use of such agents currently does not seem warranted.

Safety Netting

You tell Mr F you think he has IBS and symptoms will wax and wane. Treatments are to manage the problem of flare-ups. A follow-up appointment should be made within the next 2 months to assess his symptoms and consider if any further interventions are required. You also tell him if symptoms worsen or he notices any blood in his stools he needs to come back straight away.

AIDE MEMOIRE

Likely Diagnoses
Anxiety

May often present with only physical symptoms. These can be variable but include headache, insomnia, back pain and GI symptoms such as diarrhoea.

Coeliac Disease

Symptoms are often nonspecific but adult patients will have persistent gastrointestinal symptoms that include steatorrhoea, bloating and abdominal pain accompanied with unintentional weight loss. Prolonged fatigue (often due to anaemia) and persistent mouth ulcers can also be present. It can occur at any age but has two peaks of onset: shortly after weaning and in people in their 20s and 30s.

Excess Alcohol

Temporary effects of short-term alcohol poisoning lead to loss of coordination, confusion, slurred speech, vomiting and occasionally diarrhoea. Dehydration symptoms usually appear a few hours after drinking and include headache and dizziness.

Inflammatory Bowel Disease

Crohn's disease and ulcerative colitis are characterised by relapse and remittance, and in both conditions GI disturbance is very common – either as persistent diarrhoea or bloody diarrhoea associated with urgency and tenesmus. Both exhibit lower abdominal pain. In Crohn's disease, the most common place for it to start is at the end of the small intestine (ileum) causing RLQ pain. In ulcerative colitis, the pain is more common in the left lower quadrant. Over time weight loss can be observed. Both are associated with extraintestinal symptoms, affecting between 25% and 40% of patients, and include arthritis, mouth ulcers, red eye and fatigue (due to anaemia). Other nonspecific symptoms such as malaise and fever can be present. Young adults (20–40 years of age) are most affected.

Irritable Bowel Syndrome

IBS is characterised by lower abdominal pain or discomfort, although left lower quadrant pain is more typical than RLQ pain. Pain is accompanied by abdominal bloating and changes to bowel habit. Pain or discomfort is often relieved by defaecation. People with IBS can present with 'diarrhoea predominant', 'constipation predominant' or alternating symptom profiles. During bouts of diarrhoea, mucus tends to be visible on the stools. Patients might also complain of increased stool frequency but pass normal or pellet-like stools. Other features such as lethargy, nausea, backache and bladder symptoms are common in people with IBS and may be used to support the diagnosis. As in IBD, young adults (20–40 years of age) are most affected.

Possible Diagnoses
Diabetes

Diarrhoea is a common symptom of diabetes and is more common in people who have had diabetes for a long time. In an undiagnosed diabetic, other more prominent symptoms would typically be present, including polyuria, polydipsia, losing weight and tiredness.

Medicines

A great number of medicines can cause diarrhoea. Commonly implicated medicines include angiotensin-converting enzyme (ACE) inhibitors, magnesium salts, selective serotonin reuptake inhibitors (SSRIs), antiepileptics, antibacterials and antivirals. Laxative abuse also needs to be considered.

Traveller's Diarrhoea

People travelling to foreign countries often experience diarrhoea, especially those visiting low- and middle-income countries. It is usually an acute and self-limiting condition although infections associated with giardia can last longer than 2 weeks and infection can recur.

Critical Diagnoses
Addison's Disease

This a rare condition affecting those 30–50 years of age. Symptoms can be nonspecific and common to other conditions. Early symptoms include low mood, fatigue, muscle weakness, weight loss and loss of appetite, increased urination and increased thirst. Over time these symptoms worsen and other symptoms such as diarrhoea, abdominal pain, nausea/vomiting, dizziness, cramps and darkening of the skin can occur.

Colorectal Carcinoma

Unexplained weight loss, anaemia, rectal bleeding, abdominal pain, a change in bowel habit, occult blood in faeces and palpable rectal or abdominal masses are symptoms which should be viewed with caution, especially in people who are middle aged or older.

■ MCQs

1. In which ONE of the following conditions is blood in the stool least likely?
   (a) Bacterial gastroenteritis caused by Shigella
   (b) Colorectal cancer
   (c) IBD
   (d) IBS
   (e) Traveller's diarrhoea

2. ACE inhibitors are known to cause diarrhoea. Which ONE of the following ACE inhibitors is least likely to cause this adverse drug reaction?
   (a) Captopril
   (b) Enalapril
   (c) Lisinopril
   (d) Quinapril
   (e) Trandolapril
3. Which ONE of the following groups of laxatives is most associated with laxative abuse?
   (a) Bulk-forming
   (b) Lubricant
   (c) Osmotic
   (d) Stimulant
   (e) Stool softeners
4. Acute diarrhoea can lead to dehydration. Which ONE of the following is NOT a symptom of mild dehydration?
   (a) Lassitude
   (b) Light-headedness
   (c) Nausea
   (d) Postural hypotension
   (e) Tachycardia
5. Acute gastroenteritis is the most common cause of diarrhoea in all age groups and is usually viral in origin. Which ONE of the following pathogens is most likely to cause diarrhoea?
   (a) Astrovirus
   (b) Bacillus cereus
   (c) Coronavirus
   (d) Cytomegalovirus
   (e) Norovirus

Answers

1. d; 2. e; 3. d; 4. e; 5. e

KEY POINTS: IRRITABLE BOWEL SYNDROME

- The cause/s of irritable bowel syndrome are still not fully understood but probably involve biological, social and psychological factors.
- Key symptoms are alternating diarrhoea and constipation associated with lower quadrant pain and bloating.
- Intermittent but chronic
- Treat predominant symptoms with a combination of laxatives, antidiarrhoeals and antispasmodics.

WEBSITES

NICE Guidance 61
www.nice.org.uk/guidance/cg61
Irritable Bowel Syndrome Group
http://www.ibsgroup.org
IBS Network
https://www.theibsnetwork.org/

CASE 15: LOWER ABDOMINAL PAIN

PRESENTATION

Mr C, who is approximately 30 years old, presents to you on a Friday morning complaining of stomach pain. He tells you the pain is in an area below and to the right of his belly button and started hurting about 4 h ago.

PROBLEM REPRESENTATION

A 30-year-old man presents with a 4-h history of acute RLQ pain.

HYPOTHESIS GENERATION (LIKELY, POSSIBLE AND CRITICAL DIAGNOSES)

Right lower abdominal pain is mainly associated with GI, urological and gynaecological origin. It can also be associated with referred pain. Given that we are dealing with a male patient, we can discount gynaecological causes, which are:

- Dysmenorrhoea – primary and secondary
- Ectopic pregnancy
- Fibroids
- Mittelschmerz (ovulation pain)
- Ovarian cyst
- Ovarian torsion
- Pelvic inflammatory disease
- Salpingitis

  Based on the acute nature of his symptoms and his age, a number of conditions are more likely and should be considered first.

Likely Diagnoses

- Appendicitis (also critical diagnosis)
- Constipation
- IBD
- IBS
- Pyelonephritis

Possible Diagnoses

- Abdominal wall haematoma
- Diverticulitis
- Hernia
- Kidney stones

Critical Diagnoses

- Appendicitis
- Carcinoma
- Intestinal obstruction
- Perforated ulcer
- Testicular torsion

CONTINUED INFORMATION GATHERING

Initial thoughts on the most likely diagnoses have so far been based on location and his age. We now need to better understand the pain he is experiencing, for example, its onset, severity and quality.

He confirms that the pain started this morning quite suddenly and describes the pain as constant, aching and bothersome. You ask him to rate the pain on a scale of 0–10 to try and assess the severity. He rates the pain as a 7.

The severity of the pain seems to rule out constipation.

Of the remaining likely diagnoses, appendicitis seems a plausible differential diagnosis given the severity of the pain, which is constant, combined with RLQ pain.

You ask about associated symptoms to help rule out other causes and rule in appendicitis. Mr C says he has had no other symptoms but does feel off-colour. This suggests IBD and IBS are less likely (GI symptoms are common), as is pyelonephritis, with UTI symptoms being prominent.

Feeling off-colour may mean he has systemic symptoms. A temperature check reveals he has a low-grade fever. This symptom would be consistent with appendicitis.

Based on information to date, your suspicions of this being appendicitis are now stronger even though he is older than most people who get appendicitis.

PROBLEM REFINEMENT

To further support your differential diagnosis, asking about previous history will be helpful. In appendicitis, no previous history should be present. Mr C confirms this is the first time he has had such symptoms. This also helps to further rule out causes such as complications of ulcers, diverticulitis, IBD and IBS.

At this point you suspect appendicitis. Checking against the list of possible diagnoses that have yet to be

considered, abdominal wall haematoma and hernias are associated with older age. Nausea and vomiting are also seen with abdominal wall haematoma, diverticulitis and kidney stones. It seems these other possible causes can reasonably be discounted.

If you are competent to perform a physical examination, this should also be done. Findings of RLQ tenderness would support appendicitis as the diagnosis.

> ⚡ **RED FLAGS**
>
> The critical diagnoses that need to be considered do not fit the age profile of our patient; carcinoma, intestinal obstruction and perforated ulcer are associated with older people and testicular torsion in younger men. Other symptoms beside pain are also common in all conditions other than testicular torsion – however, pain here is in the testes rather than right lower quadrant.

MANAGEMENT

Self-care Options

Not applicable.

Prescribing Options

A second opinion from a medically qualified practitioner should be sought urgently, and onward referral to Accident &Emergency arranged if appendicitis is still considered likely.

Safety Netting

You tell Mr C you suspect he has appendicitis, will arrange for a second opinion, and if the doctor also suspects appendicitis, then you are going to admit him to the hospital.

AIDE MEMOIRE

Likely Diagnoses

Appendicitis

For appendicitis, RLQ pain has the highest positive predictive value, although migration from periumbilical to RLQ pain and fever also suggest appendicitis. The pain of appendicitis is described as colicky or cramp-like but after a few hours becomes constant. Movement tends to aggravate the pain and nausea/vomiting might also be present. It is most common during adolescence.

Constipation

Constipation is a symptom of many abdominal conditions. In addition to a reduced bowel movement, associated lower abdominal discomfort/pain is often present.

Inflammatory Bowel Disease

Crohn's disease and ulcerative colitis are characterised by relapse and remittance. Both exhibit lower abdominal pain. In Crohn's disease, the most common place for it to start is at the end of the small intestine (ileum) causing RLQ pain. In ulcerative colitis, the pain is more common in the left lower quadrant. For both conditions GI disturbance is very common – either as persistent diarrhoea or bloody diarrhoea associated with urgency and tenesmus. Both are associated with extraintestinal symptoms, affecting 25%–40% of patients, and include arthritis, mouth ulcers, red eye and fatigue (due to anaemia). Other nonspecific symptoms such as malaise and fever can be present. Young adults (20–40 years of age) are most affected.

Irritable Bowel Syndrome

IBS is characterised by lower abdominal pain or discomfort, although left lower quadrant pain is more typical than RLQ pain. Pain is accompanied by abdominal bloating and changes to bowel habit. Typically, symptoms will have been present for some time, and in primary care a diagnosis is suggested if symptoms have persisted for 6 months or longer. People with IBS can present with 'diarrhoea predominant', 'constipation predominant' or alternating symptom profiles. During bouts of diarrhoea, mucus tends to be visible on the stools. Patients might also complain of increased stool frequency but pass normal or pellet-like stools. IBS is most commonly seen in younger adults (less than 40 years of age) and affects women more than men.

Pyelonephritis

Unilateral flank pain that can be felt in the RLQ associated with nausea, vomiting and fever are typical presenting symptoms in association with lower UTI symptoms. Onset is often sudden.

Possible Diagnoses
Abdominal Wall Haematoma

Abdominal wall hematomas are an uncommon cause of acute abdominal pain mostly affecting those over 60 years of age. A typical presentation is localised sharp sudden pain that does not radiate. It is associated with nausea and vomiting. Predisposing factors include increasing age, trauma, exercise and valsalver movements.

Diverticulitis

Diverticulitis is usually associated with intermittent left lower abdominal pain and tenderness on physical examination, but it can manifest as RLQ. Other symptoms include bloating, fever, nausea/vomiting and bowel changes, including rectal bleeding. In acute presentations, the pain tends to be constant and severe. It is most commonly seen in those aged over 50 years.

Hernia (Inguinal)

In general, hernias are reducible and have an expansible cough impulse. Patients notice a bulge in the groin which becomes more obvious when upright. Pain/discomfort or burning in the groin is experienced. They are more commonly seen on the right side, are seen with increasing age and are most common in people aged 75–80 years.

Kidney Stones

Urinary calculi (stones) can occur anywhere in the urinary tract, although most frequently stones get lodged in the ureter. Pain is abrupt in onset and starts in the loin, radiating around the flank and RLQ. Pain is very severe and colicky in nature. Attacks are spasmodic and tend to last minutes to hours and often leave the person prostrate with pain. The person is restless and cannot lie still. Symptoms of nausea and vomiting might also be present. It is twice as common in men than in women and usually occurs between the ages of 40 and 60 years.

Critical Diagnoses
Carcinoma

Carcinoma is characterised by abdominal pain (although more likely to be left lower quadrant) accompanied with appetite and weight loss, rectal bleeding, change in bowel habit and signs of anaemia.

Intestinal Obstruction

The pain is described as colicky and intermittent. Constipation is common and is the symptom with the highest positive predictive value. Abdominal distension, vomiting and loss of appetite may also be experienced. It is most commonly seen in those over 50 years of age.

Perforated Ulcer

A complication of a peptic ulcer is perforation. Symptom presentation of perforation is sudden severe epigastric pain but pain can become more generalised including the RLQ. Nausea/vomiting, light-headedness and lack of appetite may also be present. A previous history of symptoms will be present, such as dyspepsia and upper abdominal pain/discomfort. Typically, ulcers affect people over 45 years of age.

Testicular Torsion

Torsion is rare and constitutes a medical emergency. The testicular blood supply gets cut off to the testicle and if not treated right away the testicle can be lost. It mostly affects men aged under 25 years and is commonest in those aged between 12 and 18 years. The main symptom is sudden onset of severe testicular pain. Torsion is most often seen in the left testicle.

▌ M C Q s

1. Pain that radiates from the loin area to the right or left lower quadrants would be most closely associated with which ONE of the following conditions?
   (a) Appendicitis
   (b) Diverticulitis
   (c) Gastric ulcer
   (d) IBS
   (e) Renal colic
2. A woman in her 30s presents with RLQ pain. Based only on symptom location, which ONE of the following conditions is the least likely cause?
   (a) Appendicitis
   (b) Ectopic pregnancy
   (c) IBS
   (d) Primary dysmenorrhoea
   (e) Secondary dysmenorrhoea
3. Abdominal pain that causes the patient to writhe around trying to get comfortable suggests which ONE of the following conditions?
   (a) Appendicitis
   (b) Inguinal hernia
   (c) Pancreatitis
   (d) Perforated ulcer
   (e) Renal colic
4. A number of conditions with RLQ can also present with fever. Which ONE of the following conditions is least associated with fever?

   (a) Appendicitis
   (b) Diverticulitis
   (c) IBD
   (d) Kidney stones
   (e) Pyelonephritis
5. The nature of pain associated with RLQ can be useful in helping to determine the cause. Which ONE of the following is least associated with sudden onset pain?
   (a) Abdominal wall haematoma
   (b) Appendicitis
   (c) Intestinal obstruction
   (d) Kidney stones
   (e) Perforated ulcer

Answers
1. e; 2. c; 3. e; 4. d; 5. c

KEY POINTS: APPENDICITIS
- The cause is not well understood but in about half of cases it is associated with obstruction.
- Key symptoms are central abdominal pain that moves to the RLQ. Coughing and palpation worsens pain.
- Most patients present within 24 h of the onset of symptoms.

CASE 16: PAINFUL ORAL LESION

PRESENTATION
Mr K, a 19-year-old man, asks you for some advice about some ulcers he has noticed in his mouth. He says they are painful and red and have been present for a few days. He wants you to recommend some sort of gel he can put on the ulcers to relieve the pain. He is fit and healthy and has no medical problems.

PROBLEM REPRESENTATION

A 19-year-old man presents with acute onset painful oral lesions.

HYPOTHESIS GENERATION (LIKELY, POSSIBLE AND CRITICAL DIAGNOSES)

Oral ulceration is common and most forms cause varying degrees of pain. The three most common presentations are trauma, recurrent aphthous stomatitis (with three recognised clinical subtypes of minor (most common), major and herpetiform) and herpes virus group infections. Of these, herpes simplex is most associated with young children and therefore could be discounted from our initial thoughts as to the cause of Mr K's symptoms.

Likely Diagnoses

- Recurrent aphthous stomatitis
  - Minor aphthous ulcers
  - Major aphthous ulcers
  - Herpetiform ulcers
- Trauma

Possible Diagnoses

- Hand, foot and mouth disease
- Herpangina
- Herpes simplex
- Medicine-induced
- Systemic conditions that present with aphthous-like ulcers
  - Behçet's syndrome
  - Coeliac disease
  - Crohn's disease and ulcerative colitis
  - HIV (e.g., immunodeficiency)
  - Vitamin B_{12}, iron or folate deficiency
- Systemic lupus erythematosus

Critical Diagnoses

- Erythema multiforme
- Stevens–Johnson Syndrome (SJS)/toxic epidermal necrolysis

CONTINUED INFORMATION GATHERING

Whilst we know he has painful oral lesions, we need to better understand how many he has, where they are and what they look like.

He tells you that he has just two ulcers located on the inside of his lip. On inspection they are relatively small, round and greyish in appearance (Fig. 4.1). Whilst lip is a common location for trauma, the ulcers' roundness suggests that trauma is unlikely. Likewise, herpetiform ulceration seems unlikely as ulcers tend to be located toward the back of the mouth. Their size also points away from a major ulcer.

It seems we are most likely dealing with minor aphthous ulceration.

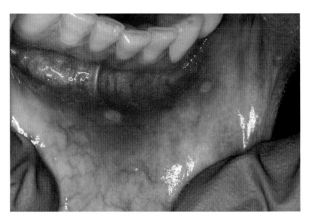

Fig. 4.1 Minor Aphthous Stomatitis. Two ulcerations located on the mandibular labial mucosa. (Source: Neville, B. W., Damm, D. D., Allen, C. M., & Chi, A. C. (2024). *Oral and maxillofacial pathology* (5th ed.). Elsevier.)

PROBLEM REFINEMENT

You ask if this is the first time he has experienced ulcers. He tells you that he has experienced similar ulcers since he was about 15 years old and gets them once or twice a year but has never sought help before as they have tended to just go on their own. He generally gets one or two each episode. Previous ulcers have also occurred on the inside of his cheek. Traumatic ulceration can now be discounted.

To further confirm your thinking and better rule out major ulcers you could ask him how long the ulcers stay in his mouth, and if he has noticed any scarring. He tells you that they usually clear up in a week or so and he has not noticed any mouth problems after they have gone; this points away from major ulcers as the cause.

Whilst the aetiology of minor ulcers is not fully understood, they have been linked with stress/anxiety. You ask Mr K if the ulcers occur at certain stressful times, e.g., exams. However, he cannot recall anything like that when he gets the ulcers.

It seems, on balance, you are still confident that he has minor aphthous ulceration.

Although unlikely, checking on whether any of the possible causes are responsible for his symptoms should be done. His age seems to rule out hand, foot and mouth disease, herpangina and herpes simplex. You ask if he has any other symptoms apart from the ulcers. He says no; this seems to rule out any systemic cause.

MANAGEMENT

Self-care Options

As minor ulcers are self-limiting, any pharmacological intervention is to provide symptomatic relief. This can be provided through anaesthetic gels/liquids, antiinflammatory mouth washes and local corticosteroid pellets. You recommend an anaesthetic gel to Mr K.

Prescribing Options

Self-care measures should be sufficient to manage his symptoms.

Safety Netting

You tell Mr K you believe his ulcers are a type called minor ulcers and they should clear up in the next 5–7 days. However, he should be told to come back if the ulcers are not improving or have not resolved after 2 weeks.

AIDE MEMOIRE

The following information relates to how these conditions present in addition to pain, which is often the predominant symptom.

Likely Diagnoses

Minor Aphthous Ulcers

These ulcers are roundish and grey-white in colour. They are small, usually less than 1 cm in diameter and shallow with a raised red rim. They occur singly or in small crops of up to five ulcers. It normally takes 7–14 days for the ulcers to heal without scarring, but recurrence typically occurs after an interval of 1–4 months.

Major Aphthous Ulcers

These account for 10%–15% of cases and are large deep ulcers (>1 cm in diameter). Crops of ulcers can occur but often coalesce to form one large ulcer. The ulcers are slower to heal than minor ulcers, typically taking 3–4 weeks to heal, and may cause scarring.

Both forms occur on nonkeratinised tissues such as the labial and buccal mucosae, floor of the mouth and cheeks and the soft palate.

Herpetiform Ulcers

Herpetiform ulcers are pinpoint and often occur in clusters (up to 100 at a time), which can coalesce. They are located in the posterior part of the mouth. Recurrence is common. They usually heal within 7–14 days.

Trauma

Trauma to the oral mucosa will result in damage and ulceration. Trauma may be mechanical (e.g., tongue biting) or thermal, resulting in ulcers with an irregular border. Patients should be able to recall the traumatic event and have no history of similar ulceration or signs of systemic infection.

Table 4.3 summarises these likely diagnoses.

TABLE 4.3	**Condition Summary of the Four Commonest Types of Painful Oral Ulcers**				
	Number	**Location**	**Size and Shape**	**Age**	**Duration**
Minor ulcers	Up to approximately five ulcers	Lips, tongue and inside cheeks	Less than 1 cm and round	10–40 years	5–10 days
Major ulcers (Fig. 4.2)	Numerous	Anywhere	Large, 1–3 cm (and of variable shape)	All ages	Up to 6 weeks
Herpetiform (Figs. 4.3 and 4.4)	Very numerous	Back of the mouth	Pinpoint and round and can coalesce	All ages	1–2 weeks
Trauma (Fig. 4.5)	Usually singular	Buccal mucosa, lower lip, tongue	Variable	All ages	7–10 days

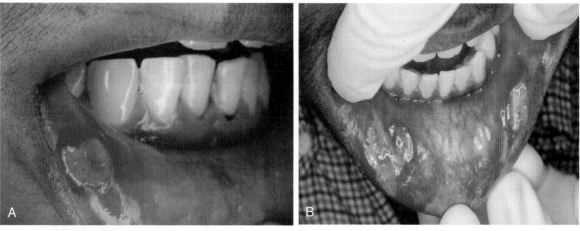

Fig. 4.2 Recurrent Aphthous Ulcers, Major. Deep crateriform ulcer (A) and scars (B). (Source: ((A) Sivapatha-sundharam, B. (2020). *Shafer's textbook of oral pathology.* (9th ed.). Elsevier.) ((B) Courtesy: Dr S. Karthiga Kannan, College of Dentistry, Zulfi Al Majmaah University, Kingdom of Saudi Arabia.))

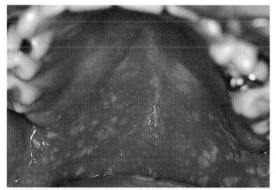

Fig. 4.3 Herpetiform Ulcer. (Source: From Crispian, S., et al. (2014). *Guía de bolsillo de enfermedades orales* (1st ed.). Elsevier.)

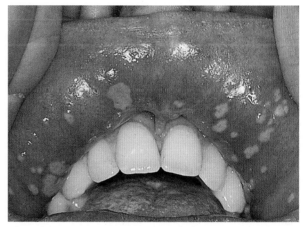

Fig. 4.4 Recurrent Aphthous Stomatitis, Herpetiform Type. There are numerous small, rounded and pinpoint ulcers, some of which are coalescing. The surrounding mucosa is lightly erythematous and the overall picture is highly suggestive of viral infection, but the attacks are recurrent and no virus can be isolated. (Source: Odell, E. W., (2017). *Cawson's essentials of oral pathology and oral medicine* (9th ed.). Elsevier.)

Possible Diagnoses

Hand, Foot and Mouth Disease

It often infects children under the age of 10 years, and most are under 5 years (95%). Small, sometimes painful ulcers can appear in and around the mouth, palate and pharynx appearing as shallow yellow-grey ulcers surrounded by an erythematous halo (Fig. 4.6). Skin rash shows macules and papules of the dorsal and palmar surfaces of the hands and feet that start pink and change to greyish blisters (Fig. 4.7).

Herpangina

Herpangina is seen mainly in children up to 10 years of age. Clinically, it presents as an acute febrile illness with a sore throat and ulcers at the back of the mouth. Nausea and abdominal symptoms can also be seen. Red spots appear within hours (up to 1 day later) in the mouth and throat. The red spots become raised into small vesicles, which form a tiny yellowish ulcer with a red rim. The ulcers are generally 1–2 mm in diameter. The ulcers take 5–10 days to heal (Fig. 4.8).

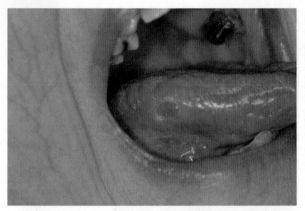

Fig. 4.5 Traumatic ulceration of the right border of the tongue related to lack of lubrication caused by dry mouth in the patient. (Source: Marchini, L., Ettinger, R., & Hartshorn, J. (2019). Personalized dental caries management for frail older adults and persons with special needs. *Dent Clin North Am.* 63(4):631-651.)

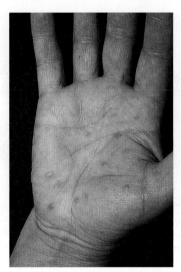

Fig. 4.7 Hand, Foot and Mouth Disease. (Source: Callen, J. P., Greer, K. E., Paller, A. S., & Swinyer, L. J. (2000). *Color atlas of dermatology* (2nd ed.). Philadelphia: W.B. Saunders.)

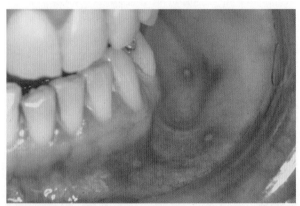

Fig. 4.6 Hand, Foot and Mouth Disease. Multiple aphthous-like ulcerations of the mucobuccal fold. (Source: Neville, B. W., Damm, D. D., Allen, C. M., & Chi, A. C,. (2023). *Oral and maxillofacial pathology* (5th ed.). Elsevier.)

Herpes Simplex

Primary herpetic gingivostomatitis is usually seen in childhood/young adults and presents with fever, sore throat and widespread superficial ulcers of the oral mucosa, especially the labial and buccal mucosa (Fig. 4.9).

Medicine-induced Ulcers

A number of case reports have described medication causing ulcers. These include cytotoxic agents, nicorandil, alendronate, nonsteroidal antiinflammatory drugs (NSAIDs; including aspirin), antimicrobials (azoles and tetracycline) and beta-blockers. Ulcers are

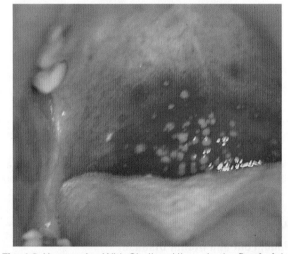

Fig. 4.8 Herpangina With Shallow Ulcers in the Roof of the Mouth. (Source: Cohen, J., Powderly, W. G. (2004). *Infectious Diseases* (2nd ed). St Louis: Mosby.)

often seen at the start of therapy or when the dose is increased.

Systemic Conditions that Present With Aphthous-like Ulcers

These conditions will present with other more prominent signs and symptoms, although oral ulceration may be one of the symptoms experienced.

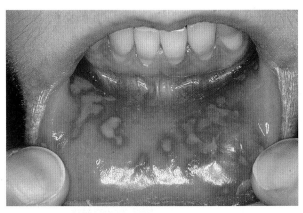

Fig. 4.9 Herpetic Gingivostomatitis, Extensive Erosions of the Oral Mucosa. (From James, W. D. et al. (2016). *Andrews' diseases of the skin* (12th ed.). Philadelphia, Saunders.)

Behçet's syndrome. This is a multisystem disorder characterised by recurrent inflammatory skin lesions, eye problems (e.g., uveitis) and oral and genital ulcers. Eye symptoms and genital lesions are more prominent than skin and oral lesions. Oral ulcers can appear anywhere in the oral cavity and tend to be large (1–3 cm).

Coeliac disease and ulcerative colitis. These are associated with unexplained gastrointestinal symptoms as predominant features. Coeliac disease is associated with diarrhoea, weight loss, abdominal pain and steatorrhoea. Unexplained fatigue (anaemia) and recurrent mouth ulcers can also occur.

In ulcerative colitis, bloody diarrhoea and abdominal pain are prominent. Fatigue, malaise and fever may also be present. Oral involvement is usually seen in people at the severe end of the spectrum.

Human immunodeficiency infection. This can cause a variety of oral ulcers, including severe necrotic ulcers affecting the buccal and pharyngeal mucosa. These ulcers are painful and can cause dysphagia.

Vitamin B₁₂, iron or folate deficiency. Anaemias tend to be insidious in onset with gradually progressive signs and symptoms. Symptoms include fatigue, weakness, headache, dizziness, pale skin and shortness of breath.

Systemic Lupus Erythematosus (SLE)

Cutaneous symptoms are common in SLE and can be the first signs in approximately 25% of people. In acute stages, a facial butterfly rash is often present. Other cutaneous symptoms are seen such as hair loss, blistering or maculopapular rashes and mucosal ulcers affecting the lips and mouth.

Critical Diagnoses
Erythema Multiforme

Erythema multiforme is a skin reaction which is characterised by the appearance of distinctive target-like lesions on the skin that can be accompanied by erosions of the oral and/or genital mucosa. Oral lesions occur on the lips and anterior oral mucosa. The lesions present as asymmetrical, erythematous, lesions. These lesions usually heal without scarring.

Stevens–Johnson Syndrome/Toxic Epidermal Necrolysis (TEN)

SJS/TEN is a rare, acute, serious and potentially fatal skin reaction in which there is sheet-like skin and mucosal loss. It is nearly always caused by medications, with antibiotics commonly implicated. Lip and/or mouth ulcers are prominent and can be severe.

▮ MCQs

1. In which ONE of the following groups are aphthous ulcers more common?
   (a) Black people
   (b) Men
   (c) Smokers
   (d) People under the age of 40 years
   (e) None of the above
2. A 24-year-old woman presents with a painful sore on the inside of her cheek. She mentions a recent allergy test which found an allergy to sodium lauryl sulphate. Which ONE of the following is the most likely diagnosis?
   (a) Cold sore
   (b) Gingivitis
   (c) Lichen planus
   (d) Mouth ulcer
   (e) Thrush
3. A 17-year-old man wants a gel for a mouth ulcer. After questioning and visual inspection, you ascertain the ulcer is on the inside of the lip, grey in colour, round and small. Based on this information, which ONE of the following is the most likely diagnosis?
   (a) Leukoplakia
   (b) Lichen planus
   (c) Major aphthous ulcer
   (d) Minor aphthous ulcer
   (e) Trauma-related ulcer

4. Which ONE of the following problems is associated with GI symptoms as well as oral ulceration?
   (a) Behçet's syndrome
   (b) Coeliac's disease
   (c) Iron deficiency
   (d) Leukoplakia
   (e) Malignancy
5. A number of conditions can present with skin lesions as well as painful ulcers. Which ONE of the following is least likely to exhibit skin involvement?
   (a) Behçet's syndrome
   (b) Erythema multiforme
   (c) Hand foot and mouth disease
   (d) SLE
   (e) Vitamin B_{12} deficiency

Answers
1. d; 2. d; 3. d; 4. b; 5. e

KEY POINTS: MINOR ULCERS

- A number of causes are implicated: stress, deficiency and genetics.
- Key symptoms are small, round, grey and painful ulcers.
- Symptoms should resolve in 10–14 days.
- Treatment is primarily symptomatic, with protectorants and anaesthetics.

WEBSITES

The Behçet's Syndrome Society
https://behcetsuk.org
The Oral Health Foundation
https://www.dentalhealth.org/

CASE 17: PAINLESS ORAL LESION

PRESENTATION

Mr H, an 80-year-old man, presents with a 3-day history of sore throat. You diagnose a viral infection and recommend increasing fluid intake and paracetamol if the pain becomes troublesome. However, during inspection of the oral cavity you notice a white lesion on the side of his tongue. You ask him if he knew that the lesion was present but he was unaware of it. He has hypertension and type 2 diabetes.

PROBLEM REPRESENTATION

An 80-year-old man presents with a painless lesion of unknown duration.

HYPOTHESIS GENERATION (LIKELY, POSSIBLE AND CRITICAL DIAGNOSES)

Painless ulcers are usually 'picked up' during routine examination. The probability of sinister pathology for Mr H needs to be considered.

Likely Diagnosis
- Oral thrush

Possible Diagnoses
- Erythema migrans (geographic tongue)
- Hairy tongue
- Lichen planus

Critical Diagnoses
- Leukoplakia
- Squamous cell carcinoma (SCC)

CONTINUED INFORMATION GATHERING

As Mr H was unaware of the lesion, it is unlikely that questions asked about the lesion will yield much useful information. It is therefore important to concentrate on the visual inspection, noting its size and shape, as well as determining if this is the only lesion present. You observe no other lesions in the oral cavity and the lesion itself is approximately 2 cm in length and a raised solid patch with no rolled edges (Fig. 4.10).

The appearance of the lesion does not suggest oral thrush, which is the most common lesion seen in the mouth. It also does not appear to be lichen planus (lace-like lesions) or SCC (rolled edges).

Given its location, it also seems geographic and hairy tongue can be discounted.

PROBLEM REFINEMENT

This leaves leukoplakia as the most likely cause. However, as thrush is an opportunistic infection, and Mr H has diabetes, you ask how he is and if he has been experiencing any problems. His answers suggest that his diabetes seems well controlled and he is adherent to his medicines. The lesion seems most likely to be leukoplakia.

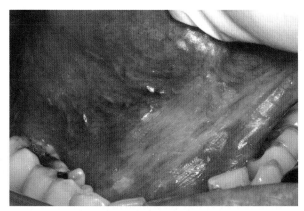

Fig. 4.10 Homogeneous Thin Leukoplakia. A thin, white plaque on the right ventral tongue. (Source: Neville, B. W., Damm, D. D., Allen, C. M., & Chi, A. C. (2024). *Oral and maxillofacial pathology* (5th ed.). Elsevier.)

You ask if he smokes and how much alcohol he drinks as these are known risk factors for leukoplakia. He tells you he is an ex-smoker and drinks but only occasionally.

A history of smoking gives more weight to your thinking that this is leukoplakia.

⚡ RED FLAGS

Not applicable.

MANAGEMENT

Self-care Options

Not appropriate.

Prescribing Options

A biopsy maybe required under a suspected cancer pathway referral. However, we have no reference in relation to how long the lesion has been present. On that basis a reassessment maybe required before onward referral.

Safety Netting

You tell Mr H that you are not sure what the cause of the mouth lesion is but you would like to see him again in 2–3 weeks to check on the problem. If it has not got any better by then, you would like to arrange a hospital visit to do some more tests.

AIDE MEMOIRE

Likely Diagnosis

Thrush

Oral candidiasis is an opportunistic fungal infection that arises in a patient with one or more local or systemic predisposing factors. Local factors include poor oral hygiene, xerostomia and the use of dentures. Systemic predisposing factors include immunodeficiency, diabetes mellitus, antibiotic use, steroid therapy (including inhaled steroids), chemotherapy or radiation therapy.

A typical presentation of oral thrush is with creamy-white, soft elevated patches that can be wiped away, leaving a painful erythematous under surface (Fig. 4.11). Lesions can occur anywhere in the oral cavity but usually affect the tongue, palate, lips and cheeks. Burning or irritation is associated with the infection rather than true pain. Patients sometimes complain of malaise and loss of appetite. In the early stages, it is minimally symptomatic.

Possible Diagnoses

Erythema Migrans (Geographic Tongue)

Tongue lesions exhibit central erythema usually surrounded by slightly elevated white-to-yellow borders,

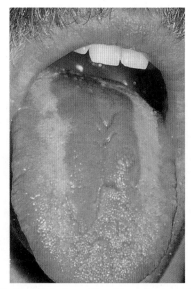

Fig. 4.11 Oral candidiasis, or 'thrush' manifests with a whitish, curd-like substance on the tongue or inside of the mouth. (Source: Christensen, B. L., Lauritsen, B., & Kockrow, E. O. (2006). *Adult health nursing* (5th ed.). Mosby.)

thus giving the appearance of continents surrounded by water (e.g., geographic tongue) (Fig. 4.12). The appearance changes over several days demonstrating a 'migrating pattern'. It is usually asymptomatic but some patients may complain of pain or burning, especially when eating spicy foods.

Hairy Tongue

Hairy tongue occurs most often in heavy smokers but also is associated with poor oral hygiene. The top of the tongue has an abnormal coating appearing in various colours, causing a hair-like appearance (Fig. 4.13). Occasionally patients may complain of a burning or tickling sensation on the tongue. Halitosis might be present.

Oral Lichen Planus

Oral lichen planus is a mucosal presentation of lichen planus that has a variety of clinical subtypes. The clinical appearance varies depending on clinical subtype. The reticular type (most common) is characterised by interlacing white lines that produce a 'net-like' pattern (Wickham's striae) (Fig. 4.14). This is most commonly located on the buccal mucosa but can be found on the tongue and lip.

In the erosive form, ulceration of the mucosa leads to pain and erythema.

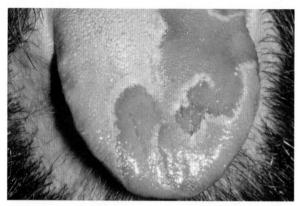

Fig. 4.12 Erythema Migrans. The erythematous, well-demarcated areas of papillary atrophy are characteristic of erythema migrans affecting the tongue (benign migratory glossitis). Note the asymmetrical distribution and the tendency to involve the lateral aspects of the tongue. (Source: Neville, B. W., Damm, D. D., Allen, C. M., & Chi, A. C. (2024). *Oral and maxillofacial pathology* (5th ed.). Elsevier.)

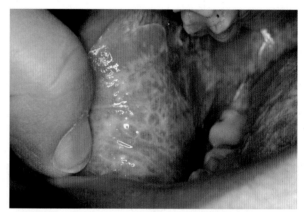

Fig. 4.14 Oral Lichen Planus. (Source: Micheletti, R. G., James, W. D., Elston, D. M., & McMahon, P. J. (2023). *Andrews' diseases of the skin clinical atlas* (2nd ed.). Elsevier.)

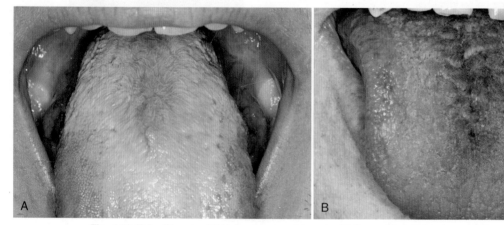

Fig. 4.13 Hairy Tongue. (A) Hairy dorsum of tongue. (B) Brown-black hairy dorsum of tongue. (Source: Woo, S. B. (2024). *Oral pathology* (3rd ed.). Elsevier.)

Critical Diagnoses
Leukoplakia

Leukoplakia is seen mostly in men with advancing age. It presents as a white lesion of the oral mucosa. Patients present with a symptomless white patch mainly on the buccal mucosa or tongue that develops over a period of weeks. The lesion cannot be wiped off, unlike oral thrush. Smoking and excessive alcohol consumption are known risk factors in its development.

It is a precancerous lesion, although epidemiological data suggest that annual transformation rate to SCC is low.

Oral Squamous Cell Carcinoma

More than 90% of oral cancers are SCC. Oral SCC most commonly presents as a nonhealing ulcer, which can be indurated/firm and have irregular margins and raised, rolled edges. Almost 60% of cases affect the tongue (32%) or tonsils (26%), although it can occur in any part of the mouth (e.g., floor of mouth (7%), gums (5%), palate (5%)). Initially asymptomatic, but as the cancer progresses the patient may experience pain, have altered speech and affected swallowing. The major risk factors for oral cavity SCC are smoking and excessive alcohol consumption.

Table 4.4 summarises how these conditions present.

TABLE 4.4 Condition Summary of Presenting Signs and Symptoms

	Number	Location	Size and Shape	Age
Thrush	Singular patch	Anywhere	Irregular and variable size	Young and elderly
Lichen planus	Diffuse	Tongue, cheek, gums	'Spiders web'	Adults
Leukoplakia	Singular patch	Tongue or cheek	Irregular and variable size	Older age
Erythema migrans (geographic tongue)	Diffuse	Top of tongue	Irregular and variable size	Any age
Hairy tongue	Diffuse	Top of tongue	Irregular and variable size	Any age but more common in older age
Carcinoma	Singular lesion	Tongue, mouth, lower lip	Irregular and variable size	Older age

MCQs

1. A 64-year-old woman asks for your advice about a lesion in her mouth. You perform a visual inspection and observe a white patch on the side of her cheek. She has no pain. Based on this information, which ONE of the following is the most likely diagnosis?
   (a) Leukoplakia
   (b) Lichen planus
   (c) Major aphthous ulcer
   (d) Minor aphthous ulcer
   (e) Trauma-related ulcer

2. Mr M, a university student, complains of a burning sensation on his tongue, that is exacerbated when eating spicy food or fizzy drinks. Upon inspection you notice several white patches on his tongue. He adds he is an asthmatic who recently had his steroid inhaler dose increased. Which ONE of the following conditions is the most likely cause?
   (a) Angular cheilitis
   (b) Cold sores
   (c) HSV oral infection
   (d) Mouth ulcer
   (e) Oral thrush

3. Known risk factors are associated with certain causes of oral ulceration. Which ONE of the following is least associated with a specific risk factor?
   (a) Carcinoma
   (b) Hairy tongue
   (c) Leukoplakia
   (d) Lichen planus
   (e) Thrush

4. Based on prevalence data, which ONE of the following would be the most likely cause of painless oral ulceration in an adult patient?
   (a) Carcinoma
   (b) Hairy tongue
   (c) Leukoplakia
   (d) Lichen planus
   (e) Thrush
5. Which ONE of the following conditions can remit and recur?
   (a) Geographic tongue
   (b) Hairy tongue
   (c) Leukoplakia
   (d) Thrush
   (e) None of the above

Answers

1. b; 2. e; 3. d; 4. d; 5. a

KEY POINTS: LEUKOPLAKIA

- The exact cause is unknown but smoking is a common risk factor.
- Key symptom is a painless white patch that cannot be rubbed off.
- Lesions are slow growing and may take months to develop.

WEBSITES

The British Dental Association
https://www.bda.org/
Oral Cancer Foundation
https://oralcancerfoundation.org/

CASE 18: RECTAL BLEEDING

PRESENTATION

A 54-year-old man (Mr Vs) presents saying he has noticed blood when he opens his bowels. He says it does not happen every time. It has been going on for a couple of weeks now but he has been too embarrassed to come in and talk about it. His medical history shows that he rarely seeks medical help and has no medical problems of note. He is currently prescribed no medication.

PROBLEM REPRESENTATION

An otherwise fit and healthy 54-year-old man presents with 2-week history of rectal bleeding.

HYPOTHESIS GENERATION (LIKELY, POSSIBLE AND CRITICAL DIAGNOSES)

The presentation may range from mild to severe, depending on the aetiology of the bleeding. Mild cases may appear as red blood streaking the patient's stool or toilet paper after wiping, and severe cases may present as a large volume, brisk bleed. This is a common presentation but may indicate a serious underlying disease.

Likely Diagnoses

- Anal fissure
- Haemorrhoids
- Gastroenteritis

Possible Diagnoses

- Angiodysplasia
- Diverticular disease
- IBD
- Medicine-induced (not applicable in this case)
- Proctitis

Critical Diagnoses

- Colon polyps
- Colorectal cancer
- Peptic ulcer

CONTINUED INFORMATION GATHERING

As he is fit and healthy and had symptoms for 2 weeks, gastroenteritis can be discounted. Early thinking is therefore to consider anal fissure or haemorrhoids as the cause. A detailed history surrounding the passage of blood is needed regarding onset, duration, amount and nature.

Mr Vs confirms the symptoms have been happening for about 2 weeks and this is the first time he has noticed such symptoms. He describes the blood as bright red in colour – that is what has been frightening him. He says the toilet bowl water is very pink tinged and the stool seems to be covered in blood.

This description seems to indicate a local aetiology given the colour of the blood and is consistent with anal fissure and haemorrhoids.

You ask if there is any pain when he defecates. He says not really, although occasionally it can be hard to pass a stool. This seems to suggest haemorrhoid as the cause rather than anal fissure.

You further ask if he has been experiencing any symptoms other than the bleeding. He says not really, although he has been getting a bit constipated and that is when he has been having difficulty going to the toilet. You ask more about his diet. He reports a relatively healthy diet with no obvious changes, and he has not eaten anything like beetroot recently.

Although haemorrhoids still seems likely, given his age and a possible change in bowel habit you are now a little concerned about possible sinister pathology.

You check his weight (normal range and BMI of 24), and check for signs of anaemia (none present).

PROBLEM REFINEMENT

His record does show that his father died of bowel cancer 8 years ago. This raises further suspicion of a sinister cause. An abdominal and rectal examination seems appropriate given your concern. Nothing abnormal is noted.

Other possible diagnoses seem not to be the cause – angiodysplasia and diverticular disease are seen in more elderly people; proctitis and IBD are associated with bloody diarrhoea and peptic ulcer with tarry stools.

⚡ RED FLAGS

You are uncertain of the diagnosis but sufficiently concerned about his symptoms to think about further investigation.

MANAGEMENT

Self-care Options
Not applicable.

Prescribing Options
No treatment should be offered at this time.

Safety Netting

You tell Mr Vs that you are not sure what might be causing the bleeding and that another test, a colonoscopy, needs to be done at the hospital to make sure that all is well. You instigate an urgent referral to the local hospital using the 2-week rule.

AIDE MEMOIRE

Likely Diagnoses
Anal Fissure

Anal fissures are common, with those aged between 15 and 40 years most affected. Symptoms often follow a period of constipation and are normally caused by straining at stool. Pain always occurs with defecation, which can be severe and sharp with pain lasting for a number of hours after defecation. Bleeding is usually of small volume and bright red. Some patients also note itching or irritation of the skin around the anus.

Gastroenteritis

Certain bacterial causes of gastroenteritis can cause bloody diarrhoea, for example *Shigella, E. coli 0157* and *Clostridium difficile*. Typically, onset is acute in a previously healthy patient. Abdominal cramps, general malaise, fever and mucus may also be seen.

Haemorrhoids

This is the most common cause of rectal bleeding in the middle-aged and older population. Symptoms experienced are dependent on the severity or type of haemorrhoid. Bright red painless rectal bleeding is the most common symptom. Blood is most commonly seen as spotting around the toilet pan, streaking on toilet tissue or visible on the surface of the stool. Itching and irritation are also commonly observed. Symptoms are often intermittent and each episode usually lasts from a few days to a few weeks. Internal haemorrhoids are rarely painful, whereas external haemorrhoids can cause pain due to the mucosal cushion becoming thrombosed. Pain is described as a dull ache that increases in severity when the patient defecates, leading to patients ignoring the urge to defecate. This can then lead to constipation, which in turn will lead to more difficulty in passing stools and further increase the pain associated with defecation.

Possible Diagnoses

Angiodysplasia

Angiodysplasia is abnormal blood vessels in the gastro-intestinal tract, which can cause bleeding. This is more common in older people and can cause painless rectal bleeding.

Diverticular Disease

Is usually associated with intermittent left lower abdominal pain and tenderness on physical examination. Other symptoms include bloating, fever, nausea/vomiting and bowel changes, including rectal bleeding. In acute presentations, the pain tends to be constant and severe. It is most commonly seen in those aged over 50 years.

Inflammatory Bowel Disease

Crohn's disease and ulcerative colitis are characterised by GI disturbance – either as persistent diarrhoea or bloody diarrhoea associated with urgency and tenesmus. Both exhibit lower abdominal pain. In Crohn's disease, the most common place for it to start is at the end of the small intestine (ileum) causing RLQ pain. In ulcerative colitis, the pain is more common in the left lower quadrant. Over time weight loss can be observed. Both are associated with extraintestinal symptoms, affecting 25%–40% of patients, and include arthritis, mouth ulcers, red eye and fatigue (due to anaemia). Other nonspecific symptoms such as malaise and fever can be present. Young adults (20–40 years of age) are most affected.

Medicine-induced

NSAIDs, anticoagulants, and antiplatelet agents are possible contributing factors to rectal bleeding.

Proctitis

Proctitis is inflammation of the lining of the rectum. Common symptoms include bloody diarrhoea, tenesmus and pain on defecation. It is associated with sexually transmitted diseases.

Critical Diagnoses

Colon Polyps

Precancerous polyps near the end of the colon can mimic bleeding from haemorrhoids. Other symptoms seen include a change in bowel habit and abdominal pain. Polyps are generally present in the colon for years before they become cancerous.

Colorectal and Anal Cancer

Rectal bleeding is observed in both cancers but bleeding can depend on the site of the tumour, for example, sigmoid tumours lead to bright red blood in or around the stool. Rectal bleeding tends to be persistent and steady though slight for all tumours. Unexplained rectal bleeding in people over 50 years of age, and those under 40 years who also have any of the following symptoms of change in bowel habit, abdominal pain, weight loss or anaemia should be referred on to a suspected cancer pathway. Occurrence is strongly related to age, with almost three-quarters of cases occurring in people aged 65 years or over.

Peptic Ulcer

Erosion of the stomach wall or upper intestine is normally responsible for GI bleeds and is often associated with NSAID intake. The colour of the stool is related to the rate of bleeding. Stools from GI bleeds can be tarry or black. If a patient is also experiencing haematemesis this would further suggest that the source of the bleed is coming from the upper GI tract.

MCQs

1. A 41-year-old woman presents with bright red painless rectal bleeding. She tells you she has no other symptoms and denies any weight loss or changes in bowel habit. Which ONE of the following is the most likely diagnosis?
   (a) Anal fissure
   (b) Colorectal cancer
   (c) Diverticulitis
   (d) Haemorrhoids
   (e) Proctitis
2. Which ONE of the following is true about haemorrhoids?
   (a) Bleeding from first degree haemorrhoids is associated with pain.
   (b) Bleeding haemorrhoids are noted as dull coloured.
   (c) Pain always occurs on defecation.
   (d) Pregnancy is a predisposing factor in causing haemorrhoids.
   (e) Second-degree haemorrhoids cannot be returned to the anal canal.

3. Haematochezia (the passage of gross blood from the rectum) usually indicates lower GI bleeding but may result from which ONE of the following?
   (a) Bleeding from the right colon
   (b) Ingestion of bismuth
   (c) Ingestion of supplemental iron
   (d) Upper GI bleeding with rapid transit of blood through the intestines
   (e) None of the above
4. Which ONE of the following usually causes painless rectal bleeding associated with no other symptoms?
   (a) Anal fissure
   (b) Angiodysplasia
   (c) Colorectal cancer
   (d) Diverticulitis
   (e) Proctitis
5. Which ONE of the following is rectal bleeding more commonly seen in younger adults?
   (a) Angiodysplasia
   (b) Colorectal cancer
   (c) Diverticulitis
   (d) IBD
   (e) Polyps

Answers
1. d; 2. d; 3. d; 4. b; 5. d

KEY POINTS: SUSPECTED CANCER

- Around 40,000 new cases of colorectal cancer are diagnosed each year in the UK.
- The 5-year survival rate is approximately 60%.
- National Institute for Health and Care Excellence (NICE) provides suspected cancer pathway referrals with 'thresholds' depending on age.

WEBSITES

Crohn's and colitis UK
https://www.crohnsandcolitis.org.uk/

CASE 19: UPPER ABDOMINAL PAIN

PRESENTATION

Mr G, a 51-year-old man, presents at lunch time asking for your help concerning a stomach ache he has had since breakfast. He wants to know if you can recommend an antacid or something similar. He expected the pain just to go away on its own, but it has been bothering him all morning.

PROBLEM REPRESENTATION

A 51-year-old man presents with a few hours' history of acute onset abdominal pain.

HYPOTHESIS GENERATION (LIKELY, POSSIBLE AND CRITICAL DIAGNOSES)

Based on the presenting symptoms and his age, the initial list of conditions to consider is relatively long, because not only is abdominal pain associated with the gastrointestinal tract but also can be cardiovascular or musculoskeletal in origin. To refine this list, it is important to establish the exact location of his 'stomach ache' as GI pain is often associated with a particular structure/organ. The patient points to an area above his umbilicus. This now allows you to base your thinking on those conditions affecting the upper abdomen, and initially discount those conditions that are almost exclusively lower abdominal presentations (e.g., diverticulitis, IBD or IBS). We are therefore dealing with:

Likely Diagnoses

- Dyspepsia
- Gastrooesophageal reflux disease (GORD)
- Peptic ulcer

Possible Diagnoses

- Abdominal wall tear
- Biliary colic
- Hepatitis
- Pancreatitis (acute-mild)
- Splenic enlargement

Critical Diagnoses

- Appendicitis
- Atypical angina
- Myocardial infarction
- Perforated ulcer

CONTINUED INFORMATION GATHERING

At present we only have limited information on his symptoms. Knowing more about the specific location, the nature of the pain and associated symptoms should help differentiate between the three likely causes.

He tells you the pain is aching and started an hour or so after breakfast and is now pretty much constant and is localised to an area around his sternum. He reports no other symptoms.

Knowing the location of pain is not very discriminatory as all three of our likely diagnoses present with mid upper abdominal symptoms. However, the fact that he has not described any other symptoms is useful. For example, heartburn is a strong predictor of GORD and in dyspepsia, symptoms other than pain frequently occur, such as bloating, flatulence and nausea.

Therefore, given the predominant symptom is constant pain, which came on sometime after eating, then a differential diagnosis of peptic ulcer is possible, which is further supported because of his age.

Further exploration of his symptoms in relation to it being a possible ulcer is required.

PROBLEM REFINEMENT

Exploring risk factors will help support your differential diagnosis. For example, his lifestyle choices such as smoking, alcohol consumption, dietary choices and stress may be contributing to the symptoms.

He tells you he smokes and has a gin and tonic most nights, but he thinks his diet is pretty good, although like most people he does eat fast food sometimes. It appears he has one or more known risk factors associated for ulcers (smoking and alcohol).

Enquiry into previous symptom history should be asked as one would expect he has suffered similar symptoms in the past if ulcer was the cause. He does say he has been experiencing intermittent symptoms over the last few weeks but has ignored them, just putting it down to food he has eaten. Whilst not confirmatory, this does show this is not the first episode.

A medication history should also be taken as a number of medicines are known risk factors for developing ulcers, most notably NSAIDs, but also bisphosphonates, corticosteroids and SSRIs. However, Mr G is not taking any medicines from his doctor.

Hepatitis, pancreatitis and splenic enlargement present with a range of symptoms other than pain; colic the pain is more severe than reported and an abdominal wall tear would not show a history of similar symptoms. These can be excluded from our thinking.

At this point uncertainty exists to the diagnosis, but an ulcer cannot be ruled out.

⚡ RED FLAGS

Mr G has not reported any 'ALARM' symptoms (anaemia, loss of weight, anorexia, recent onset of progressive symptoms, melaena) so malignancy can be ruled out. As with possible causes, as he has no other symptoms then cardiovascular problems and perforated ulcer are not the cause. Appendicitis cannot be fully ruled out as early presentations can start with centralised pain before moving to the RLQ, although given he has had similar symptoms in the past it does seem unlikely.

MANAGEMENT

Self-care Options

The motivation of Mr G to stop smoking should be assessed as smoking doubles your chances of developing an ulcer. If he is receptive to stopping smoking, then nicotine replacement therapy can be offered. He believes his diet is reasonable but you could provide him literature on healthy eating.

Prescribing Options

You decide to give Mr G a trial of a month's course of a proton pump inhibitor to see if this controls his symptoms.

Safety Netting

You tell Mr G that you are uncertain of the exact cause of his symptoms and would like to try a trial of a proton pump inhibitor and ask him to return in a month to see how he is. If symptoms have not been controlled, then a test to see if he as a stomach infection needs to be done. You also tell him that if his symptoms worsen or the pain moves to below his belly button in the next few hours then he needs to see someone straight away as there is an outside chance that his symptoms may be appendicitis.

AIDE MEMOIRE

Likely Diagnoses

Dyspepsia

Patients with dyspepsia present with a range of symptoms commonly involving, vague abdominal discomfort (aching) above the umbilicus associated with excessive belching, bloating, flatulence, a feeling of fullness. Occasionally nausea and/or vomiting is experienced.

Gastrooesophageal Reflux Disease

Retrosternal heartburn is the classic symptom of GORD but some people experience sensation of food stuck in the throat. Atypical symptoms of GORD include cough and hoarseness.

Peptic Ulcer

Typically, the patient will have well-localised, midepigastric pain described as 'constant', 'annoying' or 'gnawing/boring'. In gastric ulcers, the pain is usually triggered by food (and not relieved by antacids) and experienced shortly after eating. In duodenal ulcers, the pain occurs 2–5 h after meals, which is relieved by food and often awakens a person at night. Gastric ulcers are also more commonly associated with weight loss and GI bleeds than duodenal ulcers. Peak incidence of duodenal ulcers is between 45 and 64 years of age, whereas the incidence of gastric ulcers increases with age.

Possible Diagnoses
Abdominal Wall Tear

Pain, which can be severe, is experienced generally after strenuous activity. Pain is exacerbated when stretching the muscles.

Biliary Colic

Biliary colic classically presents with sudden persistent severe epigastric pain. Pain typically lasts longer than 30 minutes but can last hours but at a lower intensity. Colic often occurs in the evening, especially after eating a heavy meal. In some people, it can awaken them in the early hours of the morning. The pain can radiate to the tip of the right scapula. Nausea and vomiting are common. The incidence increases with increasing age and is most common in people over 40 years of age. It is also more prevalent in women than in men.

Hepatitis

Dull right upper quadrant pain is associated with general malaise, fever, fatigue, nausea, dark urine, pale stools and yellowing of the skin.

Pancreatitis (Acute-Mild)

A mild attack can present with steady epigastric pain that can radiate to the back. Patents generally will have fever, nausea/vomiting with associated abdominal tenderness and elevated heart rate. It is commonly seen in those that misuse alcohol (25% of cases) or suffer from gallstones (50% of cases).

Splenic Enlargement

Often asymptomatic but sometimes causes symptoms such as left upper abdominal pain/discomfort associated with a feeling of fullness without eating or after eating small amounts of food. Anaemia, fever and weight loss may be present.

Critical Diagnoses
Appendicitis

Pain often starts around the umbilicus before moving to the RLQ. The pain of appendicitis is described as colicky or cramp-like but after a few hours becomes constant. Movement tends to aggravate the pain and nausea/vomiting might also be present. It is most common during adolescence.

Atypical Angina

Atypical angina does not manifest with the same symptoms as classical angina. Symptoms associated with atypical angina include fatigue, sweating, belching, nausea/vomiting, rapid breathing and upper abdominal pain.

Myocardial Infarction

Classic symptoms are severe chest pain, which travels from left arm to neck, shortness of breath, sweating, anxiety and nausea/vomiting. However, upper abdominal pain can be the presenting symptom of an acute myocardial infarction.

Perforated Ulcer

A complication of a peptic ulcer is perforation. Symptom presentation of perforation is sudden severe epigastric pain but pain can become more generalised including the RLQ. Nausea/vomiting, light-headedness and lack of appetite may also be present. A previous history of peptic ulcers will be present such as dyspepsia, upper abdominal pain/discomfort. Typically, ulcers affect people aged over 45 years.

Gastric Cancer

Early symptoms of stomach cancer include persistent pain, dyspepsia-like symptoms, loss of appetite and fatigue. As the cancer becomes more advanced other symptoms of unexplained weight loss, dysphagia, vomiting, melaena, anaemia, jaundice is experienced. Typically, ulcers affect people aged over 65 years.

■ MCQs

1. Which ONE of the following is not a risk factor in developing peptic ulcer?
   (a) Alcohol consumption
   (b) Aspirin
   (c) Exercise
   (d) *Helicobacter pylori* infection
   (e) Smoking
2. Which ONE of the following symptoms is least associated with duodenal ulcers?
   (a) Epigastric pain
   (b) Onset 2–3 h after eating
   (c) Pain worse at night
   (d) Pain relieved by eating
   (e) Weight loss
3. Which ONE of the following symptoms associated with epigastric pain would most likely instigate a general practitioner referral?
   (a) A feeling of fullness
   (b) Bloating
   (c) Dysphagia
   (d) Nausea
   (e) Retrosternal pain
4. Which ONE of the following conditions that causes abdominal pain is associated with referred pain?
   (a) Gastritis
   (b) Hepatitis
   (c) Myocardial infarction
   (d) Pancreatitis
   (e) Splenic enlargement

5. Which ONE of the following conditions is the least likely cause of upper abdominal pain?
   (a) Duodenal ulcer
   (b) Dyspepsia
   (c) Gastric ulcer
   (d) Hepatitis
   (e) Renal colic
6. Patients with peptic ulcers are at increased risk of a number of complications. Which ONE of the following is not a complication?
   (a) Haemorrhage
   (b) Pancreatitis
   (c) Perforation
   (d) Peripheral vascular disease
   (e) Short bowel syndrome

Answers

1. c; 2. e; 3. c; 4. c; 5. d; 6. d

KEY POINTS: PEPTIC ULCER

- Caused by a breakdown of the gastric or duodenal mucosa often due to *H. pylori* infection or NSAID use
- Key symptoms are constant epigastric burning or gnawing pain.
- With appropriate treatment ulcers heal in 4–8 weeks.

WEBSITES

GutsUK
https://gutscharity.org.uk/

5

Skin

CASE 20: FACIAL RASH IN A CHILD

PRESENTATION

A father of a 5-year-old boy presents to the pharmacy on a Saturday morning. His son has a rash on his face that came on quickly over the last day or so. His son is at home as he is a bit off-colour. He has not taken his son's temperature.

PROBLEM REPRESENTATION

A 5-year-old boy presents with a 24-h history of acute onset facial rash with malaise.

HYPOTHESIS GENERATION (LIKELY, POSSIBLE AND CRITICAL DIAGNOSES)

Despite not having an empirical measure of temperature, it does sound like the child has mild systemic symptoms. On that basis, it seems reasonable that the most likely causes to consider would be those of infective origin that can affect the face.

Likely Diagnoses

- Chicken pox
- Cold sore (herpes simplex)
- Erysipelas
- Erythema infectiosum
- Impetigo

Possible Diagnoses

- Atopic dermatitis
- Angular cheilitis (usually elderly)
- Contact dermatitis
- Hand, foot and mouth disease
- Insect bites
- Molluscum contagiosum
- Pityriasis alba

Critical Diagnoses

- German measles (rubella)
- Measles

CONTINUED INFORMATION GATHERING

Normally, a visual inspection of the rash would be performed but as his son is at home we will have to rely on the parent's description. You ask him to describe where on the face the rash is and what it looks like.

He tells you that the rash is concentrated around his son's nose and looks red and angry and seems to be weeping a little (Fig. 5.1).

The location of the rash most closely fits with impetigo; erysipelas and erythema infectiosum affect the cheeks – erysipelas has a characteristic butterfly distribution on the cheeks and erythema infectiosum is also known as 'slapped cheek disease'; chicken pox lesions are widespread and not localised; and cold sores are usually confined to the lips.

The nature of the rash also seems a best fit for impetigo. Erysipelas and erythema infectiosum have maculopapular rash and chicken pox and cold sores are vesicular.

PROBLEM REFINEMENT

Impetigo tends to itch and so you ask if he knows if his son's rash itches. He tells you his son has been scratching. This suggests the rash is itchy, which is consistent with impetigo and further rules out erysipelas.

His son seems to have mild constitutional symptoms, which although unusual in impetigo, are not unknown.

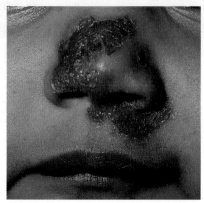

Fig. 5.1 Impetigo Contagiosa. (Source: Weston, W. L., Lane, A. T., & Morelli, J. G. (2007). *Color textbook of pediatric dermatology* (4th ed.). St. Louis, MO: Mosby.)

However, one would expect more marked constitutional or prodromal symptoms with chicken pox, erysipelas and erythema infectiosum. With cold sores, there is also some warning before lesion eruption, although this may be difficult to determine from the parent.

Based on location, look of the lesion, presence of itch and mild constitutional symptoms you are now confident that his son has impetigo despite him not being present.

> ⚡ **RED FLAGS**
>
> Measles and German measles show prodromal symptoms, which our patient has not exhibited. You could check the vaccination status of the child.

MANAGEMENT

Self-care Options

As impetigo is infectious, you give general advice on hygiene:
- Avoid sharing towels
- Regular hand washing

Prescribing Options

It seems he has relatively localised lesions, and so topical fusidic acid or mupirocin three times a day for 5 days would seem appropriate. Alternatively, hydrogen peroxide cream could be tried.

Safety Netting

You tell the parent his son has impetigo and emphasise the self-care measures due to its infectious nature. His son should be kept away from school until lesions are healed,

dry and crusted over or until 48 h after starting treatment. You tell him his son needs antibiotics but if his rash has not cleared up after 5 days use then he needs to bring him in to be looked at. Further treatment might be necessary, for example, systemic antibiotics (e.g., flucloxacillin).

AIDE MEMOIRE

Likely Diagnoses
Chicken Pox

Before the rash develops, the patient might experience up to 3 days of prodromal symptoms that could include fever, headache, and sore throat. The rash typically begins on the face, stomach and back before spreading to other parts of the body. Initially, lesions appear as small red lumps that rapidly develop into vesicles, which crust over after 3 to 5 days. New lesions tend to occur in crops for the first 4 days, so at the height of infectivity lesions appear in all stages of development. The vesicles are often extremely itchy. Chicken pox is highly contagious, from a few days before the onset of rash until all lesions have crusted over.

Cold Sore (Herpes Simplex)

Prodromal symptoms of itching, burning, pain or tingling symptoms typically occur from 6 to 48 h before lesion eruption. They appear as blisters and vesicles with associated redness on the vermillion border of the lip (Fig. 5.2 and Fig. 5.3). These crust over, usually within 24 h, tend to be itchy and painful and might bleed. Lesions spontaneously resolve in 7–10 days. Many patients can

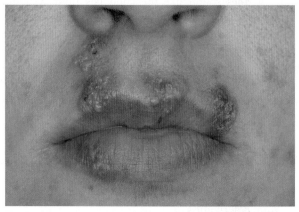

Fig. 5.2 Recurrent Herpes Labialis (Cold Sore) Due to Reactivation of Herpes simplex virus type 1 (HSV-1). (Source: Marsh, P.D., Lewis, M.A.O., Williams, D., & Martin, M.V. (2009). *Oral microbiology* (5th ed.). Churchill Livingstone.)

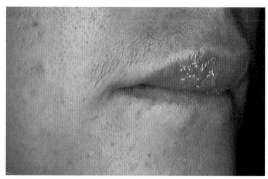

Fig. 5.3 Herpes Simplex (Cold Sores). These begin with tingling skin and sensitivity, and they erupt with tight vesicles, then pustules, and then a crust. Lesions commonly appear on the upper lip. (Source: Hurwitz, S. (1993). *Clinical pediatric dermatology: A textbook of skin disorders of childhood and adolescence* (2nd ed.). Philadelphia: Saunders.)

identify a trigger, with UV light reported to induce cold sores in 20% of sufferers. Recurrence is common and lesions tend to occur in the same location.

Erysipelas

Usually abrupt in onset and often accompanied by fevers, chills, and shivering. It predominantly affects the lower limbs, but when it involves the face, it can have a characteristic butterfly distribution on the cheeks and across the bridge of the nose (Fig. 5.4). The affected skin has a very sharp, raised border. It is bright red, firm and swollen. It may be finely dimpled (like an orange skin).

Erythema Infectiosum

Erythema infectiosum is also called 'slapped cheek disease' or 'fifth disease'. It predominantly affects children between the ages of 3 and 15 years. Cold-like symptoms appear a couple of days before the rash appears. Typically, the rash appears on the cheeks and presents as red and inflamed marks (like the person has been slapped) (Fig. 5.5). Itch is often present, and the rash can spread to the arms and legs.

Impetigo

Impetigo is a superficial, highly contagious bacterial skin infection affecting the superficial layers of the epidermis. There are two clinical forms; a non-bullous form accounting for about 70% of cases, and a bullous form. The non-bullous form is mostly located on the face or extremities. It tends to start with a single red macule that develops in to a pustule or vesicle, which then ruptures releasing exudate that dries and crusts over in to a characteristic honey colour. It can spread rapidly usually as a result of autoinoculation. Lesions may be mildly itchy. The bullous form presents similarly

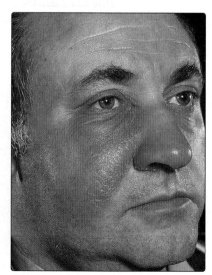

Fig. 5.4 Erysipelas of the Right Cheek Due to a Streptococcal Infection. (Source: Gawkrodger, D. (2017). *Dermatology: An illustrated colour text* (6th ed.). Elsevier.)

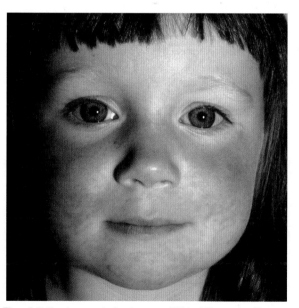

Fig. 5.5 Erythema Infectiosum (Fifth Disease). (Source: Habif, T. P. (2016). *Clinical dermatology: A color guide to diagnosis and therapy* (6th ed.). St. Louis, MO: Mosby.)

except that bullae (1-2 cm in diameter) are present, are often more widespread and systemic symptoms of malaise, fever, and lymphadenopathy are often present.

Possible Diagnoses
Atopic Dermatitis
Atopic dermatitis is common in children, typically presenting in infancy and early childhood and may persist into adulthood. Lesion distribution varies based on age. Infants and younger children often have lesions on the extensor surfaces of extremities, cheeks and scalp. Older children and adults often present with patches and plaques on the flexor surfaces (antecubital and popliteal fossa). Lesions are red and dry, and itch is a prominent feature. Personal and family history of atopy is usual.

Angular Cheilitis
Commonly both angles of the mouth are affected. Redness, fissuring, and soreness are typical (Fig. 5.6). It can be painful and occasionally bleed. Most often seen in older people.

Contact Dermatitis
A variety of morphological presentations – causing redness, dryness and lichenification–can be seen that are associated with itch. Irritant and allergic forms develop following exposure to an allergen/irritant.

Hand, Foot and Mouth Disease
Prodromal symptoms of fever, malaise, loss of appetite and possibly sore throat can be seen a day or two before lesions appear. Greyish blisters appear on the sides of the fingers, hands and feet. Small blisters can develop in and around the lips and mouth. These can be painful.

Insect Bites
Typically, papular urticaria is experienced after being bitten. Crops of very itchy red papules and vesicles of variable size are observed. Systemic symptoms are not present.

Molluscum Contagiosum
Most commonly affects children. It is usually asymptomatic. The lesions are small flesh-coloured or pearly white, small papules with a central punctum that is diagnostic (Fig. 5.7). Typically, they appear in crops of fewer than 20 lesions. The most common locations are on the face, chest, armpit, upper legs and genital area.

Pityriasis Alba
Most commonly seen in children and young adults. The rash can be mildly itchy and appears as pink/pale, scaly, poorly-defined or irregular patches which fade to leave pale areas on the skin (Fig. 5.8). The face is commonly affected but the rash can be seen on the body, arms and legs. These pale areas are more noticeable in people with skin of colour, and more pronounced after exposure to the sun. It often goes unnoticed when it first starts, but it is the loss of pigment that triggers people to seek medical advice.

Critical Diagnoses
German Measles (Rubella)
Prodromal symptoms of fever, malaise, sore throat, runny nose and mucosal petechiae are noticed before the rash begins on the face and spreads to the neck,

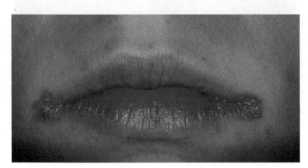

Fig. 5.6 Angular Cheilitis. (Source: Ibsen, O. A. C., & Phelan, J. A. (2023). *Oral pathology for the dental hygienist: With general pathology introductions* (8th ed.). Saunders.)

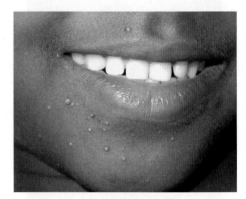

Fig. 5.7 Molluscum Contagiosum. Skin-coloured papules distributed on the face. (Source: Halpern-Felsher, B. (Ed.). (2023). *Encyclopedia of child and adolescent health* (1st ed.). Academic Press.)

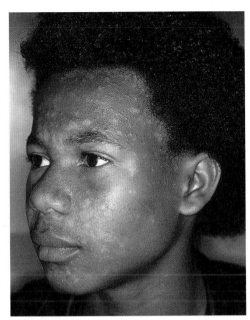

Fig. 5.8 Pityriasis Alba, Demonstrating Hypopigmented Macules of the Face. (Courtesy, James E. Fitzpatrick, MD.)

trunk and extremities. Tender or swollen glands almost always accompany rubella, most commonly behind the ears and at the back of the neck.

Measles

Prior to rash, prodromal symptoms of fever, malaise, conjunctivitis, cough and coryza are experienced followed by the appearance of Koplik's spots. A maculopapular rash then starts on the face and behind the ears before moving on to the trunk and extremities.

MCQs

1. The mother of a 2-year-old toddler seeks your advice about her son. He has had a recent fall off his scooter, leaving him with a couple cuts and grazes across his knee and face. However, the cuts and grazes around his face and chin appear to be weeping a yellow colour. Which ONE of the following is the most likely diagnosis?
   (a) Angular cheilitis
   (b) Chicken pox
   (c) Hand, foot and mouth disease
   (d) Nonbullous impetigo
   (e) Scarlet fever

2. The mother of a 6-year-old child tells you her son has a rash on his upper trunk that appeared about 5 days ago, which has now spread to his face and limbs. His mother further explains he is scratching the rash a lot, especially at night. You find out he experienced general cold-like symptoms prior to the rash appearing. Which ONE of the following is the most likely cause of these symptoms?
   (a) Chickenpox
   (b) Impetigo
   (c) Measles
   (d) Rubella
   (e) Urticaria

3. A mother of a 3-year-old toddler asks for your advice. She says he has had a high temperature for the last 3 days, and she has noticed a rash on his upper trunk. She also says she has noticed numerous tiny little spots on the inside of the mouth and tongue. Which ONE of the following is the most likely cause of these symptoms?
   (a) Chicken pox
   (b) Measles
   (c) Mumps
   (d) Rubella
   (e) Scarlet fever

4. A mother of a 5-year-old daughter wants some advice. Her daughter has developed a rash on her face. Based solely on this information, which ONE is the most likely condition causing the rash?
   (a) Atopic dermatitis
   (b) Erythema infectiosum
   (c) Pertussis
   (d) Pityriasis rosea
   (e) Psoriasis

5. The mother of a 6-year-old son asks for some cream to get rid of a rash on his face. The lesions are randomly distributed over his face, nonitchy and are raised. Based solely on this information, which ONE of the following is the most likely cause of the rash?
   (a) Chicken pox
   (b) Hand, foot and mouth disease
   (c) Molluscum contagiosum
   (d) Nonbullous impetigo
   (e) Scarlet fever

Answers

1. d; 2. a; 3. b; 4. b; 5. c

KEY POINTS: IMPETIGO

- *Staphylococcus aureus* and/or *Streptococcus pyogenes* bacterial infection
- Key symptoms are localised rash that exhibits honey-yellow crusting.
- Resolution in 5–10 days with antibiotic treatment

CASE 21: GENERALISED PRURITUS

PRESENTATION

Mrs J, a 71-year-old woman who is well known to you, asks for your advice. She has been bothered with generalised itchy skin for the last 2–3 months, which is causing sleeping difficulties. She says the itching started about the same time as when they came back from an extended winter break in Spain. She takes atorvastatin for hyperlipidaemia and seems to have a residual tan from her holidays.

PROBLEM REPRESENTATION

A 71-year-old woman presents with a 3-month history of generalised itching interfering with sleep.

HYPOTHESIS GENERATION (LIKELY, POSSIBLE AND CRITICAL DIAGNOSES)

Generalised itching is a common presentation and can be debilitating, affecting quality of life. Where skin lesions are absent, generalised itch is often caused by dry skin, although in up to 50% of patients, no identifiable cause can be found. It can also indicate an underlying internal cause. Internal causes are many, and may stem from a metabolic or haematologic cause, endocrine dysfunction or certain forms of cancer. In the elderly population, dry skin is a common cause of pruritus, especially in the winter and should be prominent in your thinking as to the cause of Mrs J's symptoms. However, her age and change in skin pigmentation should raise suspicions for an underlying systemic condition.

Likely Diagnosis

- Dry skin (xerosis)

Possible Diagnoses

- Aquagenic pruritus
- Diabetes

- Haematologic disorders
  - Iron deficiency
  - Polycythaemia vera
- Infection
- Liver disease
- Medicines
- Neurologic (e.g., multiple sclerosis)
- Pregnancy (not applicable)
- Psychological (e.g., anxiety/depression)
  - Scabies
- Sjögren's syndrome
- Thyroid dysfunction

Critical Diagnoses

- Malignancy
- Renal failure

CONTINUED INFORMATION GATHERING

At this point, you examine the skin to confirm the absence of any lesions and to assess skin integrity. You find no visible lesions and the skin, in places, shows superficial scaling thus supporting dry skin as the cause of Mrs J's itching.

She has been on an extended holiday (but only) to Spain. Infections causing pruritus are mostly associated with low- and middle-income countries, implying this is not the cause. She does take a statin – a known group of medicines that can cause itching. You check her medical and drug history. The atorvastatin was prescribed 2 years ago and there have been no recent dose changes, suggesting this also is not the cause of her itching.

You ask if any particular part of the body seems more affected. Mrs J reiterates that the itch is widespread. This finding points away from liver disease where itch is often worse on the palms and soles. With regard to liver disease, you also note no yellowing of the sclera or jaundice. You also ask if the itching is worse after contact with water to check for aquagenic pruritus or polycthaemia vera. Mrs J says she has not noticed her symptoms being made worse by water.

Itching associated with dry skin still seems likely but other conditions still need to be considered.

Problem Refinement

At this point you ask about any constitutional symptoms she may have noticed such as weight changes, fatigue, night sweats, temperature intolerances and polyuria or polydipsia, as this might point to thyroid dysfunction, diabetes, Sjögren's syndrome, renal disease or malignancy.

Mrs J says she is tired all the time but has put that down to her poor sleep recently. Almost all systemic causes (except Sjögren's syndrome) can show fatigue and this does not help much in establishing the cause.

Finally, you ask about her general well-being and personal life to look for any changes in mood or disproportionate worry that might suggest a psychological cause of itch. She reports nothing untoward.

The diagnosis still seems to point to dry skin as the cause but her symptom of tiredness could be a sign of underlying systemic illness and requires further investigation.

⚡ RED FLAGS

Mrs. J shows no unexplained weight loss (cancer or renal failure) or neurological deficit (multiple sclerosis).

MANAGEMENT

Self-care Options

First, strategies to keep the skin from drying out should be tried. Mrs J should minimise her time in the shower or bath, and apply moisturising creams immediately after. Irritants, if known, should be avoided.

Prescribing Options

Emollients should be prescribed to help the itching. A full blood count and measurement of thyroid-stimulating hormone, fasting glucose, alkaline phosphatase, bilirubin, creatinine and blood urea nitrogen undertaken to check for a systemic cause.

Safety Netting

You tell Mrs J that you believe her dry skin is part of the natural ageing process. You tell her that the emollient creams should control her symptoms but you will run some tests to make sure that nothing else is the matter. You say that if these tests come back normal, and her skin is still itching in a couple of weeks, then an antihistamine could be tried.

AIDE MEMOIRE

Likely Diagnosis
Dry skin (xerosis)

Signs and symptoms of dry skin will vary between individuals but are characterised by abnormally dry, itchy and scaly skin. The skin can feel tight and uncomfortable. In moderate/severe cases, the skin can crack and fissure. It can exhibit seasonality and is often worse in the winter.

Possible Diagnoses
Aquagenic Pruritus

Patients complain of an intense pricking itch on contact with water or change of skin temperature, but do not develop a rash. The thighs and upper arms are most commonly affected. It is more common in middle-aged women.

Diabetes

Generalised pruritus is a rare symptom that occurs at the onset of diabetes.

Haematologic Disorders

Iron deficiency. Symptoms experienced are associated with the speed at which anaemia develops. Most commonly, patients show fatigue, dyspnoea, headache and restless leg syndrome. Less commonly, symptoms include heart palpitations, tinnitus, hair loss and generalised itchiness.

Polycythaemia Vera. In approximately 20%–50% of patients, itch is precipitated by taking a hot bath or shower. This can be used as a 'provocative test'. Other symptoms such as headache, dizziness, fatigue, sweating more than usual, blurred vision and dyspnoea predominate. It is more common in older age groups.

Infection

A number of infective causes can present with generalised pruritus as their initial presentation and include hepatitis C, HIV/AIDs and some local/endemic infections such as Chikungunya fever and river blindness. Substance misuse or sexual history might implicate HIV or hepatitis C infection, and foreign travel for endemic infections.

Liver Disease

Pruritus is a common symptom in several forms of liver disease, although itch is usually secondary to cholestasis. When itch is present, it can be generalised, but is typically worse on the palms and soles. Therefore, other signs of liver disease need to be looked for such as jaundice, dark urine, pale faeces, fatigue, spider naevi and nausea.

Medicines

Many medicines can cause itch. Commonly implicated medicines are opioids and antibiotics. Other classes of medicines include angiotensin-converting enzyme (ACE) inhibitors, calcium channel blockers, Selective serotonin reuptake inhibitors (SSRIs), antiepileptics, biologics, statins and chloroquine.

Neurologic (e.g., Multiple Sclerosis)

Multiple sclerosis typically presents before the age of 50 years but diagnosis is challenging due to variable presentation. Symptoms include eye pain accompanied with partial or unilateral vision loss, paraesthesia, muscle weakness, urinary symptoms, cognitive dysfunction, mobility problems and fatigue. Pruritus has been reported but is unusual.

Pregnancy

Pruritus is seen in the last trimester and disappears 2–3 days postpartum. Most women will have an obvious associated cholestatic jaundice. If jaundice is not present, then liver alkaline phosphatase enzymes will be raised.

Psychological (e.g., Anxiety/Depression)

Some patients describe an intense urge to scratch or pick at the skin, without an associated skin disease or other underlying cause – known as functional itch disorder. This has been associated with mental health disorders and worsening stress.

Scabies

Skin lesions can be minimal or absent but present with generalised severe itch.

Sjögren's Syndrome

The two main symptoms are dry eyes and mouth but other symptoms such as joint pain, cough, fatigue, vaginal dryness and dry skin leading to pruritus can be experienced. It is more common in women and those aged over 40 years.

Thyroid Dysfunction

Pruritus is a rare manifestation and of little diagnostic value. Unexplained weight changes, heat/cold, sleep issues and gastrointestinal disturbances are common presentations.

Critical Diagnoses
Malignancy (e.g., Lymphoma, Leukaemia, Multiple Myeloma)

Lymphoma is most strongly associated with pruritus affecting up to 30% of patients. Unexplained weight loss, night sweats, unexplained fevers, fatigue or lymphadenopathy can be experienced but pruritus notoriously predates other symptoms by months. Lymphoma, although more common in older people, is one of the cancers seen in younger adults.

Renal Failure

Pruritus can be an early feature of renal failure although few patients present this way. Lethargy, night-time cramps, weight loss, urine output changes and gastrointestinal disturbances are seen. In time, more than 50% of patients with chronic renal disease, and up to 80% of patients on dialysis, have pruritus.

█ MCQs

1. Which ONE of the following statements regarding primary biliary cirrhosis is true?
   (a) It is rarely asymptomatic.
   (b) Pruritus is always generalised.
   (c) Pruritus is the commonest symptom.
   (d) Pruritus is thought to be caused by an accumulation of bile acids in the skin.
   (e) Transaminases are highly elevated.

2. Which ONE of the following is not a typical symptom of kidney failure?
   (a) Hallucinations
   (b) Insomnia
   (c) Itching
   (d) Nausea
   (e) Restless legs

3. A 56-year-old woman presents with skin itching, sweating, weight loss and fatigue. Which ONE of the following conditions is most likely?
   (a) Hyperthyroidism
   (b) Hypothyroidism
   (c) Leukaemia
   (d) Opioid adverse reaction
   (e) Renal failure

4. A 34-year-old woman is experiencing generalised itch. Based on age and sex, which ONE of the following conditions is most likely?
   (a) Aquagenic pruritus
   (b) Liver disease
   (c) Polycythaemia vera
   (d) Sjögren's syndrome
   (e) Thyroid disease

5. Itch associated with lymphoma is thought to be caused by which ONE of the following?
   (a) Cytokines irritating nerve endings
   (b) Decreased platelets
   (c) Inability to metabolise phosphates
   (d) Purine build up in the blood
   (e) Renal failure

Answers

1. d; 2. a; 3. a; 4. e; 5. a

KEY POINTS: AGE-RELATED DRY SKIN

- Caused by abnormality of the barrier function of the skin
- Key symptoms are itching skin with a rough or scaly texture often on the lower legs.
- Mainstay of treatment are emollients

CASE 22: HAIR LOSS

PRESENTATION

Mrs J, a 27-year-old woman, presents to you complaining of hair loss. She says she has noticed her hair falling out more than usual over the last 4–6 weeks and big clumps of hair are left in the shower. She is visibly upset.

PROBLEM REPRESENTATION

A 27-year-old woman presents with a 6-week history of noticeable hair loss.

HYPOTHESIS GENERATION (LIKELY, POSSIBLE AND CRITICAL DIAGNOSES)

Most causes of hair loss are associated with the hair growth cycle, which consists of three stages: anagen, catagen and telogen. In the anagen stage, the cells in the hair bulb divide rapidly creating new hair growth. The catagen stage is a transitional short phase, where a hair stops growing and detaches itself from the blood supply and is termed a club hair. The final, telogen stage, begins with a resting period, where a club hair rests in the root whilst new hair begins to grow beneath it. After this time, the resting club hairs fall out to allow a new hair to grow. Hair loss is therefore due to a decrease in hair growth (anagen hair loss) or an increase in hair shedding (telogen hair loss), as well as conversion of thick terminal hairs to thin vellus hairs (androgenetic alopecia). The features of hair loss depend on the cause. Androgenetic alopecia is the commonest cause of hair loss in both men and women. It affects more people the older they are, and in women of Mrs J's age, only a small proportion will have hair loss associated with an androgenetic cause. Therefore, other causes need to be equally considered.

Likely Diagnoses

- Anagen effluvium
  - Alopecia areata
  - Medicine-induced
- Androgenetic alopecia (male and female pattern hair loss)
- Telogen effluvium

Possible Diagnoses

- Inflammatory skin diseases
  - Lichen planopilaris
  - Folliculitis decalvans
- Systemic disease
  - Iron deficiency
  - Lupus erythematosus
  - Secondary syphilis
  - Thyroid dysfunction
- Tinea capitis
- Traction alopecia

Critical Diagnosis

- Trichotillomania

CONTINUED INFORMATION GATHERING

An assessment of hair loss with regards to severity and location is needed; is it limited to specific regions (patterned), presence of bald patches (patchy) or effecting the whole scalp (diffuse). Taking a medical and family history is also necessary.

Mrs J reiterates that she is seeing more and more hair falling out – she says her hairbrush is full of hair – something that did not use to happen. She does not describe any specific bald patches. Your observations are that she seems to have a full head of hair. She tells you she takes the contraceptive pill (last 5 years) and her father is quite bald (he is 61 years old). Given there is no visible hair loss, either patchy or diffuse, this seems to rule out female pattern baldness and alopecia areata, which are associated with obvious marked hair loss. Whilst hormonal medicines can cause hair loss this seems unlikely in this case. At this point telogen effluvium seems more likely.

PROBLEM REFINEMENT

Further exploration of her personal history is required. If an event triggered her hair loss, this will have occurred a number of months before hair loss was observed. Questioning around any events a few months prior to Mrs J noticing hair loss does not reveal any obvious causes.

It appears there is no identifiable cause for her perceived hair loss. At this point, the diagnosis still points towards telogen effluvium. A hair pull test could be performed to help confirm your thinking (see Box 5.1).

You perform this test and find it to be positive (e.g., >10% of hair pulls away). At this point you believe telogen effluvium is the likely cause. Checks to rule out possible causes need to be made by asking about other symptoms experienced. Mrs J reports no other scalp problems and denies any skin rashes or systemic symptoms. This seems to rule out inflammatory skin conditions and tinea and systemic causes.

⚡ RED FLAGS

Hair loss seems diffuse and there are no signs of asymmetrical hair loss as seen in trichotillomania.

MANAGEMENT

Self-care Options

Mrs J should be reassured that regrowth usually occurs. She should try and handle her hair gently, and avoid vigorous combing and brushing.

Prescribing Options

No medication is currently warranted.

Safety Netting

You tell her that you cannot determine any specific cause for her hair loss, and some blood tests might help see if there are any reasons for the hair loss. You tell her you will check for anaemia and thyroid function. If blood results are normal, it would be worth reassessing Mrs J's hair loss in 4–6 weeks. If anaemia or thyroid dysfunction has been identified, then follow upblood tests should be instigated; 4 weeks for haemoglobin levels and 6 weeks for thyroid-stimulating hormone levels.

AIDE MEMOIRE

Likely Diagnoses
Anagen Effluvium

Alopecia areata. It is associated with autoimmune conditions, such as vitiligo, diabetes, thyroid disease, rheumatoid arthritis and discoid lupus erythematosus. It affects men and women equally, and, although it can occur at any age, the most common presentation is in children and young adults. It is characterised by sudden onset nonscarring hair loss, which ranges from a single oval patch to multiple patches that can become confluent. It often results in unpredictable hair loss. In most cases, hair falls out in a few small patches, but occasionally it can present with diffuse widespread thinning and shedding (alopecia totalis). The classic finding is a smooth, hairless patch surrounded by so-called exclamation point hairs (short broken hairs which taper proximally) that may be seen around the margin, or in any part of the patch. The hair may regrow partially or completely in 80% of initial episodes.

Medicine-induced hair loss. Acute hair shedding leading to diffuse alopecia is a typical side effect of cancer chemotherapy and scalp radiation. Hair loss is acute and severe and may produce loss of most of the scalp hair, eyebrows and eyelashes.

Androgenetic Alopecia

This is the most common type of progressive hair loss. It is caused by a combination of genetic and hormonal factors; dihydrotestosterone is the main hormone responsible for androgenetic alopecia in genetically susceptible individuals. Dihydrotestosterone induces a change in the hair follicles on the scalp; they become thinner, shorter and lighter, until the follicles shrink completely and stop producing hair. Onset can be at any age following puberty and increases with age but typically affects a higher proportion of men and from a younger age than women. In men, the frontal hairline is thinner; hair loss occurs at the crown of the scalp and hair recession is seen at the temporal aspects of the scalp. In women, hair loss primarily occurs at the crown with the frontal hairline is preserved.

Telogen Effluvium

Excessive shedding results from a large number of hair follicles moving into the resting phase (telogen). It most often presents in women with plenty of hair. They often describe hair coming out in handfuls with an increased number of hairs in their hairbrush or shower, and sometimes thinning of the hair in the scalp. On examination, a positive hair pull test should be noted but no bald patches should be seen as acute telogen effluvium does not usually produce visible alopecia.

In many cases, the shedding is preceded 2–6 months earlier by an 'event' such as childbirth, weight loss, fever, injury or stressful event. The time, and therefore the event when hair shedding started, is usually remembered well by patients. Underlying medical conditions (e.g., hyperthyroidism and hypothyroidism) and medicines (e.g., hormones (contraceptives), anticonvulsants, anticoagulants, beta-blockers, ACE inhibitors and lithium) are often implicated.

Possible Diagnoses

Inflammatory Skin Diseases

Folliculitis decalvans. It is a rare cause of hair loss often around the crown. It usually affects middle-aged men. Besides hair loss, it may cause mild itch, discomfort or pain. It is also known as tufted folliculitis because of the 'toothbrush' appearance in longstanding cases, where multiple hair shafts emerge from a single hair follicle (Fig. 5.9).

Lichen planopilaris. This is also rare. It usually affects young adult women and typically presents as smooth white multiple patches of hair loss that can merge to form large irregular patches (Fig. 5.10). Itch, discomfort and pain may also be present.

Systemic disease

Iron deficiency. This is the most common form of anaemia. It presents with a wide range of signs and symptoms. The most common are dyspnoea, fatigue, headache, pallor, dry skin and hair loss.

Systemic lupus erythematosus. It presents with a wide range of symptoms that vary from person to person. Symptoms often flare up and remit. The most common symptoms are extreme fatigue, fever, joint pain and skin lesions (often a butterfly-shaped rash on the face that covers the cheeks and bridge of the nose). It can also cause

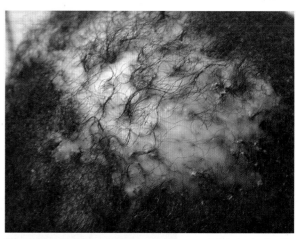

Fig. 5.9 Folliculitis Decalvans. (Source: Micheletti, R. G., James, W. D., Elston, D. M., & McMahon, P. J. (2023). *Andrews' diseases of the skin clinical atlas* (2nd ed.). Elsevier.)

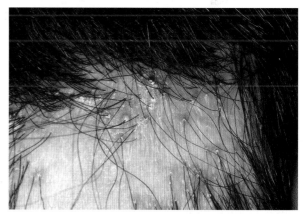

Fig. 5.10 Lichen Planopilaris. (Source: James, W. D., Elston, D. M., & McMahon, P. J. (2018). *Andrews' diseases of the skin clinical atlas.* Elsevier.)

hair loss. Hair loss may be an early sign of lupus; there are two forms of alopecia – a scarring form that causes permanent hair loss and nonscarring form that tends to show gradual hair thinning, especially on the hair line, and is not permanent.

Secondary syphilis. This is a generalised infection that presents with systemic and cutaneous symptoms, which over time resolve spontaneously. Patchy hair loss is one manifestation of cutaneous symptoms.

Thyroid dysfunction. Thyroid dysfunction, especially hypothyroidism can produce hair loss. Other symptoms are prominent and include fatigue, cold intolerance, weight gain, impaired concentration and dry skin.

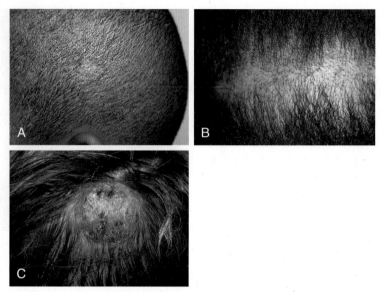

Fig. 5.11 Tinea Capitis. (A) Seborrheic pattern. (B) Black-dot pattern. (C) Kerion presenting as a tender boggy mass in the scalp. (Source: High, W. A., & Prok, L. D. (Eds.). (2021). *Dermatology secrets* (6th ed.). Elsevier.)

Tinea Capitis

The first signs of infection are the appearance of a well-circumscribed round patch of alopecia that is associated with itch and scaling. Common areas of involvement include the occipital, parietal and crown regions. Inspection of the area might reveal erythema and 'black dots' on the scalp as a result of broken off hair stubs (Fig. 5.11). Children are most likely to be affected.

Traction Alopecia

This is a form of unintentional hair loss associated with specific social, cultural and cosmetic practices. Patients (primarily women) wearing wigs, tight braids or using curling rollers are at risk (Fig. 5.12). Hair loss usually occurs in the frontotemporal area. It is reversible if the tension on the hair is removed.

Critical Diagnosis
Trichotillomania

This is a psychiatric disorder that refers to patients who have an impulsive desire to twist and pull scalp hair, but often deny it. Hair loss is patchy, and scarring may be present. Patients present with uneven broken hairs in the most frequently pulled areas.

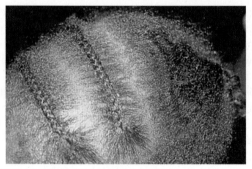

Fig. 5.12 Traction Alopecia. (Source: Cohen, B. A. (2013). *Atlas of pediatric dermatology* (4th ed.). Elsevier Limited.)

MCQs

1. A 45-year-old female patient with a past medical history of hypothyroidism presents to your clinic complaining of hair loss. The patient states the hair loss started 2 weeks ago. The hair loss is described as diffuse. A hair pull test is performed from different parts of the scalp and is positive. A closer look at the hairs shows a dark bulb at the bottom. Which ONE of the following is the most likely type of alopecia in this patient?
   (a) Alopecia areata
   (b) Anagen effluvium
   (c) Female pattern hair loss
   (d) Telogen effluvium
   (e) None of the above

2. What proportion of a person's hair is in the telogen phase at any given time?
   (a) About 10%
   (b) About 20%
   (c) About 30%
   (d) About 40%
   (e) More than 50%
3. Scalp hairs have a finite life cycle. Under normal conditions, how long do scalp hairs survive?
   (a) Less than 6 months
   (b) 1 year
   (c) 2 years
   (d) 3 years
   (e) Approximately 5 years
4. Hair loss in men is extremely common, although it is more common in White men than Black men. Which ONE of the following is the approximate proportion of White men that will have hair loss by the time they are 30 years old?
   (a) 20%
   (b) 30%
   (c) 40%
   (d) 50%
   (e) >50%
5. Many medicines are implicated in causing hair loss. Which ONE of the following is most likely to cause hair loss?
   (a) Ibuprofen
   (b) Clopidogrel
   (c) Dabigatran
   (d) Omeprazole
   (e) Ramipril

Answers

1. d; 2. a; 3. d; 4. b; 5. d

KEY POINTS: TELOGEN EFFLUVIUM

- Temporary hair loss due to a 'shock' causing resting hair to fall out
- Key symptom is diffuse hair loss.
- Regrowth usually occurs on removal of the trigger.

WEBSITES

Alopecia UK
https://www.alopecia.org.uk/
The British hair and nail society
https://bhns.org.uk/

CASE 23: ITCHY RASH ON THE HAND

PRESENTATION

Mr RS, a Caucasian man in his late 20s/early 30s, presents late on Friday afternoon. He complains of bothersome itchy skin and a rash he has had on his hand for the last few days.

PROBLEM REPRESENTATION

An adult man presents with acute onset rash on the hand with associated itching.

HYPOTHESIS GENERATION (LIKELY, POSSIBLE AND CRITICAL DIAGNOSES)

For our patient, the conditions to consider in the first instance, based on his age and those that predominantly affect the hands, are:

Likely Diagnoses

- Dermatitis
- Insect bites
- Pompholyx (dyshidrotic eczema)
- Scabies

Possible Diagnoses

- Bullous pemphigoid
- Hand, foot and mouth disease
- Keratolysis exfoliativa
- Lichen planus
- Palmoplantar psoriasis
- Tinea manuum

Critical Diagnosis

- Not applicable

CONTINUED INFORMATION GATHERING

We need to ask further questions about the rash, specifically questions exploring the look and distribution of rash and intensity of itch.

Mr RS tells you the rash itches a lot, but he has not noticed the rash elsewhere. Examination reveals redness to the hand, especially between the fingers. (Fig. 5.13). The skin appears dry and rough and appears to have been scratched, which is confirmed by the patient.

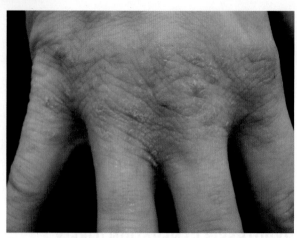

Fig. 5.13 Scabies (Hand). (Source: Marcdante, K., & Kliegman, R. M. (2019). *Nelson essentials of pediatrics* (8th ed.). Elsevier.)

At this stage, all likely conditions being considered can present with such symptoms, although insect bites tend to show more obvious papules and vesicles.

To explore if dermatitis is the cause, knowing if Mr RS has a positive previous personal history of rash or if the rash appeared as a specific result of exposure would be useful.

He tells you this is the first time he has experienced such symptoms on his hand and cannot remember handling or using anything different recently either at work, which is as an National Health Service patient transport officer, or at home. He also says he cannot recall any similar rashes elsewhere away from his hands.

These answers point away from dermatitis. It also seems unlikely insect bites are to blame as he has already said he cannot remember any event that he associates with the start of the rash. Additionally, insect bites are not usually associated with redness in between fingers.

PROBLEM REFINEMENT

Questions around the severity and timing of the itch would be useful to see if his symptoms are due to scabies or pompholyx – both have intense itching, but itch associated with scabies is usually more pronounced at night. He says it is really itchy and it has been difficult to sleep properly because of the itching.

A check on family members or close contacts showing similar symptoms should be explored due to scabies being infectious. He tells you he lives on his own and does not know if any of friends have similar symptoms.

However, as he is an National Health Service worker involved in patient transport, it is plausible that this is how he may have caught scabies through occupational exposure.

Based on all findings, it appears that the differential diagnosis is now leaning towards scabies. Confirmation of the diagnosis through microscopy of skin scrapings could be performed but normally the diagnosis is made on clinical findings alone.

Prior to any actions being taken, it is worth considering if his symptoms could be attributed to any of the possible causes. These can be discounted on age (pemphigoid; hand, foot and mouth disease; lichen planus), intensity of itch (keratolysis exfoliative, lichen planus) or rash involvement elsewhere (palmoplantar psoriasis, tinea manuum).

⚡ RED FLAGS

Not applicable.

MANAGEMENT

Self-care Options

You tell Mr RS that all his bedding, clothing and towels need to be washed on high temperatures as they may harbour the scabies mite. He also needs to know that all close personal contacts within the last month should also get treatment.

Prescribing Options

Permethrin cream is first-line treatment. You tell Mr RS that the cream should be applied to the whole body from the neck downwards.

Safety Netting

You explain to Mr RS that you suspect he has scabies and if the rash and/or itching persists 2 weeks after using permethrin then he needs to be reassessed. Further permethrin treatment may be needed. He should also be told to return sooner if symptoms worsen as secondary bacterial infection due to scratching is possible.

AIDE MEMOIRE

Likely Diagnoses
Dermatitis

Dermatitis affecting the hands presents as skin that is hot, itching, scaly/rough and possibly painful. Hand function may be impaired due to fissuring and cracking of the skin. Sometimes small water blisters can be seen on the palms or sides of the fingers.

Insect Bites

Typically, papular urticaria is experienced after being bitten. Crops of very itchy red papules and vesicles of variable size are observed. Systemic symptoms are not present.

Pompholyx (Dyshidrotic Eczema)

Pompholyx is a specific type of eczema that causes small, itchy blisters to develop on palms and sides of the fingers (Fig. 5.14). It can affect people of any age, but it is most often seen in adults under 40 years.

Scabies

Intense generalised itching, which is often worse at nights, is the most common symptom. Itching can interfere with sleep. Associated rash mainly affects the hands and wrists but can be seen in axillae, thighs and buttocks. It exhibits erythematous papules and due to scratching excoriation, scratch marks are common. Scabies is more common in the elderly, children and adolescents, and is often seen as family outbreaks or where close physical contact for the delivery of personal care is required such as care homes.

Possible Diagnoses
Bullous Pemphigoid

Pemphigoid is a rare blistering autoimmune disorder that usually affects people over the of age 70 who have neurological disease, particularly stroke, dementia and Parkinson's disease. It causes severe itch and usually large bullae that rupture forming crusted erosions. A dermatitis-like rash may be present for weeks before any blisters appear. Any part of the skin can be involved, but the most common sites are body folds, hands and feet.

Hand, Foot and Mouth Disease

This is seen mostly in young children (95% are under 5 years of age). Cold-like symptoms can be seen prior to developing a skin rash on the palms of the hands and soles of the feet. Rash can show macules and papules that start pink and change to greyish blisters. Itch is not a prominent feature. Small, sometimes painful, ulcers can appear in and around the mouth, palate and pharynx, appearing as shallow yellow-grey ulcers surrounded by an erythematous halo.

Keratolysis Exfoliativa

Keratolysis exfoliativa presents with superficial blisters on the palms of the hands that burst, leading to peeling of the skin. The peeling is not painful, and the skin is not usually itchy (Fig. 5.15). The peeling may get worse during the summer or after frequent hand washing or exposure to water, and recurrence is common. Some people also notice peeling on their feet.

Lichen Planus

The rash appears as a shiny, slightly raised pink or purple-red small lesions and can show fine white streaks (Wickham's striae) on their surface. The rash can be anywhere but most affects the insides of the wrists, around the ankles and on the lower back (Fig. 5.16). Itch

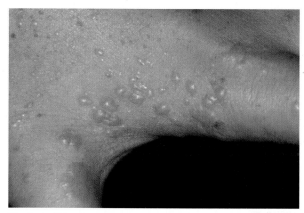

Fig. 5.14 Pompholyx. (Source: Micheletti, R. G., James, W. D., Elston, D. M., & McMahon, P. J. (2023). *Andrews' diseases of the skin clinical atlas* (2nd ed.). Elsevier.)

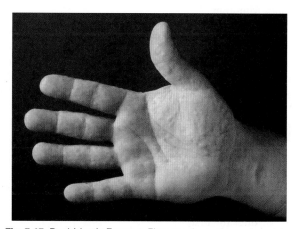

Fig. 5.15 Dyshidrotic Eczema. Firm papules and pseudovesicles on the palms and volar sides of fingers. Annular collarette-like scaling in the dyshidrosis lamellosa sicca (keratolysis exfoliativa) variant. (Source: Bolognia, J. L., Schaffer, J. V., & Cerroni, L. (2018). *Dermatology: 2-Volume Set* (4th ed.). Elsevier.)

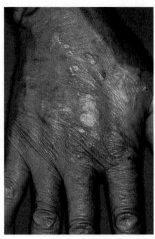

Fig. 5.16 Lichen Planus on the Dorsal Surface of the Hand. Wickham's striae can be easily identified in the upper right lesion. Note the flat-topped lesions. (Source: Bolognia, J. L., Jorizzo, J. L., Schaffer, J. V. (2012). *Dermatology* (3rd ed.). Elsevier, 2012, with permission.)

may be absent but it is usually present and can be severe. Lichen planus usually occurs in adults aged 40–60 years and affects all ethnicities equally.

Palmoplantar Psoriasis

The skin of the palms and/or soles tends to be red and inflamed, exhibiting pustules. Symmetrically distributed lesions are common. Over time, the skin becomes thickened and fissured leading to painful and itchy skin. The condition is persistent and recurrent.

Tinea Manuum

Symptoms include itchy raised lesions on the back of the hands. The palms can also be affected but is often seen as dry skin that may itch or cause pain. Many people have athlete's foot (tinea pedis) and transfer the infection to their hands after scratching their feet.

■ MCQs

1. Permethrin is the medicine of choice to treat scabies. Which ONE of the following statements about its use is not true?
   (a) A second application is always required 2 weeks after the first.
   (b) All members of their household and any other close personal contacts (even if asymptomatic) should also be treated.
   (c) Permethrin is applied to the whole body from the chin and ears downwards.
   (d) Permethrin should be washed off after 8 to 12 h.
   (e) The treatment should be applied to cool dry skin.

2. Scabies must be transmitted by skin-to-skin contact. Which ONE of the statements is not consistent with transmission?
   (a) Scabies is frequently sexually acquired.
   (b) Scabies is transmitted through close/prolonged skin contact.
   (c) Symptoms begin 1–2 weeks after primary infestation.
   (d) The mites can live away from a host for an average of 24–36 h.
   (e) Transmission through casual contact, such as a handshake, is unlikely.

3. Pompholyx is a condition that can be confused with scabies. Which ONE of the following signs and/or symptoms is not associated with pompholyx?
   (a) It is usually asymmetrical.
   (b) It tends to affect the centre of the palms.
   (c) Palms may be red and wet with perspiration.
   (d) The vesicles usually persist for 3 to 4 weeks before disappearing spontaneously.
   (e) Tiny vesicles develop several hours after itching develops.

4. Keratolysis exfoliativa is a skin condition in which there is peeling of the palms. Which ONE of the following is not associated with keratolysis exfoliativa?
   (a) It is most common in young adults.
   (b) It is usually more common during the summer months.
   (c) It presents initially with blisters over the palms.
   (d) It tends to recur every few weeks.
   (e) Patients typically complain of asymptomatic peeling on the palms.

5. Scabies is caused by infestation with the parasite *Sarcoptes scabiei*. Which ONE of the following is not commonly associated with scabies?
   (a) All body parts can be affected.
   (b) Itching can take several days to develop.
   (c) Intense pruritus
   (d) Papules
   (e) Spread by direct contact

Answers

1. a; 2. c; 3. a; 4. c; 5. a

WEBSITES

PEM Friends
https://www.pemfriendsuk.co.uk/

CASE 24: MACULOPAPULAR RASH

PRESENTATION

The parents of a 7-year-old boy bring in their son to see you. He has been poorly for the last 2 days and complained originally of a sore throat, but this is getting better. However, he now has a temperature and today they have noticed a rash. He is normally fit and healthy and has no medical problems.

PROBLEM REPRESENTATION

A 7-year-old boy presents with a 2-day history of acute onset constitutional symptoms with associated new rash.

HYPOTHESIS GENERATION (LIKELY, POSSIBLE AND CRITICAL DIAGNOSES)

Skin conditions presenting with macules (flat skin lesion ≤1 cm in diameter) and papules (an elevated, solid skin lesion ≤1 cm in diameter) are common. A maculopapular rash can be defined as a smooth skin rash or redness covered by elevated bumps. They are also referred to as morbilliform eruption or exanthematous eruption (exanthema). They can be characterised as acute (less than 4 weeks), subacute (4–8 weeks) or chronic (>8 weeks). They represent a diagnostic challenge but are commonly caused by infections in children and allergy in adults. As we are dealing with a 7-year-old child, our first thoughts on those conditions that are a common cause of his symptoms are:

Likely Diagnoses

- Erythema infectiosum (fifth disease)
- Hand, foot and mouth disease
- Roseola infantum (sixth disease, exanthem subitum)

Possible Diagnoses

- Allergies
- Drug eruptions
- Erythema multiforme
- Infectious mononucleosis
- Infectious causes from endemic regions
  - Dengue fever
  - West Nile fever
  - Zika virus
- Rubella (German measles)
- Rubeola (Measles)
- Scarlet fever

Critical Diagnoses

- Cutaneous lupus erythematosus
- HIV (very rare in this age group)
- Juvenile idiopathic arthritis
- Kawasaki disease
- Rubella complications
- Rubeola complications

CONTINUED INFORMATION GATHERING

The fact that he presents with fever followed by rash is not particularly helpful in narrowing down the cause of his symptoms as all three conditions being considered have this in common. We could look to the fact that he had prodromal symptoms before the rash (sore throat) to shape our thinking. Erythema infectiosum and hand, foot and mouth disease can present with viral-like symptoms, including sore throat whereas roseola does not. It is also worth remembering that certain possible causes (e.g., German measles and scarlet fever) can have sore throat too.

Based on this information, our questioning strategy is now one of determining if the cause is hand, foot and mouth disease or erythema infectiosum and should focus on the distribution of rash and changes over time.

The parents say they first noticed the rash on his belly but it is now also over his chest. This does not fit with either condition being considered, and casts doubt on our thinking. We may need to consider other possible causes.

PROBLEM REFINEMENT

Further exploration around the nature of the rash and if any other symptoms have been noticed should be conducted. Inspection of the skin shows the rash blanches on pressing and feels rough to the touch; this most closely fits with scarlet fever. You know scarlet fever effects the tongue and so on inspection you would expect this to be inflamed. The tongue is indeed red and inflamed. Both blanching rash and red tongue fit with a diagnosis of scarlet fever.

Although you are reasonably confident that scarlet fever is the diagnosis, it is important to consider other causes. We know he does not take any medicines, thus eliminating a drug-induced problem and reducing the chances of erythema multiforme (50% of cases have a drug-induced history). Additionally, to eliminate conditions associated with travel, the parents should be asked about any recent holidays. They confirm no recent foreign travel.

Whilst German measles/measles are vaccine preventable, it cannot be totally ruled out from our thinking due to incomplete vaccination rates leading to very small numbers of UK confirmed cases each year. However, the parents confirm he is up to date with all vaccines.

> ⚡ **RED FLAGS**
>
> The location of the rash seems not consistent with lupus and HIV. In arthritis, joint pain and swelling would be a prominent feature. Kawasaki disease, whilst similar to scarlet fever, shows other symptoms such as conjunctivitis, cracked lips and swollen hands/feet.

MANAGEMENT

Self-care Options

To help treat the fever, over-the-counter paracetamol or ibuprofen could be recommended. The child should also be encouraged to drink fluids and consider eating soft food to help with the sore throat.

To minimise spread hygiene measures need to be put in place such as effective and frequent hand washing and avoiding sharing towels.

Prescribing Options

You prescribe penicillin 250 mg taken four times daily x 10 days.

In addition, you tell the parents that their son should not go to school for at least 24 h after starting the antibiotic. Scarlet fever is a notifiable disease, and you must notify the local health protection team.

Safety Netting

You tell the parents that their son has scarlet fever and his symptoms should resolve in approximately 1 week. A follow-up appointment should be made if antibiotics do not clear up symptoms or they worsen. This is to ensure the child is not suffering from complications; although rare, these include otitis media, sinusitis, acute rheumatic fever, glomerulonephritis, bacteraemia, pneumonia, endocarditis and meningitis.

AIDE MEMOIRE

Likely Diagnosis

Table 5.1 highlights those causes of maculopapular rash that are relatively common or notifiable.

Possible Diagnoses
Drug Eruptions (Exanthematous)

Medicines such as antibiotics, anticonvulsants and nonsteroidal antiinflammatory drugs (NSAIDs) are commonly associated with maculopapular rash and occurs within 4–12 days after starting the medicine. The rash usually first appears on the trunk before spreading to the limbs and neck. The distribution is bilateral and symmetrical. Lesions itch or may feel hot.

Erythema Multiforme

Erythema multiforme mostly affects children and young adults, and is characterised by symmetrical macules, papules or wheals on the tops of the hands and forearms, although other parts of the body can be affected. Onset is usually sudden in an otherwise healthy individual. Systemic symptoms vary, but malaise, pain in the joints (arthralgia), muscular stiffness and fever are frequent. Medication is known to be a trigger factor and includes anticonvulsants, antibiotics and NSAIDs.

TABLE 5.1 Causes of Maculopapular Rash

	CRITICAL/NOTIFIABLE				COMMON MACULOPAPULAR CONDITIONS			
	Measles (Rubeola)	German Measles (Rubella)	Scarlet Fever (Fig. 5.17)	Allergy	Glandular Fever	Erythema Infectiosum	Roseola (Fig. 5.18)	Hand, Foot and Mouth
Fever	Yes	Yes	Yes	No	Yes, but only in ~10% of people	Yes	Yes	Yes
Swollen glands	No	Yes	Sometimes	No	Yes	No	No	No
Prodromal symptoms	Cold-like symptoms, conjunctivitis, cough. Koplik's spots appear 24–48 h before rash	Sore throat, coryza, malaise, mucosal petechiae	Usually follows a sore throat or skin infection such as impetigo	No	General malaise, headache	Nonspecific viral symptoms	None	Loss of appetite, malaise. Possibly sore throat, cough and abdominal pain
Other signs and associated symptoms		Pain and swelling in joints	Strawberry tongue		Sore throat key symptom			
Location	Ears and face, progressing to trunk & limbs	Face moving quickly to neck, trunk and extremities	Almost always originates from the groin and spreads bilaterally up the trunk to the axilla.	Anywhere	Trunk	Face before moving to arms and legs	Neck, trunk and spreads to limbs	Sides of fingers, hands and feet. Small, sometimes painful ulcers can appear in and around the mouth.
Nature of rash	Blanching		Blanching and 'sandpaper'-like quality	Itchy and blanching weal's		'Slapped' cheeks, burning hot. Limb rash 'lace-like'	Blanching	Small greyish lesions on hands that peel off within a week
Age most affected	Children & adolescents	Under 12 years	Under 8 years	Any	15–24 years	5–15 years	<3 years	<10 years

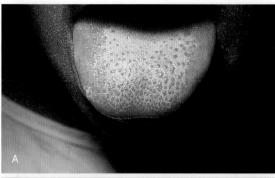

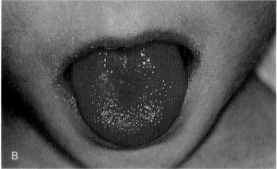

Fig. 5.17 Scarlet Fever. (A) A white strawberry tongue is usually followed by (B) a red strawberry tongue as the erythrotoxin-mediated enanthema evolves. (Source: Cohen, B. A. (2021). *Pediatric dermatology* (5th ed.). Saunders.)

Infectious Causes From Endemic Regions

Travellers are at risk of vector-borne diseases, some of which present with a rash.

Dengue fever. It is found in tropical and subtropical climates, including parts of Europe. Like West Nile fever, most people are asymptomatic. When symptoms occur, there may be a high fever often accompanied by a severe headache, muscle and joint pains, nausea, vomiting, abdominal pain and anorexia. Around the third day, a maculopapular rash develops, spreading from the trunk to the face and limbs.

West Nile fever. Most people are asymptomatic. Those who experience symptoms may exhibit flu-like symptoms, vomiting, diarrhoea or rash. In a small proportion of cases, it can lead to encephalitis. It has become more common in recent years and is seen in all continents other than Antarctica.

Zika virus. Zika virus may be symptomless, or the symptoms can be vague and mild. They last for up to a week. The most common symptoms of Zika are fever, rash, headache, conjunctivitis, joint and muscle pain. Infection during pregnancy can lead to foetal loss and preterm birth.

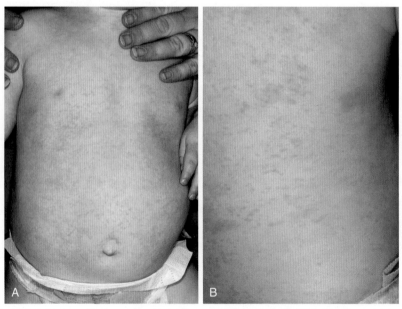

Fig. 5.18 Roseola Infantum. Erythematous blanching macules and papules (A) in an infant who had high fever for 3 days preceding development of the rash. On closer inspection (B), some lesions reveal a subtle peripheral halo of vasoconstriction. (Source: Paller, A. S., & Mancini, A. J. (Eds.). (2006). *Hurwitz clinical pediatric dermatology* (3rd ed.). Philadelphia: Saunders.)

Critical Diagnoses

Cutaneous Lupus Erythematosus

Lupus is a multisystem, inflammatory connective tissue disorder which often involves the skin. Acute lupus involves a prominent rash on the cheeks and nose ('butterfly rash'). However, subacute lupus presents with red, raised, scaly circular lesions on sun-exposed areas of the body such as the face, 'V' of the neck, scalp, arms and upper back.

HIV

Maculopapular rash especially on the face, trunk, and palms of the hand is one of the early signs. It lasts for 2–3 weeks. Other early signs and symptoms are flu-like symptoms.

Juvenile Idiopathic Arthritis

Juvenile idiopathic arthritis is seen in those under 16 years of age. The main symptom is pain and swelling of several joints (arthritis). It is used to describe several disease subtypes for which signs and symptoms vary. Systemic onset juvenile chronic arthritis (Still's disease) will present with additional symptoms of fever and rash.

Kawasaki Disease

This is a rare condition mainly affecting children under the age of 5 years. In many children, the initial symptom is a high-grade fever that typically rises and falls, and lasts for more than 5 days. It can be confused with scarlet fever as other symptoms include swollen cervical glands, strawberry tongue and rash. However other symptoms that can be seen are conjunctivitis, swollen and red hands and feet and dry, red cracked lips. If untreated approximately 25% of children will develop heart complications, which can be fatal.

Rubella

See Table 5.1. Congenital rubella syndrome can occur if pregnant women are infected during the first 20 weeks of pregnancy.

Rubeola

See Table 5.1. Pneumonia and encephalitis are known severe complications of measles.

MCQs

1. A number of infectious causes of maculopapular rash are associated with complications. Which ONE of the following is linked with heart problems?
   (a) Kawasaki disease
   (b) Rubeola
   (c) Scarlet fever
   (d) West Nile fever
   (e) Zika virus
2. Which ONE of the following may present with conjunctivitis as one of its symptoms?
   (a) Erythema infectiosum
   (b) Hand, foot and mouth
   (c) Roseola infantum
   (d) Rubella
   (e) Zika virus
3. Antiepileptics are cited as medicines that have maculopapular rash as an adverse drug reaction. Which ONE of the following antiepileptics is most associated with this?
   (a) Carbamazepine
   (b) Lamotrigine
   (c) Sodium valproate
   (d) Topiramate
   (e) Vigabatrin
4. Which ONE of the following does not present with a blanching maculopapular rash?
   (a) Drug eruptions
   (b) Erythema infectiosum
   (c) Measles
   (d) Roseola
   (e) Scarlet fever
5. Maculopapular rash is seen in each of the following conditions, but in which ONE of the following is it least common?
   (a) Drug eruption
   (b) German measles
   (c) Glandular fever
   (d) Measles
   (e) Scarlet fever

Answers
1. a; 2. e; 3. b; 4. b; 5. c

KEY POINTS: SCARLET FEVER
- Caused by *S. pyogenes*
- Key symptoms are prodromal symptoms of sore throat and fever followed by a rash on the torso that has a sandpaper-like quality.
- Symptoms should resolve in approximately 1 week.

WEBSITES

UK Government – notifiable diseases
https://www.gov.uk/guidance/notifiable-diseases-and-causative-organisms-how-to-report

CASE 25: RASH ON THE ARM

PRESENTATION

Mrs P, a middle-aged Asian woman who is known to you, asks for your advice about a rash she has on her arm that she noticed a couple of weeks ago. You know her to be hypertensive.

PROBLEM REPRESENTATION

A middle-aged woman presents with a 2-week history of rash on an extremity.

HYPOTHESIS GENERATION (LIKELY, POSSIBLE AND CRITICAL DIAGNOSES)

Based on location, we can start to narrow down the list of possibilities to some extent. For example, those most associated with the face (acne, rosacea, seborrhoeic dermatitis) or legs (cellulitis) or trunk (herpes zoster, pityriasis rosea) will be low down in our thinking. Also, based on her age, conditions mainly affecting children will also be very unlikely (e.g., roseola, lichen striatus, scarlet fever). Those conditions that mainly affect the limbs in an adult are:

Likely Diagnoses

- Dermatitis
- Discoid eczema
- Lichenoid drug eruptions
- Lyme disease
- Psoriasis
- Tinea infection

Possible Diagnoses

- Bullous pemphigoid
- Lichen planus
- Pityriasis rosea
- Pityriasis versicolor
- Prurigo nodularis
- Urticaria

Critical Diagnoses

- Cutaneous lupus
- Erythema multiforme
- Kaposi's sarcoma

CONTINUED INFORMATION GATHERING

We need to know more about the rash, for example, what it looks like, its size and if any other lesions have been noticed. Redness is difficult to place too much importance on as this can be very variable and is affected by a person's skin type – in this case we are looking at lesions on an Asian skin type, and it is well known that this can affect the look of the lesion in comparison to 'classic' symptoms on Caucasian skin types.

Examination reveals the rash is located near her left wrist, is small (<3 cm) and appears as a slightly raised pinky circular rash with fine white streaks on the surface.

Based on appearance, it appears Lyme disease and fungal infection are less likely due to the lesion not showing central clearing. The location would be unusual for discoid eczema and psoriasis. However, the white streaks on the lesion surface are seen in psoriasis but none of the other likely conditions.

Itch, to varying degrees, is associated with all but Lyme disease, and so asking about the severity of itch will help your thinking.

Mrs P says the rash is annoyingly itchy but she has tried to avoid scratching the rash. This seems to now exclude Lyme disease and further points away from psoriasis (mild or moderate itch is generally experienced). As psoriasis often shows lesion symmetry, you ask Mrs P if she has lesions on her other arm despite her not mentioning it. She denies any rashes on her other arm or elsewhere on her body. This seems to rule out psoriasis.

At this point, discoid eczema also seems less likely than dermatitis or a fungal infection as this tends to be seen on the lower legs and be bilateral. Dermatitis is often associated with exposure to irritants (contact dermatitis). With the rash being on her left wrist, a watch or bracelets may be responsible. You ask Mrs P about this but she says she always wears the same watch and does not wear jewellery here. This seems to suggest dermatitis is not the cause. This only leaves fungal infection or a drug reaction as possibilities from our list of likely causes.

We know she takes regular medication for hypertension. Her records show she has been taking nifedipine for over 18 months with no dose changes. Although it is known nifedipine can cause skin problems, it seems highly unlikely that this is the cause of her recent onset rash.

This leaves fungal infection to further consider. We know the rash is raised and itches. This is consistent with a fungal infection, but we also know that the rash is pink/purple in colour and shows no central clearing. At this point, we need to think about conditions from the possible list as the cause.

PROBLEM REFINEMENT

Given what we currently know, the conditions that 'fit' are lichen planus, pityriasis rosea and pityriasis versicolor.

Prodromal symptoms are associated with pityriasis rosea and recent travel with pityriasis versicolor. Enquiry into these two things shows Mrs P was fit and healthy prior to the rash appearing and has not been on holiday. Furthermore, if the rash was a 'herald patch', associated pityriasis rosea, then a more widespread rash on the torso should have appeared over this 2-week period.

Lichen planus now seems most likely, and her age is consistent with this presentation. In 50% of patients, oral involvement is also present. You ask Mrs P if she has noticed any white streaks in her mouth. She says she has seen some whiteness on the inside of her cheeks.

You are now relatively confident that the lesion is lichen planus.

⚡ RED FLAGS

Mrs P does not appear to have symptoms of any of the critical diagnoses, e.g., location wrong for lupus, lack of systemic symptoms associated with erythema multiforme and no bruise-like lesions of Kaposi's sarcoma.

MANAGEMENT

Self-care Options

Mrs P could try emollients to help with any dryness and the itch she is experiencing.

Prescribing Options

Lichen planus is generally self-limiting but can take up to 18 months to heal. Potent or very potent steroids are the mainstay of treatment. You recommend she use Betnovate cream twice a day, and as the lesions change colour from purple to grey/light brown to discontinue use.

Safety Netting

You tell Mrs P you believe she has lichen planus and that it will probably take many months before it resolves. Given she will be using potent steroids, it would be advisable to review her symptoms after 3 to 4 weeks.

AIDE MEMOIRE

Likely Diagnoses
Dermatitis (Contact/Allergic)

Both forms cause redness, drying of the skin and might show papules and vesicles. Itching is a prominent feature and often causes the patient to scratch, which results in broken skin with subsequent weeping. The rash in contact dermatitis tends to be well demarcated. In allergic dermatitis, milder involvement away from the site of exposure is seen on repeated exposure and can reactivate at previously exposed sites. The distribution of rash is closely associated with clothing and jewellery or exposure to certain chemicals via work exposure. In chronic exposure, the skin becomes dry, scaly and can crack and fissure.

Discoid Eczema

Characterised by discrete round, relatively small light red patches that are very itchy. Rash is often bilateral and symmetrical, occurring on the limbs, particularly the legs. It is most common in middle-aged patients.

Lichenoid Drug Eruptions

Drug eruptions are relatively common and can present in a variety of ways, including maculopapular rash (95% of causes), fixed drug eruptions, urticaria, psoriasiform and lichenoid. Lichenoid drug eruptions present with lesions that mimic lichen planus. They tend to itch and distribution can be extensive (Fig. 5.19). Commonly prescribed medicines implicated are antimalarials, beta-blockers, lithium and NSAIDs.

Lyme Disease

Early signs and symptoms of Lyme disease include flu-like symptoms and erythema migrans. The rash starts at the site of the tick bite and enlarges over a period of days, often becoming large. As it expands, it often exhibits central clearing, and is often described as looking like a bull's-eye on a dart board (Fig. 5.20). The rash is pink/red in colour, flat and may be warm to touch but does not itch.

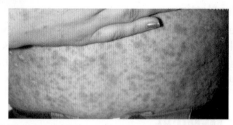

Fig. 5.19 Lichenoid Drug Eruption. Skin biopsy showed a lichenoid drug eruption. Lichenoid drug eruptions may last months after stopping the causative medication. (Source: Habif, T. P., Dinulos, J. G., Chapman, M. S., & Zug, K. A. (2024). *Skin disease: Diagnosis and treatment* (4th ed.). Elsevier.)

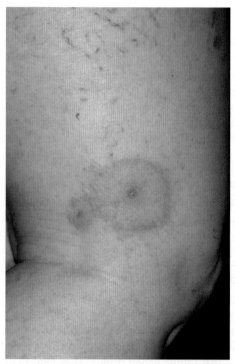

Fig. 5.20 Erythema Migrans. Characteristic lesion of Lyme disease. (Source: Dinulos, J. G. (2021). *Habif's clinical dermatology* (7th ed.). Elsevier.)

Psoriasis

Plaque psoriasis mostly affects the extensor surfaces and exhibits symmetry. Lesions are well defined, slightly raised and pinkish in colour, and are covered in fine silvery-white scales. Depending on severity, the number of plaques can range from few to many that cover large areas of the body. Itch is often experienced.

Tinea

Tinea infection can affect any part of the body. Initial presentation is of a single circular raised lesion with a scaly leading edge. Over time, multiple lesions develop which may coalesce with distribution being asymmetrical. Lesions exhibit 'central clearing' with red advancing edge and clear skin behind. Itch is common. It is most often seen in children and young adults.

Possible Diagnoses
Bullous Pemphigoid

Pemphigoid is a rare blistering autoimmune disorder that usually affects people over the of age 70 who have neurological disease, particularly stroke, dementia and Parkinson's disease. It causes severe itch and usually large bullae that rupture forming crusted erosions. A dermatitis-like rash may be present for weeks before any blisters appear. Any part of the skin can be involved, but the most common sites are body folds, hands and feet.

Lichen Planus

The rash appears as a shiny, slightly raised pink or purple-red small lesions and can show fine white streaks (Wickham's striae) on their surface. The rash can be anywhere but mostly affects the insides of the wrists, around the ankles and on the lower back. Itch may be absent but it usually itches, which can be severe. Lichen planus usually occurs in adults aged 40–60 years and affects all ethnicities equally.

Pityriasis Rosea

Prodromal symptoms of fever and headache can be experienced prior to rash. The first sign in many patients is a herald patch which is a single scaly pink patch and is seen a few days or weeks before the rash spreads. It can be mistaken for ringworm. The main rash usually appears on the torso, which is scaly and diffuse and takes 6–8 weeks to disappear (Fig. 5.21). In people who have dark skin, the patches may leave areas of darker or lighter pigmentation.

Pityriasis Versicolor

Characterised by macular lesions, which vary in colour, are usually small (less than 1 cm) but can join to form larger patches on the back, chest, and upper arms. The condition is more associated with warm climates and most people will have acquired the infection when on holiday. The rash does not itch significantly.

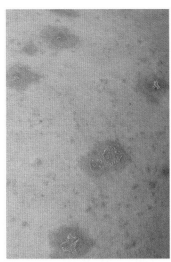

Fig. 5.21 Pityriasis Rosea. Both small, oval plaques and multiple, small papules are present. Occasionally the eruption consists only of small papules. (Source: Dinulos, J. G. (2021). *Habif's clinical dermatology* (7th ed.). Elsevier.)

Prurigo Nodularis

An intensely itchy rash that consists of small red nodules, which are variable in size and are located on the arms, legs and chest. Nodules may persist for months. It is more common in older people.

Urticaria

Acute episodes of urticaria present with circular itching weals of varying size and number that show central clearing (Fig. 5.22). They appear oedematous, and redness blanches when pressed. They can be located anywhere and tend to resolve within 24 h.

Critical Diagnoses

Cutaneous Lupus

Lupus is a multisystem, inflammatory connective tissue disorder which often involves the skin. Acute lupus involves a prominent rash on the cheeks and nose ('butterfly rash'). However, subacute lupus presents with red, raised, scaly circular lesions on sun-exposed areas of the body such as the face, 'V' of the neck, scalp, arms and upper back.

Erythema Multiforme

Erythema multiforme mostly affects children and young adults, and is characterised by symmetrical macules, papules or weals on the tops of the hands and forearms, although other parts of the body can be affected. Onset is usually sudden in an otherwise healthy individual. Systemic symptoms vary, but malaise, pain in the joints (arthralgia), muscular stiffness and fever are frequent. Medication is known to be a trigger factor and includes anticonvulsants, antibiotics and NSAIDs.

Kaposi's Sarcoma

The most common initial symptom is the appearance of small, painless, flat and discoloured patches on the skin that look like bruises. It is most seen in those with HIV infection.

MCQs

1. A young adult woman asks for your advice about a region of inflamed skin on her elbows. You look at the rash and observe it to be pale pink in colour with a slight red border. Which ONE of the following conditions is the most likely cause?
   (a) Discoid eczema
   (b) Irritant contact dermatitis
   (c) Pityriasis versicolor
   (d) Plaque psoriasis
   (e) Ringworm
2. An adult man presents with a circular red rash on his arm. On examination, the rash appears to be scaly and dry. The patient adds they find the rash extremely itchy. Which ONE

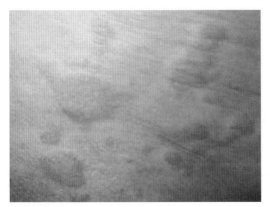

Fig. 5.22 Urticaria. (Source: DermNet. Urticaria; 2023. https://dermnetnz.org/topics/urticaria-an-overview. Accessed October 23, 2023.)

of the following conditions best explains his symptoms?

(a) Allergic contact dermatitis
(b) Discoid eczema
(c) Irritant contact dermatitis
(d) Plaque psoriasis
(e) Ringworm

3. Which ONE of the following best describes the clinical presentation of lichen planus?

(a) Clustered vesicles
(b) Golden coloured crusts
(c) Pruritic, papules and plaques
(d) Pruritic, red, large fluid-filled blisters
(e) Salmon coloured plaques with silvery scale

4. Which ONE of the following body part(s) are least affected by psoriasis?

(a) Back
(b) Elbow
(c) Knee
(d) Sacral region
(e) Scalp

5. Which ONE of the following is the cause of allergic contact dermatitis?

(a) Autoimmune reaction
(b) Delayed-type hypersensitivity reaction
(c) Direct irritant reaction
(d) Immediate hypersensitivity reaction
(e) Inflammatory reaction

Answers

1. d; 2. e; 3. c; 4. e; 5. b

KEY POINTS: LICHEN PLANUS

- Cause is unclear but is thought to be an autoimmune problem.
- Key symptoms are clusters of slightly raised small pink lesions that show fine white streaks on their surface.
- Can take up to 18 months to resolve
- Steroids are mainstay of treatment.

WEBSITES

UK Lichen Planus
https://www.uklp.org.uk/

CASE 26: RASH ON THE CHEST

PRESENTATION

Mr PR, an elderly Caucasian man, asks for some cream to help get rid of a rash he has over part of his chest. The rash started 2 days ago, and he describes it as irritating. He tells you he takes medicines for his heart, arthritis and glaucoma.

PROBLEM REPRESENTATION

An elderly man presents with a 2-day history of an irritating rash on the torso.

HYPOTHESIS GENERATION (LIKELY, POSSIBLE AND CRITICAL DIAGNOSES)

There is a large number of potential conditions that present with rash on the torso. As we know he is elderly and the rash is acute in onset, the likely conditions to consider in the first instance would be:

Likely Diagnoses

- Dermatitis
- Drug reaction
- Pityriasis rosea
- Pityriasis versicolor
- Shingles
- Tinea corporis
- Xerosis (dry skin)

Possible Diagnoses

- Psoriasis
- Seborrhoeic warts

Critical Diagnoses

- Mycosis fungoides
- Bowen's disease and squamous cell carcinoma

CONTINUED INFORMATION GATHERING

You ask him to tell you more about what he means by the rash being irritating. After chatting with Mr PR, you establish that the irritation is more soreness/pain than itch. Considering this information then, most of the initial conditions being considered seem less likely. For example, xerosis, drug reactions, pityriasis rosea and pityriasis versicolor are usually described as being

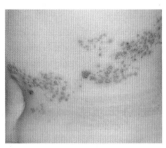

Fig. 5.23 Shingles. (Source: Brooks, D. L., & Brooks, M. L. (2012). *Exploring medical language: A student-directed approach* (8th ed.). Mosby.)

mildly pruritic. Tinea infection is characterised by moderate itching.

Dermatitis tends to show itching as a prominent feature but can also be experienced as pain. Shingles also causes pain and has been described as burning, stabbing or throbbing. On this basis, these two conditions seem more likely.

Examination of the rash will help distinguish between dermatitis and shingles. The rash is located on his left side below his armpit and has spread across on to his chest, which only happened yesterday. The rash appears red and angry with clusters of papules and vesicles (Fig. 5.23).

The examination further confirms that xerosis, pityriasis rosea and pityriasis versicolor are unlikely as they present with superficial scaling (xerosis also occasionally causes small cracks in the skin leading to pink or red patches of skin). Pityriasis versicolor and drug eruptions cause maculopapular rashes. Drug eruptions can be discounted by taking a medicine history – you establish he takes bendroflumethiazide, nifedipine, ibuprofen and pilocarpine eye drops, and has done so for the last 3 years, with no recent changes. A drug eruption is not responsible for his symptoms.

The location, distribution and look of the rash coupled with acute onset and it being painful suggests we are dealing with shingles.

PROBLEM REFINEMENT

Shingles often causes systemic upset and dermatitis does not. Asking about this will further help your thinking it is shingles. Mr PR reports he has been a bit off-colour over the last week or so. You are now reasonably confident he has shingles. To confirm your suspicions,

you ask if he has previously had chicken pox; he tells you he had chicken pox as a boy. Your working differential diagnosis is shingles.

> **⚡ RED FLAGS**
>
> Conditions listed as possible or critical do not appear to be the cause of his symptoms. All are more chronic in nature.

MANAGEMENT

Self-care Options

Mr PR already takes ibuprofen for arthritis but this does not seem to be fully controlling the pain associated with the rash. You recommend he take paracetamol as well. You also could explain to him that he can pass on the problem to others until the final vesicles have crusted over so he should avoid sharing towels and sheets. Wearing loose fitting clothing may help not to aggravate the rash.

Prescribing Options

Instigation of antiretroviral therapy is recommended up to 72 h from when the rash started. This may help with reducing the incidence of postherpetic neuralgia. You prescribe famciclovir 500 mg three times a day for 10 days.

Safety Netting

You tell him he has shingles and that a course of tablets should help clear the problem up but to come back after finishing the tablets if the rash has not gone or he is still in pain.

AIDE MEMOIRE

Likely Diagnoses
Dermatitis

Dermatitis can present as a variety of morphological presentations – causing redness, dryness and lichenification that are associated with itch, which can be intense. Personal and family history of allergic conditions is observed in atopic dermatitis. Irritant and allergic forms develop following exposure to an allergen/irritant.

Drug Reaction (Fixed)

A fixed drug eruption is defined by lesions that recur in the same area when the same medicine is given on different occasions. The rash usually starts shortly after initiation affecting hands, feet and torso. Many medicines are implicated in this type of reaction and include antibiotics, ACE inhibitors, calcium channel blockers, anticonvulsants, NSAIDs, allopurinol, benzodiazepines and sulphonamides. The rash appears as well-defined, round or oval red patches or plaques.

Pityriasis Rosea

Prodromal symptoms of fever and headache can be experienced prior to rash. The first sign in many patients is a herald patch which is a single scaly pink patch and is seen a few days or weeks before the rash spreads. It can be mistaken for ringworm. The main rash usually appears on the torso, and is scaly and diffuse and takes 6–8 weeks to disappear. In people who have dark skin, the patches may leave areas of darker or lighter pigmentation.

Pityriasis Versicolor

A mildly itchy flat rash of the torso (but can also affect the upper arms, neck and stomach) that exhibits fine skin scaling. On white skin, the affected areas usually appear darker than surrounding skin, and in dark-skinned people, the affected patches can appear pale.

Shingles

Initially, prodromal symptoms of discomfort/pain along the affected nerve are observed a day or two before the rash appears. Pain is described as burning, itching or throbbing. Additionally, some people may experience headache and fever. Shingles rash starts with maculo-papular lesions which quickly develop into fluid-filled vesicles. Some vesicles will burst and crust over. The rash is painful and itchy. The position and shape of the rash will depend on which nerves are involved. Shingles is more common in the elderly, those experiencing stress or are immunocompromised.

Tinea Corporis

Tinea infection can affect any part of the body. Tinea corporis is most often seen in children and young adults. Initial presentation is of a single circular raised lesion with a scaly leading edge. Over time, multiple lesions develop which may coalesce with distribution being asymmetrical. Lesions exhibit 'central clearing' with a red advancing edge and clear skin behind. Itch is common.

Xerosis (Dry Skin)

It affects almost everyone, to some extent, over the age of 60 years. Typically, the skin feels dry to the touch and exhibits scaly quality with superficial cracks. If severe, the skin can become red and inflamed or even fissured. Itching is usually present. Common sites are the shins and arms. Symptoms may be made worse in 'dry' climates.

Possible Diagnoses
Psoriasis

Psoriasis presents in a variety of morphological types, but it is plaque psoriasis that is most associated with affecting the torso, although typically it also affects the elbows and knees. Lesions are well defined, slightly raised and pinkish in colour that are covered in fine silvery-white scales. Depending on severity, the number of plaques can range from few to many that cover large areas of the body. Itch is often experienced.

Seborrhoeic Warts

These are also known as seborrhoeic keratoses and basal cell papillomas. They are very common, especially in older people, and appear as single or multiple lesions of variable size. Common sites are the trunk but they can also affect the face and neck. They vary in colour widely, from skin colour to black. Typically, they are asymptomatic but can itch and become inflamed or bleed if caught on clothing. They are often described as having a 'stuck-on' appearance.

Critical Diagnoses
Mycosis Fungoides

This is a rare condition affecting people over the age of 50 years. Rash, which is itchy, is slow growing and exhibits irregularly shaped patches resembling psoriasis or dermatitis. Each year in the UK, approximately 450 people are newly diagnosed with mycosis fungoides. Most affected people live a normal life span.

Bowen's Disease and Squamous Cell Carcinoma

These cancers are a result of long-term sun exposure and are therefore most common on the face, scalp and neck, hands and lower legs. Appearance is variable but often starts as slow-growing small red scaly/crusty raised areas that are usually asymptomatic but can be sore or tender, and which may bleed. Typically, they are seen in older men.

MCQs

1. The lifetime risk of developing shingles is approximately 30% and increases with age and has a number of associated risk factors. Which ONE of the following is NOT a risk factor?
   (a) Being immunocompromised
   (b) Chronic kidney disease
   (c) Diabetes
   (d) Heart failure
   (e) Rheumatoid arthritis

2. A number of complications can arise from shingles. Which ONE of the following is the complication seen most frequently?
   (a) Corneal ulceration
   (b) Peripheral motor neuropathy
   (c) Postherpetic neuralgia
   (d) Secondary infections of lesions
   (e) Skin scarring

3. The rash of shingles initially starts as maculopapular which then develops into clusters of vesicles before they burst and crust over. However, the rash can present atypically in certain patient groups. Which ONE of the following patient groups can the rash be nonvesicular?
   (a) Diabetic people
   (b) Immunocompromised people
   (c) Older people
   (d) Pregnant women
   (e) Younger people

4. Shingles is infectious until all vesicles have crusted over. Advice should be given to minimise the potential to transmit to others. Which ONE of the following pieces of advice is not usually given?
   (a) Avoid contact with people who have not had chickenpox
   (b) Avoid covering lesions
   (c) Avoid work if lesions are still weeping
   (d) Do not share towels
   (e) Wash hands frequently

5. Shingles can be prevented, and the UK does have a vaccination programme introduced in 2013. However, there are certain restrictions on who is eligible for the vaccine. Which ONE of the following groups is eligible for the vaccine?
   (a) Those aged over 50 years
   (b) Those aged over 55 years
   (c) Those aged over 60 years
   (d) Those aged over 65 years
   (e) Those aged over 70 years

Answers

1. d; 2. c; 3. c; 4. b; 5. e

KEY POINTS: SHINGLES

- Herpes zoster infection causes symptoms through reactivation of the dormant virus in an associated nerve root.
- Prodromal pain is followed by a vesicular rash following a dermatome.
- Postherpetic neuralgia is a common complication, especially in older people.
- Treatment includes pain management and antivirals, where appropriate.

WEBSITES

Shingles Support Society
https://shinglessupport.org.uk/

CASE 27: SUSPECT MOLE

PRESENTATION

A concerned female patient in her early 30s presents with a mole on her lower leg that she says has begun to change over the last couple of months. She is otherwise fit and healthy and has no medical problems. She takes the combined oral contraceptive pill for birth control.

PROBLEM REPRESENTATION

A healthy young adult woman presents with a recent history of an evolving mole.

HYPOTHESIS GENERATION (LIKELY, POSSIBLE AND CRITICAL DIAGNOSES)

A mole (melanocytic naevus) is a common benign skin lesion due to a local proliferation of melanocytes. They can be present from birth (congenital) or appear later on in life (acquired). There are various kinds of congenital and acquired moles. Those acquired later in childhood or adult life often follow sun exposure. Consideration of a new mole that develops after the age of

40 years, a mole that is different from the person's other moles (the 'ugly duckling') and moles that change should be viewed with suspicion as potentially cancerous.

Likely Diagnoses

- Atypical mole
- Benign common mole
- Freckles
- Seborrhoeic keratoses

Possible Diagnoses

- Actinic keratosis
- Angioma/haemangioma
- Angiokeratoma
- Dermatofibroma
- Lentigines

Critical Diagnoses

- Kaposi's sarcoma
- Melanoma

CONTINUED INFORMATION GATHERING

Our patient is a young adult with a suspicious mole on her leg, which is a classic site for melanoma development. To assess moles, the National Institute for Health and Care Excellence recommends using the weighted Glasgow 7-point checklist (see Box 5.2). This checklist consists of three major and four minor points. If the suspicious pigmented skin lesion scores 3 or more, the patient needs to be referred using a suspected cancer pathway referral for melanoma.

You obviously need to go through this checklist with the patient. You ask her to describe the changes she has

noticed. She tells you that her mole was always pale brown but it now seems to have gone darker compared with her other moles and she thinks it has got bigger. She does not report any itching, bleeding or redness/irritation.

PROBLEM REFINEMENT

On examination, the mole is 6 mm in diameter and relatively symmetrical and does show a two-tone appaerance (Fig. 5.24). A change in colour would score 2, and if we rely on her subjective assessment of the lesion getting bigger (a score of 2), her overall score is 4.

> ⚡ **RED FLAGS**
>
> A score of 4 would mean that the mole needs to be further assessed.

MANAGEMENT

Self-care Options

Safe sun messages need to be reinforced. It is also important to discuss with the patient the ABCDE mnemonic to help them perform self-examination to identify possible sinister changes (see Box 5.3).

BOX 5.2   The 7-Point Checklist

Major (Scores 2)
1. Change in shape
2. Change in size
3. Change in colour

Minor (Scores 1)
1. Largest diameter 7 mm or more
2. Inflammation
3. Oozing
4. Change in sensation (e.g., itch or irritation)

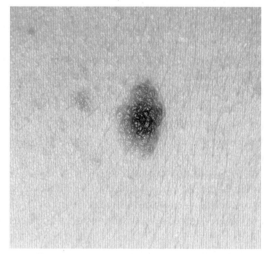

Fig. 5.24 Dysplastic/Atypical Mole. Pink, tan, brown, irregularly shaped papule with an indistinct border. (Source: Marks, J. G., Jr., & Miller, J. J. (2019). *Lookingbill and Marks' principles of dermatology* (6th ed.). Elsevier.)

BOX 5.3   The ABCDE Guide to Suspected Melanoma Recognition

Asymmetry	Ordinary moles are usually symmetrical in shape. Melanomas are likely to be irregular or asymmetrical.
Border	Moles usually have a well-defined, regular border. Melanomas are more likely to have an irregular border with jagged edges.
Colour	Moles are usually a uniform brown. Melanomas tend to have more than one colour. They may be varying shades of brown mixed with black, red, pink, white or a bluish tint.
Diameter	Moles are normally no bigger than the blunt end of a pencil (about 6 mm across). Melanomas are usually more than 7 mm in diameter.
Evolution	The symmetry, border, colour or diameter of a mole has changed over time.

Prescribing Options

Not applicable.

Safety Netting

You tell her that as the mole has changed, it would be best to get a second opinion at the hospital as melanoma cannot be ruled out at this time, although most moles turn out to be nonmalignant and are called atypical moles.

AIDE MEMOIRE

Likely Diagnoses
Atypical Moles

Atypical moles are benign pigmented lesions that look different from a common mole and exhibit some clinical features that suggest malignant melanoma. They are usually bigger, characterised by a size of >5 mm in diameter and can show irregular shape, indistinct borders and variable colours, often showing a mixture of several colours, from pink to dark brown. They tend to be flat, with a smooth, slightly scaly or pebbly surface. A number of types have been described: a halo naevus is surrounded by a depigmented halo of normal skin and is common in older children and young teenagers; a Spitz naevus is a firm, round, pink, red or reddish-brown nodule of less than 2 cm in diameter. It usually occurs on the face or legs; a blue naevus is a raised smooth lesion which is blue or blue-black in colour and less than 1 cm in diameter that occur anywhere but are common on the face; a congenital naevus (birthmark) is present from or shortly after birth, usually larger than acquired naevi and dark brown or black in colour.

Benign Common Moles

These tend to appear shortly after birth until early adulthood. They occur anywhere on the body and tend to be round/oval and symmetrical with smooth and well-demarcated borders and have an even colour of pink, tan or brown. Light-skinned individuals tend to have light-coloured moles and dark-skinned individuals tend to have dark brown or black moles. Sizes range from a couple of millimetres to several centimetres but are usually less than 6 mm in diameter. People with a greater number of naevi or atypical moles have a higher risk of developing melanoma. Benign moles tend to have an overall similar appearance, whereas an outlier with a different appearance is more likely to be undergoing malignant change, the 'ugly duckling' concept.

Freckles

These are flat poorly-defined macules usually less than 1 cm in diameter that vary in colour from light to dark brown. They become more numerous through exposure to sunlight. People with fair complexions are most likely to experience freckles.

Seborrhoeic Keratosis (Also Known as Seborrhoeic Warts or Basal Cell Papillomas)

Mostly seen in older people, these are benign, flat or raised lesions that vary in colour from light brown to jet black. Initially, they take on the colour of the person's skin but gradually darken. They have a 'stuck-on' appearance. They can occur anywhere but are more usual on the trunk and there may be multiple lesions. Over time, they can become wart-like. Occasionally, they can become inflamed, itchy or bleed but this is normally because they have been caught on clothing.

Possible Diagnoses
Actinic Keratosis

Lesions occur on parts of the body that are exposed to long-term sun exposure (e.g., head, forearms, hands).

They begin as small rough spots. Roughness is a key feature – often referred to as feeling like rubbing sandpaper. They are generally flat and brown and have well-demarcated edges. Symptoms of actinic keratosis include tenderness, itchiness and burning (Fig. 5.25). Over years, they enlarge and often become red and scaly.

Angioma and Haemangioma

These are benign vascular skin lesions that can appear at any time in life, although the most common type of angioma, the cherry angioma, is more common with increasing age. They tend to be less than 1 cm in diameter and appear as firm red to purple papules and can be over any part of the body but are rare on the hands and feet.

Angiokeratomas

These present as an asymptomatic blue-red hyperkeratotic papule anywhere on the skin and are usually <5 mm in diameter. The surface is variable in nature but tends to become warty over time.

Dermatofibromas

Dermatofibromas are benign firm, flesh-coloured nodules that are usually found on the lower legs in adults. The nodule can be brown and have a history of fairly rapid enlargement, which may suggest melanoma.

Lentigines

These vary in size but most are less than 5 mm in diameter and appear as flat brown/black sometimes irregularly shaped lesions. They can look like freckles but tend to be darker and do not fade in the winter. There are number of types of lentigo, with solar lentigo (ager spots/liver spots) being most common, and result from chronic sun exposure and occur from middle age onward. Ink-spot lentigo can cause confusion with melanoma as they are very dark/black and may have an irregular border.

Critical Diagnoses

Kaposi's Sarcoma

This is associated with HIV infection. Lesions can appear anywhere, tend to be multiple and are generally dark-coloured macules that develop into nodules or plaques.

Melanoma

Most commonly seen on the legs of women and the back in young adults, and on the face in both sexes in older adults. They are more common in fair-skinned individuals and in those with high sun exposure. Other risk factors include numerous atypical moles, a family history of melanoma and advancing age. Melanoma presents as a growing, changing area of pigmentation and on pathological grounds is seen as four types: superficial spreading melanoma, which accounts for approximately 80% of cases; nodular melanoma that is a more aggressive type; lentigo maligna melanoma often seen in older patients; and acral melanoma, found on the palms and soles and is more common in Asian populations (Fig. 5.26).

▮ MCQs

1. Which ONE of the following is the most common site for skin cancer in women?
   (a) Arms
   (b) Head
   (c) Legs
   (d) Neck and shoulders
   (e) Trunk
2. Which ONE of the following does the star rating on sunscreen mean?
   (a) Indication of UVA protection
   (b) Indication of UVA and UVB protection
   (c) Indication of UVB protection
   (d) Indication of sunburn protection
   (e) None of the above
3. Which ONE of the following may be a warning sign of melanoma?
   (a) A mole that is new or growing
   (b) A mole that is itching
   (c) A mole that is bleeding
   (d) A mole showing variable colour
   (e) All of the above
4. Sun safety is a key factor in reducing a person's chance of developing skin cancer. Which ONE of the following is true about wearing sunscreen?
   (a) It should be applied every day if you plan to be outside.
   (b) Only needs to be applied when the sun is strongest, e.g., between 11 am and 3 pm.
   (c) Reapply every 4 h.
   (d) SPF 15 is classified as a sunblock.
   (e) They only need to be used if you sunburn easily.

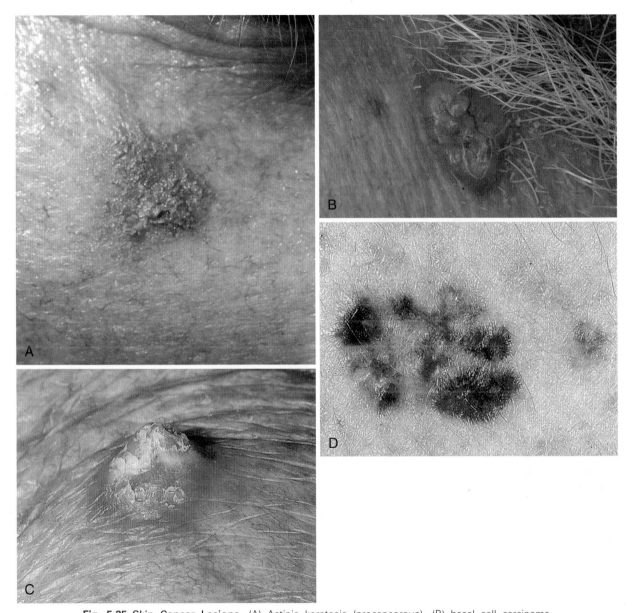

Fig. 5.25 Skin Cancer Lesions. (A) Actinic keratosis (precancerous), (B) basal cell carcinoma, (C) squamous cell carcinoma and (D) malignant melanoma (superficial spreading). (Source: Habif, T. P., Campbell, J. L., Jr., Dinulos, J. G., Chapman, M. S., & Zug, K. A. (2011). *Skin disease: Diagnosis and treatment* (3rd ed.). Saunders.)

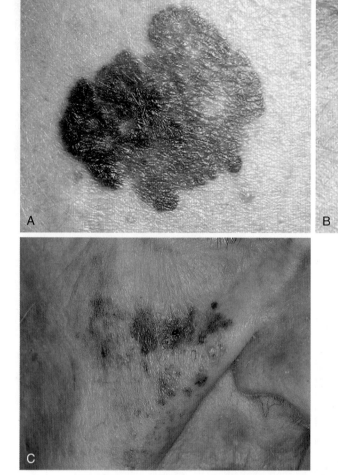

Fig. 5.26 Type of Melanoma. (A) Superficial spreading. (B) Nodular. (C) Lentigo maligna melanoma. (Source: (A) and (B) Habif, T. (2010). Nevi and malignant melanoma. In T. Habif (Ed.), *Clinical dermatology* (5th ed.). Mosby.; (C) Courtesy of Kalman Watsky MD.)

5. The British Association of Dermatologists advise people not to use sunbeds as are they associated with all health risks. Which ONE of the following is not a known health risk?

(a) Eye irritation
(b) Premature skin ageing
(c) Skin cancer
(d) Sunburnt skin
(e) Worsening psoriasis

Answers

1. c; 2. a; 3. e; 4. a; 5. e

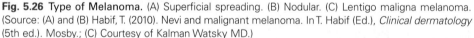

KEY POINTS: MELANOMA

- Outlook depends on the stage of the cancer when diagnosed – the earlier detected (e.g., stage 1 and 2), the higher the 5-year survival rate
- Healthcare professionals and patients should monitor moles for changes in size, shape, borders, colour and surface characteristics and for bleeding, ulceration, itching and tenderness.
- Excise melanomas whenever feasible

WEBSITES

Cancer research UK
https://www.cancerresearchuk.org/about-cancer/melanoma
Sunscreen and sun safety
https://www.nhs.uk/live-well/seasonal-health/sunscreen-
   and-sun-safety/

CASE 28: TORSO RASH IN A CHILD

PRESENTATION

Mrs R, a regular patient, asks for your advice about her daughter, 'A', who is 4 years old. She tells you that her daughter has developed a few spots on her chest and they appear to be itchy, as she has seen her scratching at them.

PROBLEM REPRESENTATION

A 4-year-old girl presents with acute onset itchy rash of unknown duration on the torso.

HYPOTHESIS GENERATION (LIKELY, POSSIBLE AND CRITICAL DIAGNOSES)

It is reasonable to first consider those conditions that predominantly affect children such as:
- Atopic dermatitis
- Chicken pox
- Erythema infectiosum (fifth disease)
- Hand, foot mouth disease
- Impetigo
- Infantile seborrhoeic dermatitis
- Measles
- Molluscum contagiosum
- Pityriasis alba
- Roseola infantum (sixth disease)
- Rubella (German measles)
- Scarlet fever
- Warts

This list however can be shortened considerably when we consider that the rash appears to be limited to the trunk and itches. Based on location, atopic dermatitis; hand, foot and mouth disease; infantile seborrhoeic dermatitis and molluscum contagiosum seem unlikely

as they tend not to be on the trunk. Regarding itch, fifth disease, measles, pityriasis alba, rubella, scarlet fever, sixth disease, warts and molluscum contagiosum do not itch.

Based on these exclusions, it appears only chicken pox and impetigo are childhood conditions that itch and can affect the torso.

In addition, rashes (which itch and can be on the torso) that can affect both children and adults need to be considered.
- Bullous pemphigoid
- Drug eruptions
- Dermatitis
- Papular urticaria
- Polymorphic light eruption
- Scabies
- Shingles

From these conditions, those considered initially would be:

Likely Diagnoses
- Chicken pox
- Dermatitis
- Impetigo
- Papular urticaria

Possible Diagnoses
- Bullous pemphigoid
- Drug eruptions
- Polymorphic light eruption
- Scabies
- Shingles

Critical Diagnosis
- Not applicable

CONTINUED INFORMATION GATHERING

A visual inspection of the rash would be helpful as the four conditions being considered do present differently; chicken pox lesions are typically vesicular but rapidly crust over and the distribution is discrete; impetigo is also characterised by vesicles that then rupture and weep with the exudate drying to a brown, yellow sticky crust; dermatitis tends to show small patches of dry skin, but inflamed skin can be red and exhibit some papular/vesicular lesions; and papular urticaria presents with crops of lesions.

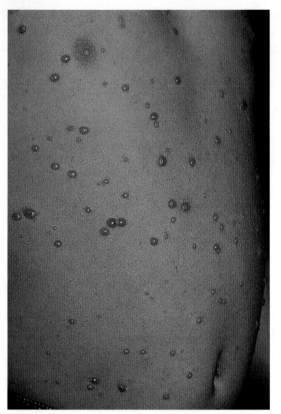

Fig. 5.27 Chicken Pox. (Source: White, G. (2004). *Color atlas of dermatology* (3rd ed.). Churchill Livingstone.)

Inspection of 'A's spots show a mixture of vesicles and red lesions that have crusted over, which appear to be only on her chest. The look of the rash fits well with chicken pox (Fig. 5.27).

PROBLEM REFINEMENT

In chicken pox, children often experience prodromal symptoms a few days before the rash develops and commonly include fever, headache and sore throat. Such symptoms are not seen in impetigo or various forms of dermatitis.

You find out that the child is a little irritable, but her mother says she has been a bit off-colour over the last few days. It appears that 'A' has been experiencing mild constitutional symptoms and you are now confident that the differential diagnosis is indeed chicken pox, even though the spots are only on the chest.

Before thinking about management, you need to make sure that the possible causes are not responsible. To exclude medicine-related rash, Mrs R can be asked if her daughter takes any medicines. She tells you she does not. Shingles is only possible if the person has previously had chicken pox. Although you think the girl's rash is chicken pox, you ask if she has had this before. Her mother says she has not had chicken pox before. Scabies, polymorphic light eruption and bullous pemphigoid all tend to present in different locations and so can also be discounted.

⚡ RED FLAGS
Not applicable.

MANAGEMENT

Self-care Options
You advise Mrs R of some measures to control the itching and help stop 'A' from scratching the lesions. This includes dressing in loose clothes, cutting her nails and possibly placing socks on her hands at night. Cooling creams/lotions can be applied and paracetamol given for any pain or discomfort.

Prescribing Options
An antihistamine (chlorphenamine) could be offered.

Safety Netting
You tell Mrs R you think 'A' has chicken pox and it is likely that the rash will spread to her back and face over the next few days, and that it is highly contagious until all lesions have crusted over. She therefore needs to keep 'A' off school until all the spots have crusted over.

You advise that if her symptoms have not cleared up after a couple of weeks then you would like to see her again.

AIDE MEMOIRE

Likely Diagnoses
Chicken Pox
Before the rash develops, the patient might experience up to 3 days of prodromal symptoms that could include fever, headache and sore throat. The rash typically begins on the face, stomach and back before spreading to other parts of the body. Initially, lesions appear as small red lumps that rapidly develop into vesicles which crust

over after 3 to 5 days. New lesions tend to occur in crops of three to five for the first 4 days, so at the height of infectivity lesions appear in all stages of development. The vesicles are often extremely itchy. Chicken pox is highly contagious, from a few days before the onset of rash until all lesions have crusted over.

Dermatitis

Various types of dermatitis (allergic and irritant contact dermatitis and atopic) present with a variety of morphological presentations, causing redness, papules/vesicles, dryness and lichenification that are associated with itch. Personal and family history of allergic conditions is observed in atopic dermatitis. Irritant and allergic forms develop following exposure to an allergen/irritant.

Impetigo

It presents mainly on the face, around the nose and mouth, but can affect other parts of the body. It usually starts as a small red itchy patch of inflamed skin that quickly develops into vesicles that rupture and weep. The exudate dries to a brown, yellow/honey-coloured sticky crust. In a small proportion of patients, a bullous form can develop where the rash is accompanied with fluid-filled bullae.

Papular Urticaria

Typically, papular urticaria is experienced after being bitten. Crops of very itchy red papules and fluid-filled vesicles of variable size are observed. It is most commonly seen on legs, arms and face. Systemic symptoms are not present.

Possible Diagnoses

Bullous Pemphigoid

This is a rare skin condition usually affecting elderly people. It presents as large fluid-filled blisters that rupture forming crusted erosions but with a history of skin itching predating the rash. The limbs and trunk are most affected.

Drug Eruptions

The commonest causes of drug eruptions are those that produce maculopapular rashes. They usually start on the trunk. The rash tends to feel hot, burn or itch. Almost any medicine can be implicated but is commonly seen with antibiotics and anticonvulsants.

Polymorphic Light Eruption

An itchy or burning rash appears within hours, or a few days after exposure to sunlight. It can take many different forms (polymorphic). The rash usually appears on the parts of the skin exposed to sunlight and exhibits seasonality, occurring in spring and early summer and usually disappearing completely in winter.

Scabies

Classically affecting interdigital spaces in the hands, feet and wrists but also the trunk, thighs and buttocks. Intense generalised itching which is often worse at night is the most common symptom. It exhibits erythematous papules and due to scratching, excoriation and scratch marks are common.

MCQs

1. Which ONE of the following conditions is characterised with mildly itching ill-defined pink rough patches that fade?
   (a) Atopic dermatitis
   (b) Erythema infectiosum
   (c) Measles
   (d) Pityriasis alba
   (e) Scarlet fever
2. Which ONE of the following conditions is characterised by a history of dry skin and visible flexural eczema?
   (a) Atopic dermatitis
   (b) Infantile seborrheic dermatitis
   (c) Pityriasis alba
   (d) Plaque psoriasis
   (e) Polymorphic light eruption
3. Which ONE of the following conditions is often improved through light exposure?
   (a) Actinic keratosis
   (b) Atopic dermatitis
   (c) Pityriasis alba
   (d) Plaque psoriasis
   (e) Polymorphic light eruption
4. A 6-year-old boy presents with rash on his leg. Based solely on location, which ONE of the following is most likely?
   (a) Atopic dermatitis
   (b) Chicken pox
   (c) Impetigo
   (d) Molluscum contagiosum
   (e) Roseola infantum

5. An 8-month-old baby presents with rash on the torso. Based only on this information, which ONE of the following is the most likely?
   (a) Atopic dermatitis
   (b) Chicken pox
   (c) Impetigo
   (d) Molluscum contagiosum
   (e) Roseola infantum

Answers

1. d; 2. a; 3. d; 4. a; 5. e

KEY POINTS: CHICKEN POX
• Caused by the herpes varicella zoster virus
• Key symptoms of prodromal malaise followed by widespread itchy vesicular rash
• Usually resolves within 2 weeks

6

Pain Problems

CASE 29: BACK PAIN

PRESENTATION

Mr H, a 44-year-old man, attends your walk-in clinic complaining of a sore back and wants to know what painkillers would be best. Mr H is unknown to you. He tells you he has been taking paracetamol (two tablets (1000 mg) four times a day) but that is not really helping to relieve the pain. A medical history reveals he has psoriasis and uses Dovonex when needed.

PROBLEM REPRESENTATION

A 44-year-old man presents with back pain unresponsive to simple analgesia.

HYPOTHESIS GENERATION (LIKELY, POSSIBLE AND CRITICAL DIAGNOSES)

Low back pain is usually nonspecific (90%–95% of cases) but can have significant neurological defects (5%–10% of cases) or be associated with serious spinal disease (<1% of cases). Pain in the lower back can also originate from nonspinal causes, such as pain associated with menstruation (dysmenorrhoea) or pelvic pathology, which can be discounted in this case.

Likely Diagnoses
- Nonspecific (simple) low back pain
- Sciatica

Possible Diagnoses
- Ankylosing spondylitis
- Kidney stones
- Osteoarthritis (OA)
- Osteoporosis

- Pancreatitis
- Shingles
- Stenosis
- Urinary tract infection/pyelonephritis

Critical Diagnoses
- Cauda equina syndrome
- Infection
- Malignancy (usually metastases)
- Vertebral fracture

CONTINUED INFORMATION GATHERING

On presentation, we only know that he has low back pain, which has failed to respond adequately to simple analgesia. Questions directed toward knowing about the exact site, duration and nature of his symptoms are needed.

Mr H tells you he has had the symptoms for about a week now and the pain is located toward the bottom of his back just above his bottom and that the pain is pretty much there all the time. He describes it as a dull ache, a bit like toothache. It appears we are dealing with an acute episode of back pain, and those of a chronic nature can be ruled out. From this description it seems nonspecific (simple) low back pain is the likely cause. Sciatica is a commonly encountered problem and frequently associated with radiating pain. You ask Mr H if the pain moves away from this area at any time. He says that this does not happen. This seems to rule out sciatica.

PROBLEM REFINEMENT

To further confirm your thinking, you ask him if he can recall any event that might have triggered it, as it is often possible to identify the cause of symptoms (e.g., from lifting, recent or excessive physical activity). However, Mr H cannot recollect a specific event that triggered his symptoms. Simple low back pain is usually not associated with other symptoms. You ask Mr H about other symptoms. He says that beside the pain he has a bit of stiffness but nothing else.

At this point, the information gathered is relatively unremarkable but consistent with simple back pain.

> ## ⚡ RED FLAGS
> There appears to be no signs or symptoms that raise concerns. Conditions causing chronic pain or sinister pathology would exhibit signs and symptoms other than pain. He is also relatively young and therefore at low risk of developing more serious pathologies.

MANAGEMENT

Self-care Options

Mr H should keep mobile and, where possible, maintain normal day-to-day activities.

Prescribing Options

Paracetamol seems to be ineffective, so alternative pain relief is required. Treatment with a nonsteroidal antiinflammatory drug (NSAID) for 7–10 days is widely advocated. A check to make sure he is suitable to take oral NSAIDs is needed. He tells you he takes occasional antacids for heartburn. NSAID use could precipitate/worsen heartburn but does not preclude short-term use, providing you inform him he needs to take them after food. Topical NSAIDs could be offered as an alternative if Mr H is concerned about oral NSAIDs.

Safety Netting

You tell Mr H you think his back pain is probably due to some type of activity that has involved overstretching his muscles. You tell Mr H that it may be a few weeks before he fully recovers. If after a month he is still in pain or he finds his symptoms worsening, then he needs to be reassessed.

AIDE MEMOIRE

Likely Diagnoses
Nonspecific Acute Low Back Pain

Nonspecific low back pain may also be referred to as 'mechanical', 'musculoskeletal' or 'simple' low back pain.

Pain in the lower lumbar or sacral area is usually described as aching or stiffness. Depending on the cause, pain might be localised (e.g., lumbosacral strains after physical activity) or more diffuse (e.g., from postural backache after sitting incorrectly for a prolonged period). In cases of acute injury, the symptoms come on quickly and there will be a reduction in mobility. Bad posture when seated and poor lifting technique when performing day-to-day tasks, such as cleaning or gardening, are very common predisposing factors. Highest prevalence rates of low back pain are seen in people aged between 35 and 55 years.

Sciatica

Sciatica typically occurs in healthy middle-aged adults. Pain is acute in onset and radiates to the leg. Pain starts in the lower back and as it intensifies radiates into the lower extremity. If disc herniation is minimal, pain is dull, deep and aching. Pain spreads from the lumbar spine to the upper part of the leg. If the disc ruptures or herniates under strain, then pain is usually lancinating in quality, shooting down the leg like an electric shock. Valsalva movements, for example, coughing, sneezing or straining at stool, often aggravate pain. Numbness, tingling and muscle weakness in the distribution of a nerve root suggest nerve root compression. To confirm the diagnosis, a positive result of a straight leg raising test should be seen.

Possible Diagnoses
Ankylosing Spondylitis

Almost all cases occur before the age of 40 years, and it is two to three times more common in men and tends to run in families. Symptoms gradually worsen over a period of several months to several years. Patients commonly exhibit fatigue and have marked stiffness on awakening with pain that can alternate from side to side of the lumbar spine. Pain may awaken the person at night and worsens at rest but improves with physical activity. Pain can be made worse by bending, lifting and prolonged sitting in one position. Up to 40% of patients may also show inflammation of the eye.

Kidney Stones

Pain is abrupt in onset and starts in the loin, radiating around the flank and can be experienced in the right lower quadrant. Pain is very severe and colicky in nature. Attacks are spasmodic and tend to last minutes to hours and often leave the person prostrate with pain. The person is restless and cannot lie still. Symptoms of nausea and vomiting might also be present. It is twice as common in men than in women and usually occurs between the ages of 40 and 60 years.

Osteoarthritis

It is associated with advancing age, affecting up to one-third of people over 65 years of age and is twice as common in women. It can be localised to a single joint or involve multiple joints and most commonly affects the hands, knees, hips, neck and low back. It is characterised by pain of insidious onset that progressively increases over months or years and is exacerbated by exertion and relieved by rest. The affected joints are painful when used and may show a restricted range of motion. Stiffness in the affected joint can occur in the morning but usually only lasts for 15–30 min.

Osteoporosis

Often osteoporosis is asymptomatic and goes undiagnosed until a fragility fracture occurs, although nonspecific pain and/or localised tenderness is present if there is vertebral fracture. The condition is most common in postmenopausal women.

Pancreatitis

A mild attack can present with steady epigastric pain that can radiate to the back. Patents generally will have fever, nausea/vomiting with associated abdominal tenderness and elevated heart rate. It is commonly seen in those that misuse alcohol (25% of cases) or suffer from gallstones (50% of cases).

Shingles

Prior to the rash developing, pain can be experienced along the affected dermatome. This is typically stabbing or throbbing and can be severe.

Spinal Stenosis

Spinal stenosis usually develops slowly over time and is most common in people over the age of 50 years. It causes back and leg pain. Symptoms include low back pain, which can develop into sciatica-like pain that typically worsens with standing or walking and gets better with leaning forward. Weakness in the leg/s can be experienced as the stenosis worsens.

Urinary Tract Infection/Pyelonephritis

Unilateral flank pain that can be felt in the lower quadrant associated with nausea, vomiting and fever are typical presenting symptoms in association with lower urinary tract infection symptoms. Onset is often sudden.

Critical Diagnoses
Cauda Equina Syndrome

When the cauda equina nerve bundle is compressed, it can result in low back pain and sciatic nerve pain in both legs, bowel and/or bladder incontinence and loss of feeling in the inner thighs.

Infection (Osteomyelitis)

Symptoms of osteomyelitis include bone pain, general malaise and presence of high-grade fever. There may be local swelling, redness and warmth at the site of the infection. Patients also usually exhibit a loss of range of motion, limp or have a reluctance to weight bear.

Malignancy

A history of unexplained weight loss, presence of anaemia, and leg weakness might be seen in addition to low back pain. It is more prevalent in patients over 50 years of age. Patients normally have symptoms for months before diagnosis due to the slow growing nature of the tumour.

Vertebral Fracture

Fractures occur due to trauma of high impact (e.g., car accidents, sports injuries).

Moderate to severe pain will be experienced that is worsened with movement. Often injuries involve nerve involvement leading to bowel/bladder dysfunction, numbness, tingling or weakness in the limbs.

■ MCQs

1. Low back pain is generally understood to become 'chronic'. Which ONE of the following would back pain be classed as chronic?
   (a) 4 weeks
   (b) 6 weeks
   (c) 8 weeks
   (d) 12 weeks
   (e) 16 weeks

2. What proportion of the population will develop low back pain at some time in their lives?
   (a) 20%
   (b) 35%
   (c) 50%
   (d) 70%
   (e) 90%
3. Which ONE of the following is not a risk factor for developing chronic back pain?
   (a) Depressive symptoms
   (b) Heavy smoking
   (c) Nonsmoker
   (d) Obesity
   (e) Previous history of low back pain
4. Which ONE of the following symptoms is most suggestive of nerve root pain?
   (a) Localised pain in the lumbar region
   (b) Mild to moderate pain
   (c) Radiation of pain to foot
   (d) Reduced straight leg raising causing back pain
   (e) Weakness in both feet
5. Which ONE of the following statements is true of OA?
   (a) Inflammation is a key pathological finding.
   (b) Morning stiffness usually lasts less than 30 min.
   (c) OA commonly affects small joints.
   (d) Pain is eased by movement.
   (e) Pain is usually worst in the morning.
6. A 60-year-old man presents complaining of persistent lower back pain that radiates to the lower leg for the last 2 weeks. He tells you that the pain in the leg is a sharp shooting pain. He says he has been less active than normal and watching TV than usual. Which ONE of the following conditions best explains his symptoms?
   (a) Ankylosing spondylitis
   (b) OA
   (c) Sciatica
   (d) Scoliosis
   (e) Simple lower back pain

Answers

1. d; 2. d; 3. c; 4. c; 5. b; 6. c

KEY POINTS: NONSPECIFIC (SIMPLE) LOW BACK PAIN

- Not associated with an underlying cause – usually associated with musculoskeletal strain
- Key symptoms are pain and stiffness.
- Acute cases should resolve within 12 weeks.

WEBSITES

BackCare
http://www.backcare.org.uk/
National Axial Spondyloarthritis Society
https://nass.co.uk/

CASE 30: FACIAL PAIN

PRESENTATION

A 26-year-old woman (Miss K) presents with intermittent frontal headaches and pain on the left-hand side of her lower face near the jaw line. She says the problem has been going on now for a number of months. She describes the headaches and facial pain as aching and dull. She has been taking ibuprofen when the pain is bothersome, and it seems to help. She has no medical problems and takes no regular medication.

PROBLEM REPRESENTATION

A healthy 26-year-old woman complains of chronic aching unilateral facial pain and headache, which seems responsive to NSAIDs.

HYPOTHESIS GENERATION (LIKELY, POSSIBLE AND CRITICAL DIAGNOSES)

There are a number of conditions which have unilateral facial pain as a predominant symptom:

Likely Diagnoses

- Dental abscess or dental caries
- Postherpetic neuralgia
- Sinusitis
- Temporomandibular disorders (TMDs)
- Trigeminal neuralgia (TGN)

Possible Diagnoses

- Atypical facial pain
- Cluster headache
- Glossopharyngeal neuralgia
- Poststroke pain (not applicable in this case)
- Salivary gland disorders

Critical Diagnoses

- Giant cell arteritis (GCA)
- Glaucoma – acute
- Multiple sclerosis
- Tumours of nasopharynx

CONTINUED INFORMATION GATHERING

As Miss K describes her pain as aching and is chronic in nature. We can use this information to narrow down the list of likely diagnoses. The nature of her pain seems to point away from TGN (lancing); dental pain (throbbing); and postherpetic neuralgia (burning). When considering the duration of symptoms, this seems to further rule out dental problems, as they tend to have acute presentations.

Given the location of the facial pain – lower face near the jaw line – this seems to point toward TMD rather than sinusitis from the remaining likely causes.

At this point, knowing more about the pain, such as when does the pain occur, how long does it last, the exact location and its severity would be useful.

She tells you that her jaw pain is pretty much constant but not too bad, although it worsens when she chews. Her headaches are across her forehead and sometimes she says they spread across the rest of her head and toward the back of her neck.

Jaw pain that worsens on mastication, and the location of her headache, further points toward TMD.

The absence of nasal symptoms would further rule out sinusitis from your thinking. Miss K reports no nasal obstruction or loss of smell, two key symptoms associated with sinusitis.

PROBLEM REFINEMENT

To further test your differential diagnosis of TMD, other important features are restricted mandibular movement and noises from the TMD joints during jaw movement.

She tells you she has to be careful with what food she eats and always takes small bite-sized pieces of food as she does struggle to fully open her mouth and she hears clicking in her jaw sometimes when chewing.

Her symptoms are consistent with a diagnosis of TMD.

> ### ⚡ RED FLAGS
>
> Miss K has no symptoms that cause concern such as unilateral nasal symptoms (tumours), severe pain (cluster headache, glaucoma), visual changes (glaucoma, giant cell arteritis) and no neurological deficits (multiple sclerosis).

MANAGEMENT

Self-care Options

Although TMD is not life-threatening, it can be detrimental to quality of life because the symptoms can become chronic and difficult to manage. You ask how she is getting on with day-to-day activities and she reports that she is able to do everything. NSAIDs are the most effective medications, and Miss K has previously used ibuprofen and seems to get relief so should be encouraged to continue to use them. She could also be advised to try a soft diet.

Prescribing Options

A trial of amitriptyline or gabapentin could be offered to Miss K.

Safety Netting

Miss K should be told you think she has TMD and generally symptoms will improve over time and that she has been doing the right thing taking ibuprofen. If she agrees to a trial to manage neuropathic pain, then she should be reviewed after 8 weeks to assess the response.

AIDE MEMOIRE

Likely Diagnoses
Dental Abscess or Dental Caries

The main symptom is sudden onset unilateral pain in the affected tooth, which can be intense and throbbing. Other symptoms include pain on biting the tooth, tooth sensitivity to heat and cold, unpleasant taste in the mouth, fever and malaise. Associated swelling in the jaw, trismus (inability to open the mouth) or lymphadenopathy may indicate a spreading infection.

Postherpetic Neuralgia

Shingles often affects the trigeminal nerve and approximately 10% of people will experience postherpetic neuralgia, which may persist for months, although it usually resolves within a few weeks. It gives rise to either a continuous burning sensation that varies in intensity or an intermittent sharp or lightening pain that can be triggered by touch (akin to TGN). It is most commonly seen in elderly or immunocompromised people.

Sinusitis

Sinusitis is defined as inflammation of the paranasal sinuses caused by predominantly viral pathogens (e.g., common colds) but can be followed by a bacterial infection. It can affect any age group although it is more common in adults. Symptoms that are highly suggestive of sinusitis are nasal obstruction and discharge, and facial pain that can be severe. Other symptoms include frontal headache, fever, loss of smell and tenderness over the cheekbones. The pain can be bilateral but often has a unilateral predominance. The pain can also increase on lying down or bending over.

Trigeminal Neuralgia

TGN is defined as sudden, usually unilateral, severe brief stabbing recurrent episodes of pain in the distribution of one or more branches of the trigeminal nerve, most commonly the second (maxillary) and third (mandicular) branches. Attacks typically last seconds with refractory periods between attacks. Multiple attacks are common (e.g., people often have 10–30 attacks daily). Pain is often described as an electric shock. Pain can be triggered by simple tasks such as brushing teeth, air moving across the face (e.g., being out in the wind) or light touch to the skin of the face. It is more common in people over 50 years of age.

Temporomandibular Disorders

TMD is most common among people between the ages of 20 and 40 years, especially women. Symptoms include pain or tenderness in the face, jaw joint area, neck and shoulders and in or around the ear. Pain worsens on chewing, speaking or opening the mouth (where restricted jaw movements are often seen). Clicking noises are heard during mandibular movements. Patients with TMD also report headaches and otological symptoms. It can affect the person's quality of life because the symptoms can become chronic and difficult to manage.

Possible Diagnoses

Atypical Facial Pain

This tends to be diagnosis by exclusion. It is most common in women 30–50 years of age who have a history of psychological illness (e.g., stress, depression or anxiety). Pain, which is variable in nature, tends to be unilateral and experienced around the jaw and ear. Heat, cold or touch may trigger the pain.

Cluster Headache

Presents with short-lasting (15 min to 3 h) severe unilateral orbital or temporal pain that causes the patient to be restless (e.g., pacing the floor) due to pain severity. Associated nasal congestion, conjunctivitis/eye watering, drooping and swelling of one eyelid and facial flushing and sweating may be observed. Attacks often start at night. Typically, people experience bouts of attacks (clusters) that last week to months followed by lengthy periods of remission. It is more common in men.

Glossopharyngeal Neuralgia

The glossopharyngeal nerve supplies sensation to the posterior third of the tongue and oropharynx, which means pain is experienced at the back of tongue, tonsils and neck. Most patients will report one-sided throat pain (pain can be deep in the ear if there is vagus nerve compression). Other than location, glossopharyngeal neuralgia has the same characteristics as TGN and can be aggravated by swallowing, coughing and touching the ear. Glossopharyngeal neuralgia is a rare condition (e.g., 100 times less common than TGN).

Poststroke Pain

Pain is experienced on the same side as the stroke and can affect the whole side of the face or be periorbital. Pain, described as aching, burning or pricking sensation, is continuous and can develop months after the stroke. Touching the face can aggravate the pain.

Salivary Gland Disorders

Tumours, duct blockage and subsequent infection of the salivary glands elicit pain in the trigeminal nerve.

The pain is intermittent and characteristically occurs just before eating. There may be associated tenderness of the involved salivary gland.

Critical Diagnoses
Giant Cell Arteritis

Sudden onset continuous unilateral temporal headache is the predominant symptom in most patients. Scalp tenderness (classically pain on combing hair), visual changes and jaw pain are common symptoms. Less common symptoms include fever and upper respiratory infection (URTI) symptoms. Approximately half of patients have a history of polymyalgia rheumatica.

Glaucoma – Acute

Seen with increasing age, primary angle closure glaucoma may be acute, subacute or chronic. Acute cases are medical emergencies and present with abrupt onset severe eye pain with associated headache, nausea and vomiting. The eye appears red, the cornea can be cloudy and the patient experiences halos around lights. Eye examination shows the pupils are fixed and a decrease in visual acuity is seen.

Multiple Sclerosis

Multiple sclerosis may mimic TGN and cause intermittent lancing facial pain. It should always be considered, particularly in a younger adult who has neurological deficits (e.g., abnormal reflexes, muscle weakness, decreased sensation).

Tumours of Nasopharynx

These are rare forms of cancers. They are more common in those people over 50 years of age. Suspicion should be raised in those with persistent unilateral symptoms of nasal obstruction, nasal congestion and discharge, frequent nose bleeds and facial swelling.

▮ MCQs

1. Which ONE of the following medicines is not commonly used to treat neuropathic pain?
   (a) Amitriptyline
   (b) Duloxetine
   (c) Fluoxetine
   (d) Gabapentin
   (e) Pregabalin

2. Which ONE of the following symptoms is not a recognised feature of classical TGN?
   (a) Light touch provokes pain.
   (b) Pain occurs across two divisions of the trigeminal nerve.
   (c) Severe shooting pain lasts around 30 sec.
   (d) The initial attack of the pain was clearly memorable.
   (e) The pain occurs in conjunction with facial flushing.

3. Which ONE of the following medicines used in TGN is currently considered first line?
   (a) Carbamazepine
   (b) Lamotrigine
   (c) Oxcarbazepine
   (d) Phenytoin
   (e) Pregabalin

4. Which ONE of the following conditions is more likely to cause bilateral facial pain?
   (a) Glaucoma
   (b) Glossopharyngeal neuralgia
   (c) Sinusitis
   (d) TGN
   (e) TMD

5. Which ONE of the following conditions is least likely to be triggered by heat/cold or touching the face?
   (a) Atypical facial pain
   (b) Dental pain
   (c) Poststroke pain
   (d) TGN
   (e) TMDs

Answers
1. c; 2. e; 3. a; 4. c; 5. e

KEY POINTS: TEMPOROMANDIBULAR DISORDERS

- The causes are complex and multifactorial, involving anatomical and psychosocial factors and associated with the chewing system.
- Pain, popping or locking with jaw opening and limited jaw range of motion are key symptoms.
- Usually nonprogressive but often becomes chronic in nature
- Specialist investigation will be required if medicines fail to resolve symptoms.

WEBSITES

The Migraine Trust
https://migrainetrust.org/
TMJ Association
https://tmj.org/

CASE 31: FOOT PAIN

PRESENTATION

Mr O, a 33-year-old man, presents with a painful foot. He tells you that he has been experiencing a dull ache around the back of the heel that seems to be worse when he walks. He wants some help as he has been unable to go to the gym for the last week as his heel is too painful to exercise on. He is generally fit and healthy and takes no medicines from his doctor.

PROBLEM REPRESENTATION

A 33-year-old man presents with a 7-day history of acute onset heel pain impacting on his day-to-day activities.

HYPOTHESIS GENERATION (LIKELY, POSSIBLE AND CRITICAL DIAGNOSES)

The foot is traditionally divided into three regions: the hindfoot, the midfoot and the forefoot. Knowing the location of pain enables us to narrow down the possibilities that need to be considered. Mr O has presented with pain toward the back of his foot located around and behind his ankle; we are therefore dealing with conditions associated with heel pain, which could be:

Arthritic
Infectious
- Osteomyelitis

Mechanical causes
- **Heel pain – plantar**
  - Calcaneal stress fracture
  - Heel pad syndrome
  - Heel spur
  - Plantar fasciitis
- **Heel pain – Posterior**
  - Achilles tendonitis

- Ankle sprain
- Haglund's deformity
- Retrocalcaneal bursitis
- Sever's disease (children and adolescents)
- **Heel pain – midfoot**
  - Sinus tarsi syndrome

Neuropathic
- Nerve entrapment
- Tarsal tunnel syndrome

Tumour

Given the location and his age, we may be dealing with:

Likely Diagnoses
- Achilles tendonitis
- Ankle sprain
- Haglund's deformity
- Retrocalcaneal bursitis

Possible Diagnoses
- Arthritic conditions
- Calcaneal stress fracture
- Heel pad syndrome
- Heel spur
- Nerve entrapment
- Plantar fasciitis
- Sinus tarsi syndrome
- Tarsal tunnel syndrome

Critical Diagnoses
- Osteomyelitis
- Tumour

CONTINUED INFORMATION GATHERING

To differentiate between the likely causes of Mr O's heel pain we need to know more about the pain. Specifically, how the pain began and what intensifies it. Mr O tells you that he noticed the pain after a gym session. The pain was not obvious at the time but came on after being at the gym. He noticed the discomfort when he was walking home. Since then the pain is pretty much constant but not severe, but troublesome enough that he has not been able to go to the gym apart for a swim. He cannot recall any specific things which make the pain worse but he does know that he cannot put his weight fully on his foot, for example, if he tried to run, as the pain increases.

This description fits most closely with tendonitis or bursitis rather than ankle sprain or Haglund's deformity. In an ankle sprain, the level of pain and disability would generally be greater, and his symptoms would have been present for longer with Haglund's deformity.

PROBLEM REFINEMENT

You ask him if you can inspect the heel to look for any signs of swelling, lumps or bruising. There are no obvious signs of injury. Again, this seems to point away from sprains and deformity. You ask him to stand on his tip toes to see if the pain increases. He tells you that it does. You are now confident it is either Achilles tendonitis or retrocalcaneal bursitis but cannot differentiate between the two. Other possible causes seem unlikely, as he has no symptoms of burning, tingling or numbness (discount neuropathies) and acute presentation means arthritis, heel pad atrophy, heel spur or sinus tarsi syndrome can be excluded.

> ### ⚡ RED FLAGS
> Osteomyelitis (no systemic symptoms) and malignancy (short duration) do not need to be considered.

MANAGEMENT

Self-care Options

Mr O should be told that until the pain subsides, he should not do exercises that put excessive load on his heel.

Prescribing Options

Analgesia can be given in the short term. Using an NSAID to tackle any inflammation seems appropriate.

Safety Netting

You tell Mr O you are unsure of the diagnosis but are confident his symptoms are due to inflammation and an antiinflammatory should settle his symptoms, but if symptoms persist for more than 2 weeks he should be reassessed and, if appropriate, referred for physiotherapy.

AIDE MEMOIRE

Likely Diagnoses
Ankle Sprains

Ankle sprains are common injuries in all populations and are the most prevalent sports-related problem. Almost all present with lateral collateral ligament damage through excessive foot inversion. In addition to pain, swelling and bruising is common and is associated with limited weight bearing. An ankle sprain is usually obvious from the history, although in a small number of cases the patient may not recall a specific event that triggered symptoms.

Achilles Tendonitis and Achilles Tendon Rupture

Achilles tendonitis most commonly occurs in runners who have suddenly increased the intensity or duration of their runs. Pain typically begins as a mild ache across the heel with pain radiating up the calf when standing on tip toes. If the Achilles ruptures, there is immediate sharp pain which can be associated with swelling and an inability to bear weight on the leg.

Haglund's Deformity

Haglund's deformity is a bony enlargement on the back of the heel. The soft tissue near the Achilles tendon becomes irritated when the bony enlargement rubs against shoes. The symptoms include pain, swelling and redness at the back of the heel accompanied by a noticeable bump on the back of the heel. Mild cases usually involve episodic pain after long periods of inactivity.

Retrocalcaneal Bursitis

Retrocalcaneal bursitis is the inflammation of the bursa located between the calcaneus and the anterior surface of the Achilles tendon. Patients experience pain at the back of the heel, especially when pressure is placed on the heel (e.g., running uphill, standing on tip toes). Tenderness and swelling at the back of the heel may be present. The pain usually gets worse as the day goes on.

Possible Diagnoses
Arthritic Conditions

Typically presents with insidious onset which affects (symmetrically) the small joints. Pain, stiffness and swelling are key clinical features. Stiffness tends to be worse in the morning and pain worsened after periods of inactivity. Foot involvement normally affects the metatarsophalangeal joints. In early stages, the hindfoot may also be painful.

Calcaneal Stress Fracture

Calcaneal stress fracture is the second most common stress fracture in the foot. It is caused by repetitive overload to the heel. Patients often report onset of moderate/severe heel pain after an increase in weight-bearing activity or change to a harder walking surface. The pain initially occurs only with activity, but often progresses to include pain at rest (i.e., continuous pain). Examination may reveal swelling or ecchymosis. Point tenderness at the fracture site is usually indicative of a calcaneal stress fracture.

Heel Pad Syndrome

This is a chronic inflammation of the heel pad. Symptoms experienced are a generalised warm dull throbbing pain felt over the weight-bearing area of the heel, developing over a few months. Pain is typically worse in the morning. It often results from trauma or heavy heel strike and is also commonly seen in the elderly as their fat pads atrophy.

Heel Spur

A heel spur occurs when a calcium deposit grows between the heel and arch of the foot. They can be associated with intermittent or chronic pain particularly when walking, jogging or running. A sharp pain like a knife in the heel is experienced when standing up in the morning, which is then replaced by a dull ache in the heel throughout the rest of the day. Swelling, inflammation and warmth are seen over the affected area. They are often associated with plantar fasciitis.

Plantar Fasciitis

It is characterised by sharp, localised pain on the underside of the heel on initiation of activity, for example, with the first weight-bearing steps in the morning and after long periods of rest, although pain is often present continuously. Local tenderness is often observed. It most commonly affects people aged 40–60 years.

Nerve Entrapment (Medial and Lateral Plantar)

Symptoms include almost constant pain, whether walking or sitting. Pain increases with load bearing and just standing is often difficult. The pain is aggravated by high-impact activities such as running.

Sinus Tarsi Syndrome

Presents as persistent pain at the lateral side of the ankle and is secondary to traumatic injuries to the ankle, such as ankle sprain or overuse. Pain is most severe when standing or walking on uneven surfaces.

Tarsal Tunnel Syndrome (Jogger's Foot)

This presents as nocturnal burning heel pain/heel arch, tingling and numbness, which is made worse by weight bearing such as standing or walking. Patients typically find some relief by removing their shoes, foot elevation and massage.

Critical Diagnoses
Osteomyelitis

Symptoms of osteomyelitis include bone pain, general malaise and presence of high-grade fever. There may be local swelling, redness and warmth at the site of the infection. Patients also usually exhibit a loss of range of motion, limp or have a reluctance to weight bear.

Tumour

These are a very rare cause of heel pain and should be suspected in cases of heel pain that is persistent and unresponsive to treatment.

▮ MCQs

1. A 37-year-old man has recently taken up running to lose weight. He develops a sudden, persistent inferior heel pain radiating to the medial arch. Which ONE is the most likely diagnosis?
   (a) Baxter's neuropathy
   (b) Calcaneal stress fracture
   (c) Jogger's foot
   (d) Morton's neuroma
   (e) Plantar fasciitis
2. Which ONE of the following conditions is most likely to present with systemic symptoms?
   (a) Arthritis
   (b) Heel spur
   (c) Osteomyelitis
   (d) Retrocalcaneal bursitis
   (e) Tumour
3. Which ONE of the following conditions is more associated with older people?
   (a) Ankle sprains
   (b) Heel pad atrophy

(c) Heel spur
(d) Plantar fasciitis
(e) Retrocalcaneal bursitis

4. Which ONE of the following conditions can be as a consequence of repeated previous injuries?
(a) Haglund's deformity
(b) Nerve entrapment
(c) Retrocalcaneal bursitis
(d) Sinus tarsi syndrome
(e) Plantar fasciitis

5. Which ONE of the following conditions can see pain worsen as day progresses?
(a) Arthritis
(b) Heel pad atrophy
(c) Heel spur
(d) Plantar fasciitis
(e) Retrocalcaneal bursitis

Answers

1. e; 2. c; 3. b; 4. d; 5. e

KEY POINTS: ACHILLES TENDONITIS

- Usually related to direct injury
- The key symptom is pain at the back of the heel.
- Improvement should be seen in 12 weeks.
- Rest, painkillers and physiotherapy are the main interventions.

WEBSITES

CASE 32: FRONTAL HEADACHE

PRESENTATION

Mrs T, a 68-year-old woman, presents to you on a Saturday morning complaining of a persistent headache toward the front of her head which came on about 2 days ago. She has been taking paracetamol (two tablets (1000 mg) four times per day) but the pain is not being fully controlled. She asks you for a stronger painkiller.

PROBLEM REPRESENTATION

A 68-year-woman presents with a 2-day history of frontal headache uncontrolled by paracetamol.

HYPOTHESIS GENERATION (LIKELY, POSSIBLE AND CRITICAL DIAGNOSES)

As Mrs T's headache is the predominant symptom and frontal and acute in nature, our thinking is therefore initially focused on:

Likely Diagnoses

- Cluster headache
- Eye strain
- Glaucoma
- GCA
- Migraine
- Sinusitis
- TGN

Possible Diagnoses

- Acute illnesses (e.g., otitis media)
- Medication overuse headache
- Tension-type headache

Critical Diagnoses

- Carbon monoxide (CO) poisoning
- Glaucoma
- GCA
- Meningitis
- Raised intracranial pressure
- Severe hypertension

CONTINUED INFORMATION GATHERING

First, we need to establish the specific location of pain. You find out that the pain is located toward the front and both sides of her head. The location of her pain seems to point away from those conditions that affect the face, namely TGN, eye strain, sinusitis, cluster headache and glaucoma.

Based solely on location it appears that migraine and GCA are more likely. Establishing the nature of the pain and its severity should be determined. She says the pain is constant and debilitating. This description could equally apply to migraine and GCA and is not particularly discriminatory. However, the constant nature of the symptoms further rules out causes with intermittent pain, (e.g., cluster headache, TGN), and the debilitating nature excludes eye strain and sinusitis.

PROBLEM REFINEMENT

You now ask further questions on associated symptoms to try and differentiate between migraine and GCA.

Mrs T says apart from feeling generally a bit poorly she has not noticed anything specific such as nausea. Given nausea is experienced by most migraine sufferers, the absence of such symptom casts doubt on migraine being the cause.

As Mrs T is 68, her age also means migraine is less likely. It seems we may be looking at GCA as the cause of her symptoms. New onset headache is a cardinal symptom of GCA, and this appears to be a new headache for Mrs T. You ask Mrs T if she has had such symptoms before, to which she says no. GCA can present with a wide range of symptoms and include vision problems, jaw pain and systemic symptoms. Mrs T seems to be showing signs of possible systemic symptoms (e.g., off-colour).

You suspect she might have GCA and given the consequences of a late or misdiagnosis of GCA you decide to manage her headache as GCA.

> ⚡ **RED FLAGS**
>
> As giant cell arteritis is a medical emergency, there is no need to review for other red critical conditions.

MANAGEMENT

Self-care Options

Not applicable.

Prescribing Options

An urgent referral is required. As Mrs T reports no eye symptoms (visual loss or double vision) she should be given oral prednisolone 40 mg per day in consultation with a specialist. This is usually performed through a local GCA pathway, for example: https://www.newcastle-hospitals.nhs.uk/content/uploads/2021/02/GCA_Fast_Track_Pathway.pdf).

A definitive diagnosis will be through secondary care follow-up and involve erythrocyte sedimentation rate and C-reactive protein testing (both would be raised).

Safety Netting

You tell Mrs T you think she has GCA and that steroids will help but you need to arrange for her to go to hospital for more tests to confirm your diagnosis.

AIDE MEMOIRE

Table 6.1 summarises the presentation of conditions where headache is a predominant symptom (excludes medication overuse headache and severe hypertension).

■ MCQs

1. Migraine is known to be caused by various triggers. Which ONE of the following are known triggers?
   - (a) Chocolate
   - (b) Flickering lights
   - (c) Red wine
   - (d) Stress
   - (e) All of the above
2. From the following conditions, which ONE has features of rigid neck, high fever and altered mental status?
   - (a) Cluster headache
   - (b) Meningitis
   - (c) Migraine
   - (d) Tension-type headache
   - (e) TGN
3. A patient is experiencing a pulsating pain that has gradually increased in intensity over the last 3 h. The pain has started on the left forehead but is now present on both temples and the whole forehead. This is highly suggestive of which ONE of the following?
   - (a) Brain tumour
   - (b) Cluster headache
   - (c) Haemorrhage
   - (d) Migraine
   - (e) Tension-type headache
4. Which ONE of the following is a predisposing factor to developing migraine?
   - (a) Early onset menarche
   - (b) Family members who have migraines
   - (c) High blood pressure
   - (d) Obesity
   - (e) Smoking
5. A number of headaches are serious and potentially life-threatening. Which ONE of the following is NOT a life-threatening condition?
   - (a) CO poisoning
   - (b) GCA
   - (c) Hypertension with associated headache, fits and visual changes
   - (d) Meningitis
   - (e) Subarachnoid haemorrhage

Answers

1. e; 2. b; 3. d; 4. b; 5. b

TABLE 6.1 Summary of Presenting Signs and Symptoms for Conditions with Headache

	Duration	Timing and/or Nature of Pain	Location	Severity	Precipitating Factors	Who Is Affected	Associated Symptoms
Cluster headache	15 min to 3 h	Attacks occur at same time of day (often night). Intense boring pain	Unilateral orbital and/or temporal	Severe	Alcohol	Adults. Three to five times more common in men	Eye redness, nasal congestion, facial flushing and sweating
Carbon monoxide	Constant during exposure	Throbbing	Diffuse	Mild	None	All ages	Nausea, vomiting, vertigo, alteration in consciousness
Eye strain	Days	Aching	Frontal	Mild	Close vision work	All ages	Eye soreness, increased sensitivity to light; neck stiffness
Giant cell arteritis	Hours to days	Pain constant	Around temples, often both sides	Severe	History of polymyalgia rheumatica	Elderly, especially women	Temporal artery tenderness sometimes noticed, e.g., when brushing hair. Double vision and visual loss (30%). Pain on chewing. Systemic symptoms of fever, fatigue and weight loss
Glaucoma	Hours	Often in the evening and sudden onset	Unilateral and orbital	Severe	Darkness	Older adults	Red eye, blurred vision, impaired visual acuity, halos around lights. Nausea and vomiting
Meningitis	Hours to days	Migraine-like	Generalised	Severe	None	Children and adolescents	Neck rigidity, sudden high fever, altered mental or neurological changes besides nausea, vomiting along with the inability to tolerate light or loud sounds
Migraine	4–72 h	Throbbing pain	Usually unilateral	Moderate to severe	Food, menstrual cycle, stress and family history	Adults. Three times more common in women.	Nausea. Dislike of bright lights and loud noise. Reversible aura

Continued

TABLE 6.1 Summary of Presenting Signs and Symptoms for Conditions with Headache—cont'd

	Duration	Timing and/or Nature of Pain	Location	Severity	Precipitating Factors	Who Is Affected	Associated Symptoms
Neck pain and cervical spondylosis	Usually comes and goes	Aching	Back of head and can travel forward	Mild to moderate	None	Older adults	Pain may get worse on neck movement
Raised intracranial pressure	Days to months	Constant. Worse in the mornings	Variable	Moderate	Movement or straining	Older adults	Blurred vision, vomiting, changes in behaviour
Sinusitis	Days	Dull ache (though can be throbbing) that starts off being unilateral	Frontal	Mild to moderate	Pain can worsen on bending forward; recent history of an upper respiratory tract infection	Adults	Nasal blockage/discharge; reduction in sense of smell; localised tenderness
Subarachnoid haemorrhage	1–5 min up to 1 h	Variable	Occipital	Severe	None	Adults	Neck stiffness, visual disturbance, vomiting
Tension-type Headache	Hours to days	Symptoms worsen as day progresses. Nonthrobbing pain	Bilateral and most often at back of head	Mild to moderate	Stress due to changes in work or home environment	All ages	None
Trigeminal neuralgia	Seconds to minutes	Lancing/electric shock-like pain at any time	Unilateral, Face	Severe	None	Adults	In some people, nasal congestion or discharge, facial sweating and conjunctivitis

WEBSITES

Polymyalgia rheumatica and cell arteritis UK
https://pmrgca.org.uk/

CASE 33: KNEE PAIN

PRESENTATION

Mr K, a 35-year-old man, wants some advice about managing knee pain. He has been experiencing pain behind his right knee for the last 3 days since playing football with his friends. He has been having difficulty getting up and downstairs and changing gear in the car is difficult as the knee is painful. He has been taking paracetamol regularly to help with the pain. This seems to be helping but he is still in pain. He is generally fit and well but does have asthma, for which he uses salbutamol when needed.

PROBLEM REPRESENTATION

A 35-year-old man with asthma presents with a 3-day history of unilateral posterior knee pain affecting normal activities.

HYPOTHESIS GENERATION (LIKELY, POSSIBLE AND CRITICAL DIAGNOSES)

In generating a list of possible conditions to consider, knowing the general location and age of the patient is helpful to narrow down what we need to think about.

Thinking about age, conditions most associated with children and adolescents will be an unlikely cause of his symptoms, so the following conditions can initially be discounted:

- Patellar subluxation
- Tibial apophysitis (Osgood–Schlatter lesion)
- Jumper's knee (patellar tendonitis)
- Osteochondritis dissecans

If we then consider those conditions which are predominantly anterior in location, these too can be dismissed from our thinking. For causes of anterior knee pain, see Table 6.2.

We are therefore dealing with the following conditions:

Likely Diagnoses

- Anterior cruciate ligament (ACL) tear
- Hamstring tendinopathy
- Hyperextension injury

Possible Diagnoses

- Arthritis
- Baker's cyst
- Posterior cruciate ligament (PCL) tear

Critical Diagnosis

- Not applicable

CONTINUED INFORMATION GATHERING

It will be important to better understand exactly how the injury occurred and when the pain and swelling started. Mr K tells you that it just happened. He tried to get the ball, which meant he had to turn sharply back on

Outer Knee Pain	Pain at the Kneecap	Inner Knee Pain	Medial Pain Below the Knee	Pain Below the Knee
Iliotibial Band Syndrome	Patellofemoral Pain Syndrome	Medial Collateral Ligament Sprain	Medial Plica Syndrome	Patellar Tendonitis
Lateral Meniscus Tear	Chondromalacia Patella (runner's knee)	Medial Meniscus Tear	Pes Anserine Bursitis	Infrapatellar Bursitis
Lateral Collateral Ligament Injury	Housemaid's Knee			
Dislocated Patella	Bipartite Patella			

TABLE 6.2 Causes of Anterior Knee Pain

himself and as he did this his foot seemed to stay rooted to the floor, so his leg went one way and his foot the other. Straight away he knew something was up as he felt pain in his knee, and he could not carry on playing football. The pain was really strong and by the time he got home his knee was pretty swollen.

Given the abrupt nature of the injury an overuse cause such as hamstring tendinopathy can be excluded. The nature of how the injury occurred would also point away from a hyperextension injury. His description seems consistent with ligament damage, especially the ACL - immediate pain and swelling; PCL damage is much less common and is seen when a direct blow occurs to the proximal tibia. As the symptoms are associated with an acute injury, forms of arthritis can be discounted, as too can Baker's cyst.

PROBLEM REFINEMENT

A physical examination should be performed if competent to do so. A number of tests can be performed to help support your diagnosis. These include the Lachman, anterior drawer and pivot shift tests. Positive findings are often seen in ACL injuries.

You do perform the Lachman test which is positive.

> **⚡ RED FLAGS**
>
> Checks for loss of sensation/weakness in the lower leg are negative, which reassures you that there is no neurovascular damage.

MANAGEMENT

Self-care Options

He is currently taking paracetamol. You could advise him to take ibuprofen to help with the uncontrolled pain and swelling, provided he can tolerate NSAIDs (given he is asthmatic).

Prescribing Options

A referral to orthopaedics seems appropriate to further evaluate the injury and assess the severity of the problem, as this will dictate future treatments.

Safety Netting

You tell Mr K that you believe he has torn his ACL but it is very difficult to know to what extent and an onward referral is needed to do more tests, such as a magnetic resonance imaging scan. You tell him surgery is often

needed and recovery from such injuries will often be lengthy over several months.

AIDE MEMOIRE

Likely Diagnoses
Anterior Cruciate Ligament Tear

The majority of ACL injuries occur from awkward quick twisting movements of the knee, particularly when the foot is stuck to the ground. It can also occur as an impact injury caused through a blow to the side of the knee. Injuries range from a minor sprain/partial tear to a complete rupture and depending on the severity can take months to fully recover from. Immediate pain and rapid swelling (within 1–2 h) are observed and the person will find it difficult to bear weight on the leg or bend the knee. At the time of the injury, there is often an audible popping noise.

Hamstring Tendinopathy

Inflammation and irritation in the tendons on the back of the thigh is a common problem. It can be seen in two areas, either high hamstring tendonitis, where the tendons attach the hamstring muscles to the hip/pelvis causing lower buttock/upper thigh pain or low hamstring tendonitis, where the tendons attach the hamstring muscles to the back of the knee causing pain behind the knee that may radiate down the back of the calf. The commonest cause is an overuse injury from repetitive sports activities. Symptoms tend to develop gradually (unlike a hamstring muscle tear) with a dull aching pain or soreness. It can lead to stiffness and a decrease in flexibility that can make normal day-to-day activities such as walking or climbing stairs more difficult.

Hyperextension Injury

A hyperextended knee is where the knee joint bends too far backwards and is most commonly caused by a sporting injury. Pain tends to be mild to moderate accompanied by swelling and bruising. Depending on the severity of injury, swelling or bruising is immediate where damage is severe (e.g., ligaments completely torn) or develop over 24–48 h if damage is minor. Instability is common and the knee joint may feel unstable when standing or walking. Knee stiffness can lead to restricted movement.

Possible Diagnoses
Arthritis

Osteoarthritis. Usually OA of the knee is related to, but not caused by, ageing and most commonly affects people over the age of 50 years. Pain is usually observed while walking or when active (if located in medial and lateral tibiofemoral areas). Other symptoms experienced can include crepitus (clicking/grinding noises), joint stiffness (often in the morning but subsides quickly after waking), knee buckling or knee locking. OA usually develops slowly, and the pain it causes worsens over time.

Rheumatoid arthritis. Rheumatoid arthritis is much less common than knee OA and usually occurs after the age of 40 years. Multiple joints are generally affected, especially the hands, feet and neck. One of the most distinguishing features of rheumatoid knee arthritis is morning joint stiffness, lasting longer than 30 min. Other symptoms include joint pain, tenderness and swelling. Symptoms typically come and go.

Baker's Cyst

A Baker's cyst results from inflammation of the popliteal bursa and can be precipitated from a knee injury or underlying conditions such as OA or inflammatory arthritis. It tends to occur in people over the age of 40 years. The first symptom with a Baker's cyst tend to notice is a small bulge behind the knee, although pain behind the knee with associated tightness and stiffness can be experienced. Pain worsens with activity or when standing for long periods but eases on rest. The cyst is most noticeable on standing and may be tender on palpation. Rarely, it can rupture and present with similar symptoms of a deep vein thrombosis.

Posterior Cruciate Ligament Tear

Posterior Cruciate Ligament Tear Given the abrupt nature of the injury an overuse cause such as hamstring tendinopathy can be excluded. The nature of how the injury occurred would also point away from a hyperextension injury. His description seems consistent with ligament damage, especially the ACL – immediate pain and swelling. PCL damage is much less common and is seen when a direct blow occurs to the proximal tibia. As the symptoms are associated with an acute injury, forms of arthritis can be discounted, as forms of arthritis can be discounted, as can Baker's cyst.

▋ MCQs

1. A 15-year-old girl presents with right knee pain. Yesterday she was practising her dismount for her gymnastic routine when she heard a loud pop while landing. Her knee was painful almost immediately after falling and her knee began to swell meaning she could not carry on. Which ONE of the following is the most likely diagnosis?
   (a) ACL tear
   (b) Lateral collateral ligament tear
   (c) Medial collateral ligament tear
   (d) Medial meniscal tear
   (e) PCL tear

2. A young male adult presents with burning pain on the lateral side of his right knee. He is a regular gym user but the pain started when he started training to run a marathon. He feels the pain while running and it now persists for some time after being at the gym. Which ONE is the most likely diagnosis?
   (a) Iliotibial band syndrome
   (b) Lateral collateral ligament injury
   (c) Lateral meniscal tear
   (d) Patellofemoral pain syndrome
   (e) Popliteus tendinopathy

3. A 66-year-old man has noticed a lump at the back of his knee. It is not painful, and he states that it has been there for 2 weeks. On examination you note a transilluminable, nonpulsatile swelling. Which ONE is the most likely cause of this presentation?
   (a) Baker's cyst
   (b) Benign neoplasm
   (c) Meniscal cyst
   (d) Popliteal artery aneurysm
   (e) Septic arthritis

4. Crepitus of the knee is a common symptom. Which ONE of the following conditions is it least likely to be observed?
   (a) Bursitis
   (b) Osgood–Schlatter's disease
   (c) OA
   (d) Rheumatoid arthritis
   (e) Patellar dysfunction

5. Which ONE of the following is not an outer knee pain problem?
   (a) Dislocated patella
   (b) Iliotibial band syndrome
   (c) Lateral collateral ligament injury
   (d) Lateral meniscus tear
   (e) Medial meniscus tear

Answers
1. a; 2. a; 3. a; 4. a; 5. e

KEY POINTS: ANTERIOR CRUCIATE LIGAMENT INJURIES

- ACL injury is a common injury usually affecting young and active individuals.
- Immediate moderate to severe pain with associated swelling is the usual presentation.
- Often requires surgery but the final outcome is dictated not just by the ACL injury but also by associated injuries to the knee joint.

WEBSITES

Chartered Society of Physiotherapy
https://www.csp.org.uk/conditions/managing-pain-home/
    managing-your-knee-pain
British Orthopaedic Association
https://www.boa.ac.uk/
Tests to assess ACL rupture
https://www.clinicaladvisor.com/slideshow/slides/tests-to-
    assess-acl-rupture/

CASE 34: MENSTRUAL PAIN

PRESENTATION

Miss KA, a 22-year-old woman, presents with period pain that she says has been getting progressively worse over the last 12–18 months. She has no medical problems.

PROBLEM REPRESENTATION

A 22-year-old woman presents with long-standing but worsening period pain.

HYPOTHESIS GENERATION (LIKELY, POSSIBLE AND CRITICAL DIAGNOSES)

Pain associated with menstruation (dysmenorrhoea) is very common, with symptoms starting before or at the time of menstruation. Dysmenorrhoea can have a negative impact on person's quality of life. It is classified as either primary or secondary dysmenorrhoea. Primary dysmenorrhoea usually occurs in adolescence shortly after menarche where pain occurs in the absence of pelvic pathology, whereas secondary dysmenorrhoea usually occurs several years after the menarche and has an identifiable pathological cause.

Likely Diagnoses

- Adenomyosis
- Endometriosis
- Primary dysmenorrhoea

Possible Diagnoses

- Fibroids
- Intrauterine device (IUD)
- Irritable bowel syndrome (IBS)
- Ovarian cyst
- Pelvic inflammatory disease (PID)
- Premenstrual syndrome (PMS)
- Polyps
- Urinary disorders

Critical Diagnosis

- Cervical and ovarian cancer
- Ectopic pregnancy

CONTINUED INFORMATION GATHERING

From the conditions being first considered, her age suggests primary dysmenorrhoea. Exploring her menstrual history and pain is important. A menstrual history should cover length of menstrual cycle, regularity and duration; characteristics of pain should include type, duration, severity and timing.

Miss KA tells you her periods are regular and last for about 5 days. She describes the pain as cramping, which start about the same time as her period but is sometimes bad enough to make her miss work.

Miss KA's symptoms appear to align with primary dysmenorrhoea.

PROBLEM REFINEMENT

To further confirm your thinking, you ask about other symptoms. She tells you that occasionally she feels a bit sick at the start of her period but that does not happen that often. You also ask if she is sexually active at the moment or uses any forms of contraception. She says she is not and uses no contraceptive methods. At this point an IUD and ectopic pregnancy can be ruled out. Her symptoms are consistent with primary dysmenorrhoea.

Given her age, the nature of the pain and lack of other symptoms then adenomyosis and endometriosis seem very unlikely. Other possible secondary causes of dysmenorrhoea (e.g., fibroids, cysts and polyps) can also be discounted as she seems to have regular periods. The lack of other symptoms seems to exclude IBS, PID, PMS and urinary disorders.

Primary dysmenorrhoea seems to be the diagnosis.

⚡ RED FLAGS

Abnormal vaginal bleeding would raise suspicion of unusual or serious pathology. Miss KA has no such symptoms.

MANAGEMENT

Self-care Options

The mainstay of treatment is NSAIDs. However, she tells you she has been taking ibuprofen (400 mg three times a day) but this has not really controlled her symptoms very well. If she has not yet tried, you could suggest using local application of heat, for example, using a water bottle, although this lacks strong evidence.

Prescribing Options

A Cochrane review (Marjoribanks et al. 2015) suggests that when NSAIDs were compared with each other, there was little evidence of the superiority of any individual NSAID. It therefore seems an alternative NSAID would be of little value. You could suggest adding in paracetamol with ibuprofen or a combined oral contraceptive pill could be tried.

She decides to take paracetamol as well as ibuprofen as she is not keen on taking the pill.

Safety Netting

You tell Miss KA that you do not think there is anything sinister about her symptoms but obviously her symptoms are severe enough to be affecting her daily living. You tell her to try the additional pain relief for the next three menstrual cycles, and if she sees no improvement, then you would like to reassess her symptoms and discuss alternative therapy.

AIDE MEMOIRE

Likely Diagnoses

Adenomyosis

Adenomyosis occurs when endometrial tissue grows into the myometrium. It can be asymptomatic but if symptoms are experienced it can cause dysmenorrhoea (sharp, cramping or severe) and heavy periods, painful intercourse, lower abdominal discomfort/pressure and bloating. It tends to occur in women over 35 years of age and in those with increased parity.

Primary Dysmenorrhoea

Crampy suprapubic pain that occurs just before menses and lasts 2–3 days after onset is characteristic. Pain may radiate to the lower back and thighs. Associated symptoms may include nausea/vomiting, fatigue and bloating. Primary dysmenorrhoea tends to improve with increased age, parity and use of oral contraceptives. Other gynaecological symptoms are not usually present.

Endometriosis

Endometriosis occurs when endometrial tissue grows outside of the uterus, most commonly on fallopian tubes, ovaries or the tissue lining the pelvis, and is the most common cause of secondary dysmenorrhoea. Pain is experienced in the lower abdomen and pelvis, which starts prior to menstruation but symptoms worsen during menses. Patients may experience pain during or after sex and period related to gastrointestinal (GI) and urinary tract symptoms. It may cause abnormal bleeding but this is uncommon. A number of risk factors have been identified in people developing endometriosis and include a family history, early menarche, nulliparity and White ethnicity. It tends to be diagnosed in women in their 30s or 40s. Table 6.3 summarises these likely diagnoses.

TABLE 6.3	Condition Summary of Signs/Symptoms for Adenomyosis, Endometriosis and Primary Dysmenorrhoea				
	Type of Pain	Pain Other Than Dysmenorrhoea	Painful Sex	When Pain	Urinary and Gastrointestinal Tract Symptoms
Endometriosis	Sharp and possibly severe	Pelvic pain	Possible	Prior to menstruation	Common
Adenomyosis	Sharp	Pelvic pain	Possible	Throughout menstruation	Unusual
Primary dysmenorrhoea	Cramping	Lower back	Unusual	Start of menstruation	Common

Possible Diagnoses
Fibroids

Fibroids are common and thought to occur in 20%–50% of women older than 30 years of age, with the incidence increasing during the reproductive years which then decline after the menopause. They are frequently asymptomatic. If symptoms are experienced, then menstrual irregularity is prominent and accompanied with dysmenorrhoea, pelvic discomfort/pain or back pain, abdominal bloating, urinary tract (frequency, urgency and incontinence) and GI symptoms (constipation). Similar risk factors are seen in fibroids as endometriosis, although Black and Asian ethnicity is a risk factor compared with White ethnicity.

Intrauterine Devices

IUDs, especially copper IUDs, may cause worsening cramping period pains. These symptoms tend to settle in 3–6 months after insertion.

Irritable Bowel Syndrome

IBS is characterised by lower abdominal pain or discomfort and bloating. Unlike causes of dysmenorrhoea, changes in bowel habit and stool consistency are very common. Symptoms of pain and discomfort are frequently relieved by defecation. Other symptoms of lethargy, nausea, backache and bladder symptoms are common. Young adults (20–40 years old) are most affected.

Ovarian Cyst (Benign)

An ovarian cyst is a fluid-filled sac that forms on or in the ovary and is often asymptomatic, but sometimes, causes intermittent lower abdominal/pelvic pain or discomfort associated with heavy periods or bleeding between periods. Other symptoms include pain during intercourse, urinary frequency and constipation.

Pelvic Inflammatory Disease

Patients are often asymptomatic or exhibit mild symptoms. Vaginal bleeding between periods and after sex can be experienced and periods themselves can be painful and heavy. Other symptoms include lower abdominal and pelvic pain, vaginal discharge, painful sex, fever and dysuria. PID is almost always caused through a sexually transmitted disease and is therefore most commonly seen in younger women, especially those with multiple sexual partners.

Premenstrual Syndrome

PMS is characterised by symptoms that cause impairment of activities of daily living or affect quality of life. Symptoms occur between ovulation and the onset of menstruation and quickly subside when menstruation begins. Symptoms are wide-ranging and frequently categorised as physical or psychological, with many women experiencing a mixture of both. Period pain has been reported but is not a typical physical symptom, and other more prominent symptoms will be experienced (see Table 6.4).

Polyps

Uterine polyps are growths attached to the inner wall of the uterus that extend into the uterine cavity. They are usually benign and asymptomatic and affect women of all ages.

Abnormal menstrual bleeding is the most common symptom and appears to increase with age. This is often irregular and unpredictable, for example, having frequent, variable length and excessively heavy periods. Intermenstrual bleeding and postcoital bleeding can also be seen. Dysmenorrhoea is uncommon.

Urinary Disorders

Interstitial cystitis (bladder pain syndrome) is a disorder where the bladder is overly sensitive and leads to pain in the pelvic area and a frequent urgent need to urinate. Painful sex is common. Symptoms can mimic endometriosis.

Critical Diagnoses
Cervical Cancer

The most common symptoms of cervical cancer include unusual vaginal bleeding, pain during sex and low back and hip pain.

TABLE 6.4 Common Symptoms of Premenstrual Syndrome		
Physical	**Behavioural/Psychological**	
Swelling	Sleep disturbances	Anxiety
Breast tenderness	Appetite changes	Depression
Aches	Poor concentration	Feeling out of control
Headache	Irritability	
Bloating/weight	Mood swings	

Ovarian Cancer

Ovarian cancer is typically seen in older people, especially from 50 years upwards. There are usually no symptoms in the early stages, and unfortunately it is often detected late. Symptoms include abdominal bloating, feeling full, loss of appetite (leading to weight loss), pelvic/abdominal pain, urinary symptoms such as frequency and urgency and IBS-like symptoms. Other symptoms can include abnormal bleeding, dyspepsia and nausea.

Ectopic Pregnancy

Symptoms associated with ectopic pregnancy include abdominal and pelvic pain, vaginal bleeding, shoulder tip pain, urinary tract and GI symptoms.

■ MCQs

1. In a case of suspected uterine fibroids, which ONE of the following symptoms is most classically associated with this diagnosis?
   (a) Dysmenorrhoea
   (b) Dyspareunia
   (c) Menorrhagia
   (d) Pain in lower abdomen
   (e) Vaginal discharge
2. Clinical manifestation of PID includes which of the following?
   (a) Dyspareunia
   (b) Fever
   (c) Lower abdominal pain
   (d) Vaginal bleeding
   (e) All of the above
3. A 62-year-old woman presents with a 3-month history of vague lower abdominal discomfort and bloating, and more recently has noticed some vaginal spotting and cystitis-like symptoms. Based on these symptoms, which ONE of the following is most likely?
   (a) Cervical cancer
   (b) Endometriosis
   (c) Fibroids
   (d) Ovarian cancer
   (e) Ovarian cyst
4. PMS has a constellation of possible symptoms. Which ONE of the following would not be expected?
   (a) Abdominal bloating
   (b) Anxiety
   (c) Constipation
   (d) Breast tenderness
   (e) Weight loss
5. Which ONE of the following is not a risk factor for PID. Which ONE of the following is not a risk factor for PID?
   (a) Frequent vaginal douching
   (b) Multiple partners
   (c) Prior episode of PID
   (d) Recent placement of an IUD
   (e) Use of a diaphragm for contraception

Answers

1. c; 2. e; 3. d; 4. e; 5. e

KEY POINTS: PRIMARY DYSMENORRHOEA

- Starts shortly after menarche once cycles are regular and is due to overproduction of uterine prostaglandins
- Classically associated with lower abdominal cramping shortly before menstruation that lasts for 48–72 h
- NSAIDs and contraceptives are the mainstay of treatment.

WEBSITES/FURTHER READING

The Ectopic Pregnancy Trust
https://ectopic.org.uk/
British Fibroid Trust
http://www.britishfibroidtrust.org.uk/
Endometriosis UK
https://www.endometriosis-uk.org/
Heat therapy for primary dysmenorrhoea
Jo, J., & Lee, S. H. (2018). Heat therapy for primary dysmenorrhea: A systematic review and meta-analysis of its effects on pain relief and quality of life. *Scientific Reports*, 8(1), 16252. https://doi.org/10.1038/s41598-018-34303-z
Nonsteroidal anti-inflammatory drugs for dysmenorrhoea
Marjoribanks, J., Ayeleke, R. O., Farquhar, C., & Proctor, M. (2015). Nonsteroidal anti-inflammatory drugs for dysmenorrhoea. *The Cochrane Database of Systematic Reviews*, 2015(7), CD001751. https://doi.org/10.1002/14651858.CD001751.pub3

CASE 35: REQUEST FOR SUMATRIPTAN

PRESENTATION

Miss M, a 28-year-old woman not known to you, presents with a headache and requests the product Migraitan (sumatriptan) that her friend has recommended. She tells you the headache has been present since yesterday and has not shown response to the paracetamol she has taken. She is otherwise fit and healthy and has no medical problems.

PROBLEM REPRESENTATION

A 28-year-old woman with a 1-day history of acute onset headache unresponsive to paracetamol.

HYPOTHESIS GENERATION (LIKELY, POSSIBLE AND CRITICAL DIAGNOSES)

Acute headache is a symptom of many conditions, either as the main presenting symptom (e.g., migraine) or one of many symptoms (e.g., infections). For our patient, the conditions to consider in the first instance would be:

Likely Diagnoses

- Eye strain
- Migraine
- Sinusitis
- Tension-type headache

Possible Diagnoses

- Acute illnesses (e.g., otitis media)
- Cluster headache
- Medicines
- Medication overuse headache
- Neck pain/cervical spondylosis
- TGN

Critical Diagnoses

- CO poisoning
- Glaucoma
- Meningitis
- GCA
- Raised intracranial pressure
- Severe hypertension or hypertension in pregnancy
- Subarachnoid haemorrhage

CONTINUED INFORMATION GATHERING

As tension-type headache causes approximately 90% of all acute headache presentations in primary care, it is logical to hypothesise that this is the most likely cause of her headache even though migraines are three times more common in women, and Miss M has requested a product specifically for the treatment of migraine.

We need to know more about her headache and asking about the location, nature and severity of the pain is needed.

Miss M reports that her headache is pretty much constant and is best described as a pounding sensation, mainly on her left side and rates the pain as 6/10. These symptoms align with migraine as it is usually one-sided, throbbing in nature and moderate to severe in nature. This differs from tension-type headache that is generally associated with nonthrobbing bilateral pain that often starts towards the back of the head and pain tends to be mild to moderate. Other likely causes, such as sinusitis and eye strain seem unlikely as no facial pain has been reported (sinusitis) and severity of pain is moderate; eye strain symptoms would generally be milder.

PROBLEM REFINEMENT

To be more confident that Miss M is suffering from a migraine we should ask questions centring on associated symptoms. Almost all migraine sufferers experience nausea, with a smaller proportion having visual or neurological symptoms prior to the headache. Further symptoms of dislike to lights and noise would support migraine as the diagnosis. Miss M tells you she is feeling sick but has no other symptoms. This is consistent with a migraine diagnosis and further rules out the other likely causes being considered.

You could ask about a previous history of similar symptoms. If this is not their first migraine attack, they will normally have a history of recurrent and episodic attacks of headache. Miss M says this is the first time she has had such a headache.

Based on her age and overall symptom presentation, you believe this is a new onset migraine.

RED FLAGS

Given her symptoms, there appears to be no indication of any sinister pathology. For example, debilitating pain is seen in glaucoma, meningitis, giant cell arteritis and subarachnoid haemorrhage and mild pain in carbon monoxide (CO) poisoning. Location also is not consistent with glaucoma, CO poisoning, meningitis or subarachnoid haemorrhage. Symptoms with raised intracranial pressure would have been long-standing.

MANAGEMENT

Self-care Options

Sumatriptan can be bought over the counter but has greater restrictions on sale compared to when prescribed by a nonmedical prescriber or doctor. In this instance, Miss M should be discouraged from buying Migraitan as she has had the symptoms for over 24 h and the effectiveness of sumatriptan will be poor. However, using simple analgesia could be recommended, for example, ibuprofen at a dose of 400 mg three times a day, to help control the pain.

Prescribing Options

None for this episode. She could be offered sumatriptan if she experiences future episodes.

Safety Netting

You tell Miss M you agree with her self-diagnosis of migraine and that her symptoms should resolve within 48 h. You tell her that if her headaches worsen to contact you straight away. In addition, if her symptoms have not settled or disappeared after 48 h, she needs to come back so that her symptoms can be reassessed.

AIDE MEMOIRE

Table 6.1 summarises the presentation of conditions where headache is a predominant symptom (excludes medication-induced headaches).

MCQs

1. A 42-year-old woman presents complaining of a headache. Based on epidemiology alone, which ONE would be the most likely cause of her headache?
   (a) Cluster headache
   (b) Eye strain
   (c) Migraine
   (d) Sinusitis
   (e) Tension-type headache
2. A 37-year-old man wants some advice about a headache he has. He reveals that the pain is toward the back of his head. Which ONE of the following is most likely based on location?
   (a) Cluster headache
   (b) Migraine
   (c) Sinusitis
   (d) Subarachnoid haemorrhage
   (e) Temporal arteritis
3. Nausea and vomiting is most associated with which ONE of the following conditions?
   (a) Cluster headache
   (b) Sinusitis
   (c) Subarachnoid haemorrhage
   (d) Tension-type headache
   (e) TGN
4. Which ONE of the following statements is most suggestive of sinister pathology?
   (a) Headache lasting 7–10 days
   (b) Headache associated with cold-like symptoms
   (c) Headache associated with the workplace environment
   (d) Headache described as vice like
   (e) Headache in children under 12 years who have no sign of infection
5. Headache is the main presenting complaint in migraine sufferers. From the following descriptions, which ONE best describes symptoms of migraine?
   (a) Pain which is unilateral and throbbing
   (b) Pain which is unilateral and lancing
   (c) Pain which is unilateral, orbital and boring
   (d) Pain which is unilateral, frontal and dull
   (e) Pain which is unilateral, orbital and severe
6. When differentiating headaches from one another it is useful to consider other symptoms to aid diagnosis, with some symptoms warranting referral. From the list of symptoms below, which ONE would indicate referral?
   (a) Pain that worsens when bending over
   (b) Pins and needles in the arms before the headache starts
   (c) Scalp tenderness at the temples
   (d) Symptoms that last longer than 3 days
   (e) Symptoms that worsen as the day progresses

Answers
1. e; 2. d; 3. c; 4. e; 5. a; 6. c

KEY POINTS: MIGRAINE

- Causes of migraine not fully understood but involves genetic and neurologic pathophysiology
- Key symptoms are one-sided throbbing headache with associated nausea.
- Acute onset with prodromal symptoms and resolution generally within 72 h of onset
- Mainstay of treatment is a combination of analgesia, antiemetics and triptans.

WEBSITES

The Migraine Trust
http://migrainetrust.org
International Headache Society
http://www.ihs-headache.org/
Organisation for the Understanding of Cluster Headache (OUCH-UK)
https://ouchuk.org/
National Headache Foundation
http://www.headaches.org/
Lifting the Burden – The Global Campaign Against Headache
https://www.l-t-b.org/

CASE 36: SHOULDER PAIN

PRESENTATION

Mr D, a 55-year-old man, presents with right shoulder pain. He says it is slowly getting worse and he is finding using his arm difficult. He tells you, it has been going on for about 3 months or so now. He has a history of cardiovascular disease and takes simvastatin and lisinopril.

PROBLEM REPRESENTATION

A 55-year-old man presents with a 3-month history of worsening shoulder pain.

HYPOTHESIS GENERATION (LIKELY, POSSIBLE AND CRITICAL DIAGNOSES)

Decreased shoulder movement can affect a person's ability to work or carry out daily activities. Patients present with pain, stiffness or weakness that can cause substantial disability. In primary care, six common causes of shoulder pain are seen, although it is not uncommon for more than one pathology to coexist.

Likely Diagnoses

- Adhesive capsulitis (frozen shoulder)
- Acromioclavicular joint disorders
- Glenohumeral instability
- Glenohumeral OA
- Referred neck pain
- Rotator cuff damage

Possible Diagnoses

- Inflammatory arthritis
- Polymyalgia rheumatica
- Referred pain other than from the neck
- Septic arthritis

Critical Diagnoses

- Malignancy (primary, metastases)
- Referred pain – myocardial ischaemia

CONTINUED INFORMATION GATHERING

His age is useful in shaping our thinking. In those under 40 years old, shoulder instability or mild rotator cuff disease are more likely and in those over 40 years old, more advanced chronic rotator cuff disease, adhesive capsulitis, types of arthritis or glenohumeral OA are seen. It seems reasonable to explore these conditions first as the cause of his symptoms.

We know when the pain started, but there is a need to establish where the pain is, the type of pain and any associated symptoms.

He tells you the pain feels like an aching sensation across his shoulder but apart from the stiffness he has no other symptoms. You explore further the stiffness he reports. He tells you that it is only recently started but he finds moving his arm difficult especially when getting dressed.

Stiffness affecting his day-to-day activities suggests a reduced range of motion. These symptoms, coupled with his age, align more with rotator cuff syndrome and frozen shoulder more than arthritic causes. It also further supports our original thinking of it not being acromioclavicular joint disorders or referred neck pain.

PROBLEM REFINEMENT

Tests for range of motion should be performed. In frozen shoulder, there should be marked reductions in all range of motion, but with rotator cuff injury this tends to be limited to overhead activities.

You get him to raise his hand as though asking a question, then ask him to touch the back of his neck with both hands and then to touch between the scapulae with both hands. The results show that he has difficulty performing all three tests. This supports a diagnosis of frozen shoulder.

You also ask about his lifestyle and occupation as rotator cuff is associated with certain activities. He tells you he works in an office and rarely exercises. This history is unremarkable but does imply that his occupation is not contributing to his symptoms.

> ⚡ **RED FLAGS**
>
> Mr D has no other symptoms so other forms of referred pain, arthritis and malignancy can be excluded.

MANAGEMENT

Self-care Options

He should be told to continue to use his arm where possible and avoid activities that worsen the pain. Mr D could be signposted to organisations that provide self-help materials (see website).

Prescribing Options

Mr D should be offered simple pain relief such as ibuprofen 400 mg three times a day.

Safety Netting

You tell Mr D you think his symptoms are caused through a frozen shoulder, and it may unfortunately persist for many weeks or months. However, you ask if he will return after 4 weeks to assess symptoms and see if conservative treatment has helped. If his symptoms are not improving, then referral for physiotherapy is an option or a steroid injection should be considered.

AIDE MEMOIRE

Likely Diagnoses
Acromioclavicular Joint Disorders

Usually secondary to trauma, so a history of an injury to the joint or performing certain activities (e.g., weightlifting) is consistent with the diagnosis. Pain, tenderness and occasional swelling are localised to the lateral tip of the shoulder. A cross-body adduction test will induce pain.

Adhesive Capsulitis (Frozen Shoulder)

This refers to a painful shoulder in which there is marked restriction in all the major ranges of motion. Often there will be a history of impaired external rotation (e.g., putting on a jacket) but the person may well not remember any event that precipitated symptoms. Pain and stiffness tend to be gradual in onset; pain can be worse at night. Frozen shoulder is said to have three overlapping phases: pain phase (last 2–9 months); stiffness phase (last 4–12 months); resolution phase (lasts in excess of 12 months). It is more common in people with diabetes and thyroid disease. It is more common in people over the age of 40 years.

Glenohumeral Instability

The glenohumeral joint has the highest range of motion of the human body and is therefore inherently unstable. This instability leads to disorders, including dislocation and subluxation. The patients are usually younger than 40 years and have a history of dislocation or subluxation events, which is often involved with collision or overhead sports. Symptoms include pain, weakness and reduced arm movement that can interfere with daily living. A positive apprehension test is consistent with the diagnosis.

Glenohumeral Osteoarthritis

Glenohumeral OA usually presents as progressive deep joint pain and loss of motion in patients older than 60 years. A history of arthritis and previous shoulder surgery are known risk factors.

Referred Neck Pain

Typically, there is pain, stiffness and tenderness of the lower neck and at the top of the scapular. Pain tends not to be worsened with movement of the shoulder. Weakness and numbness or abnormal sensations in the shoulder and arms can also be experienced.

Rotator Cuff Damage

Typically, the patients are older than 40 years and complain of pain in the top and lateral aspect of the arm with radiation no farther than the elbow. Symptoms can interfere with daily activities, such as raising the arm or doing overhead activities. Pain is often worse at night, and resisted movements are painful. An occupational history may reveal heavy lifting or repetitive movements, especially above shoulder level.

Possible Diagnoses

Inflammatory Arthritis

Typically affects the small joints of the hands and feet but can affect other joints such as the shoulder. Pain, swelling and stiffness of the joint are usual. Symptoms are symmetrical.

Referred Pain Other Than From the Neck

Usually pain is not influenced by shoulder movements. Examples of referred pain include gallbladder symptoms, where pain may refer to the right shoulder; elbow pain, particularly epicondylitis, may refer upwards to the shoulder.

Polymyalgia Rheumatica

The typical symptoms are aching and stiffness about the upper arms/shoulders, neck and hips. Symptoms develop quickly and are worse in the morning. It is most commonly seen in those over the age of 50 years. Other symptoms that may be experienced are fatigue, fever and loss of appetite. It rarely causes swollen joints.

Septic Arthritis

Sudden onset of pain in one joint, which can be severe, that is accompanied with swelling, skin reddening/heat. Constitutional symptoms and fever are also usually present.

Critical Diagnoses

Malignancy (Primary, Metastases)

Malignancy should be suspected where persistent pain is not relieved by routine measures and steadily gets worse over time. Night pain is also seen. As with other cancers, unexplained weight loss, loss of appetite and fatigue can be observed.

Referred Pain – Myocardial Ischaemia

Typically, a heart attack will be sudden onset chest pain, feeling sick, sweating, shortness of breath, anxiety and pain that may spread to the jaw, neck, shoulder and arm.

▮ MCQs

1. Which ONE of the following is the most common type of shoulder problem?
   (a) Acromioclavicular joint disorders
   (b) Frozen shoulder
   (c) Glenohumeral OA
   (d) Partial or full dislocation
   (e) Rotator cuff injuries
2. Which ONE of the following causes of shoulder pain is least associated with night pain?
   (a) Acromioclavicular joint disorders
   (b) Adhesive capsulitis (frozen shoulder)
   (c) Malignancy
   (d) Rotator cuff damage
   (e) None of the above
3. Which ONE of the following causes of shoulder pain is more commonly seen in younger people?
   (a) Acromioclavicular joint disorders
   (b) Adhesive capsulitis (frozen shoulder)
   (c) Glenohumeral OA
   (d) Polymyalgia rheumatica
   (e) Rotator cuff
4. Which ONE of the following causes of shoulder pain is least associated with constitutional symptoms?
   (a) Glenohumeral osteoarthritis
   (b) Inflammatory arthritis
   (c) Malignancy
   (d) Polymyalgia rheumatica
   (e) Septic arthritis
5. In which ONE of the following conditions would there be the greatest reduction in the range of motion?
   (a) Acromioclavicular joint disorders
   (b) Frozen shoulder
   (c) Glenohumeral OA
   (d) Polymyalgia rheumatica
   (e) Rotator cuff injuries

Answers

1. e; 2. a; 3. c; 4. a; 5. b

KEY POINTS: FROZEN SHOULDER

- Caused by inflammation and thickening of shoulder tissue
- Key symptoms are limited movement with associated pain and stiffness.
- Generally lasts months

WEBSITES

British Elbow and Shoulder Society (BESS)
https://bess.ac.uk/patient-information/

CASE 37: WRIST PAIN

PRESENTATION

Mrs V, a 44-year-old Caucasian woman, asks for your advice about wrist pain she has been experiencing for about 6 weeks. She describes the pain as soreness and aching as well as having tingling in her fingers. She reports no other symptoms and is currently taking no medication, either prescribed or over the counter.

PROBLEM REPRESENTATION

A 44-year-old woman presents with a 6-week history of wrist pain and numbness.

HYPOTHESIS GENERATION (LIKELY, POSSIBLE AND CRITICAL DIAGNOSES)

Wrist pain is classified as acute, caused by a specific sudden injury such as a sprain or fracture, or as subacute or chronic long-term pain, resulting from factors such as repetitive stress, arthritis and nerve entrapment. In this case, we can rule out sudden impact as Mrs V has had the symptoms for a number of weeks. We therefore do not need to consider fracture, joint subluxation or ligament tears.

Mrs V does describe sensory disturbances; conditions that can present with tingling should first be considered.

Likely Diagnoses

- Nerve entrapment
  - Carpal tunnel syndrome
  - Ulnar nerve entrapment
- Ganglion cyst

Possible Diagnoses

- Systemic causes
  - Gout
  - OA
  - Rheumatoid arthritis
- Tendinopathy

Critical Diagnosis

- Not applicable

CONTINUED INFORMATION GATHERING

We know Mrs V has reported soreness, aching and tingling sensations in her wrist but we need to know the specific location of these symptoms. For example, carpal tunnel affects the thumb and middle fingers; ulnar entrapment, the fourth and fifth fingers; and ganglion cyst, location whilst variable, is often experienced on the top of the wrist. Mrs V reports the pain is across the inside of her wrist and she has been getting 'pins and needles' mainly in her right little finger.

This seems to align with ulnar entrapment.

You ask further questions about the nature and timing of the pain. She reports that the pain is more discomfort than true pain and seems to be constant. This presentation seems to further support ulnar entrapment. If her symptoms were caused by carpal tunnel syndrome, then night pain is prominent.

PROBLEM REFINEMENT

To support your thinking, you perform a physical examination and find no obvious swelling or tenderness but tapping over the pisiform bone induces tingling in her little finger. You are now reasonably confident you are dealing with ulnar nerve entrapment but you check to see if her symptoms are worse at any given time or if any activities worsen symptoms.

Mrs V reports only wrist pain and has not noticed any other symptoms. This seems to rule out OA, rheumatoid arthritis, gout and tendinopathy, especially as the location of Mrs V's pain would be unusual for these conditions.

RED FLAGS

It is important to consider any nerve involvement in the entire limb, including the neck. As ulnar nerve entrapment is your working diagnosis, it would be prudent to exclude nerve compression at the elbow (cubital tunnel). Mrs V reports no symptoms above the wrist.

MANAGEMENT

Self-care Options

Treatment of ulnar nerve entrapment is aimed at the underlying cause. In many cases, the cause of the compression can be identified (e.g., through work-related behaviours or sports activities). You find out she works mostly at a desk job but has not had any changes in her work schedule. It might be worth advising her to ask for an occupational assessment of her work practice/environment to see if this is contributing to her symptoms.

Prescribing Options

For Mrs V, NSAIDs could be offered to help ease the pain, and if symptoms persist you could suggest physiotherapy.

Safety Netting

You tell Mrs V that you believe her problem is due to one of her nerves in the wrist being trapped and explain to her that the prognosis of most ulnar neuropathies is good, although symptoms often take weeks, if not months to resolve. A follow-up appointment with Mrs V should be made in 6 weeks unless her symptoms worsen.

AIDE MEMOIRE

Acute Causes (Not Applicable in This Case)

A sudden impact, for example, when a person falls forward onto an outstretched hand, can cause sprains, strains and even fractures.

Fracture

The scaphoid is the most commonly fractured carpal bone, and this usually happens after falling onto an outstretched hand. Physical examination may reveal a swollen wrist with tenderness. Swelling of the anatomic snuffbox increases the likelihood of a scaphoid facture as the scaphoid is located below the snuffbox.

Joint Subluxation

A joint subluxation is a partial dislocation of a joint. It is often the result of acute injury or repetitive action. Symptoms include pain and swelling around the joint, a loss of range of motion, temporary loss of feeling or numbness and joint instability.

Ligament Tears

As with fractures, acute traumatic injury can damage ligaments of the wrist/hand. Commonly, the triangular fibrocartilage complex is involved. Symptoms include swelling, bruising and difficulty with wrist movements. A positive (increased pain) ulnar fovea sign indicates ligament damage.

Likely Diagnoses
Nerve Entrapment

Ulnar neuropathy. This is due to compression of the ulnar nerve as it passes through the elbow or wrist. Entrapment is commonest at the elbow and is the second most common neuropathy of the upper extremity. It is most commonly seen in men over the age of 35 years. Entrapment at the elbow occurs when there is prolonged stretching of the nerve by keeping the elbow fully bent or when there is direct pressure on the nerve from leaning the elbow against a solid surface. Entrapment at the wrist can occur when there is direct pressure on the nerve, which is of long duration or repetitive in nature. It can simply occur by leaning on the elbows habitually. With repeated activity such as golf or tennis, the nerve may become entrapped by surrounding structures.

Symptoms first experienced are wrist discomfort and numbness and/or tingling in the fourth (ring) and fifth (little) fingers. However, in severe/chronic cases grip weakness or tenderness in the hand are seen.

Carpal tunnel syndrome. This is the most common entrapment syndrome affecting the upper extremities. It is more commonly seen in women and in certain occupations, for example, people who work in the sewing, cleaning and packing industries. In addition, certain conditions, such as obesity and diabetes, can increase the risk of developing carpal tunnel syndrome.

It occurs when the median nerve is compressed as it passes through the carpal tunnel. This compression can cause numbness in the thumb and the three middle fingers of your hand. Insidious pain at the wrist is often an early symptom. It can make it hard to grip an object with one or both hands. It also causes pain or numbness in one or both hands, especially at night. Shaking the wrist can relieve symptoms.

Various tests can be performed to help with the diagnosis and include the Phalen's test, Tinel's test and tourniquet test.

Ganglion Cyst

A ganglion cyst is the most common soft tissue mass in the hand affecting adults. The dorsal wrist (on the back or the upper side of the wrist) is most affected. In most cases, other than a compressible and moveable mass, there are no symptoms. Occasionally, they can cause pain and tingling in the hand if the cyst presses on a nerve. They often resolve spontaneously.

Possible Diagnoses
Systemic Causes

Osteoarthritis. OA can be seen in the metacarpophalangeal joint of the thumb. It is a very common condition that predominantly affects postmenopausal women. It presents with pain (often likened to toothache) at the base of the thumb, which is activity related, particularly gripping, using taps and doorknobs, unscrewing lids or turning keys. Pain is worse with joint use and is relieved by rest.

Rheumatoid arthritis. It can commonly involve the wrist; although if one wrist is affected, the other one usually is too. There may be prolonged morning stiffness and pain with signs of joint swelling. Pain is also usually worse when the joint is rested or inactive.

Gout. Gout is classically associated with the big toe; however, it can affect the elbow, wrist and finger joints. Gout solely affecting the wrist is rare. Symptoms associated with wrist involvement include swelling of the wrist and/or hand and hotness, redness and/or tenderness of the affected joint/s. Symptoms are sudden in onset but can last a number of weeks during each episode.

Tendinopathy

De Quervain's tenosynovitis (writer's cramp). Two major dorsal tendons of the thumb are involved: the extensor pollicis brevis and the abductor pollicis longus. These tendons run in a synovial sheath in the first extensor compartment of the hand. Inflammatory changes in the sheath and tendons result in tenosynovitis. It is more common in women, particularly those of 30–50 years of age.

The typical presentation includes radial wrist pain at the thumb base and into the distal radius (part of the radius connected to the wrist joint). Aching aggravated by activity and relieved by rest is characteristic. Patients may identify a new or repetitive hand-based activity as the cause.

Physical examination may reveal a minimally swollen wrist with local tenderness and sometimes around the soft tissues of the anatomic snuffbox. Thumb motion is invariably painful. The Finkelstein's test is confirmatory. The condition is normally self-limiting and generally resolves after a year.

▌ MCQs

1. Which ONE of the following symptoms is most associated with carpel tunnel syndrome?
   (a) Finger stiffness
   (b) Hand tremors
   (c) Numbness in the little finger
   (d) Numbness in the thumb
   (e) Sweaty palms

2. Which ONE of the following is not commonly associated carpal tunnel syndrome?
   (a) A positive Phalen's test
   (b) Burning and tingling in the fingers
   (c) Pain that is worse at night
   (d) Sweaty palms
   (e) Weak grip

3. Which ONE of the following tests is least helpful in providing a diagnosis in a patient with pain in the thumb, index finger and middle finger?
   (a) Durkan test
   (b) Finkelstein's test
   (c) Phalen's test
   (d) Tinel's test
   (e) Tourniquet test

4. Which ONE of the following structures is most affected when a person suffers a sudden impact when falling on to an outstretched hand?
   (a) Lunate
   (b) Pisiform
   (c) Scaphoid
   (d) Trapezium
   (e) Triangular fibrocartilage complex

5. Wrist pain associated with morning stiffness is commonly seen in which ONE of the following conditions?
   (a) Carpal tunnel syndrome
   (b) Joint subluxation
   (c) OA
   (d) Rheumatoid arthritis
   (e) Tendinopathy

Answers
1. d; 2. d; 3. b; 4; c; 5. d

KEY POINTS: ULNAR NERVE ENTRAPMENT

- Caused by compression of the ulnar nerve in the Guyon canal
- Key symptoms are numbness and/or tingling in the fourth and fifth fingers.
- May take weeks/months to fully resolve

7

Respiratory Problems

CASE 38: CHILD WITH CROUP-LIKE SYMPTOMS

PRESENTATION

A young mother brings her son into your clinic. She appears to be quite anxious. She explains that her son (18 months old) has been violently coughing, with difficulty in breathing all night. Although easier this morning, he is still coughing a lot and a bit breathless.

PROBLEM REPRESENTATION

An 18-month-old child presents with a 12–24-h history of respiratory difficulty.

HYPOTHESIS GENERATION (LIKELY, POSSIBLE AND CRITICAL DIAGNOSES)

Croup (laryngotracheobronchitis) is the commonest cause of inspiratory stridor and manifests itself with cough and difficult/noisy breathing. It tends to be a frightening experience for parents and the child. It is important to differentiate croup from other problems which cause upper airway obstruction, as most are medical emergencies.

Likely Diagnosis
- Croup

Critical Diagnoses
- Anaphylaxis
- Bacterial tracheitis
- Epiglottitis

- Foreign-body aspiration
  - Tracheal
  - Oesophageal
- Peritonsillar abscess
- Retropharyngeal abscess

CONTINUED INFORMATION GATHERING

We already know that the child has a cough for up to 24 h. This is diagnostically useful as cough associated with foreign-body aspiration, anaphylaxis and epiglottitis present with very sudden onset. These conditions are therefore unlikely to be the cause of his cough.

You ask her to describe what the cough sounds like and if she had noticed any other problems prior to or during the bouts of coughing that she has not mentioned.

The mother reports he has had a mild fever and a runny nose for a few days and the cough has a barking-like quality. This supports croup as the diagnosis as there is often a history of prodromal symptoms and the cough is often described as having a barking/seal-like quality. Furthermore, the presence of fever means a diagnosis of foreign body or anaphylaxis is unlikely.

A negative history of drooling will eliminate epiglottitis (this is highly sensitive and specific to epiglottitis). No drooling is reported.

Her son's symptoms appear to be a case of croup but bacterial tracheitis still needs to be eliminated.

PROBLEM REFINEMENT

If swallowing is normal, this will point strongly to a diagnosis of croup, as this is difficult in bacterial tracheitis.

The mother reports no problems swallowing. You are confident that her son has croup.

 RED FLAGS

A final check of his symptoms to rule out anaphylaxis should be made, for example, checks for angiooedema. His mother says she has not seen any swelling in and around the face.

MANAGEMENT

Self-care Options

Not applicable.

Prescribing Options

Given your assessment, the child has mild to moderate croup. Hospital admission should be considered. A single dose of oral dexamethasone (150 mcg/kg) should be given and, if symptoms persist, hospital admission should be arranged.

Safety Netting

You say to the patient's mother that you think he has croup. You will give him an injection to help with his symptoms and once he is stable, he can go home. You also signpost the parent to written material (see Websites) so the parents can help their child if he suffers from future attacks.

AIDE MEMOIRE

Likely Diagnosis

Croup

Croup is a frequent cause of respiratory distress in young children and results from inflammation and/or swelling of the larynx, trachea and vocal cords. It mainly affects children aged between 6 months and 3 years. The incidence is highest between 1 and 2 years of age and occurs slightly more in boys than girls; it is more common in autumn and winter months. Prior to the cough, upper respiratory tract symptoms, including coryza and nasal congestion/discharge, may have been present for between 12 and 72 h. Croup symptoms occur in the late evening and night and involve inspiratory stridor and cough which is described as having a barking (seal-like) quality. In between episodes of coughing,

the child may be breathless and struggle to breathe properly. Typically, symptoms improve during the day and often recur again the following night, with the majority of children seeing symptoms resolve in 48 h. For management purposes, it is classed as mild, moderate or severe:

Mild croup: no stridor at rest, barking cough

Moderate croup: moderate stridor at rest, barking cough, no or little agitation

Severe croup: significant stridor at rest with severe respiratory distress, including sternal recession. The child may appear anxious, pale and tired.

Critical Diagnoses

Anaphylaxis

Urticaria and/or angiooedema are often the first signs of anaphylaxis. The person will look and feel unwell. Airway swelling, breathlessness, wheeze and stridor will be present. Signs of shock may be present, including increased pulse rate, dizziness and looking pale and clammy.

Bacterial Tracheitis

The child usually appears very unwell with high fever, sudden onset stridor and respiratory distress. It usually follows a viral-like respiratory illness.

Epiglottitis

Onset is usually acute, with a few hours of high fever, lethargy, inspiratory stridor and rapidly worsening respiratory distress. Cough is usually minimal or absent. The child will appear anxious, pale and 'toxic', and is often sitting immobile with their chin slightly lifted and mouth open drooling saliva.

Foreign-body Aspiration

Usually there is a clear history of foreign-body inhalaion or ingestion. Where the trachea is involved, patients present with sudden choking followed by protracted cough and respiratory distress and stridor. In oesophageal cases, symptoms tend to be milder, with symptoms of difficulty in swallowing and epigastric discomfort.

Peritonsillar and Retropharyngeal Abscess

Peritonsillar or retropharyngeal abscess can present with dysphagia, drooling, stridor, dyspnoea, rapid breathing, neck stiffness, fever and unilateral cervical adenopathy. Onset is typically more gradual than with croup. Table 7.1 summarises these diagnosis.

TABLE 7.1   Condition Summary of Croup and Conditions Presenting With Croup-like Symptoms

	Croup	Tracheitis	Epiglottitis	Foreign-body Aspiration	Anaphylaxis	Abscess
Age	6 months to 3 years	Any age	2–6 years	<4 years	Any	Any
Onset	Gradual	Gradual	Sudden	Sudden	Sudden	Gradual
Fever	Low grade	High grade	High grade	None	No	Yes
Nature of cough	Barking	Barking	Muffled, guttural cough (if present)	Barking	n/a	n/a
Swallowing	Normal	Difficult	Very difficult	Variable; depends on site of impaction and degree of blockage	Variable; depends on severity	Normal
Preferred Posture	Recumbent	Sitting	Sitting upright	n/a	n/a	n/a
Drooling	No	No	Yes	No	No	Yes

MCQs

1. Which ONE of the following have been shown to be effective in the treatment of mild croup in children?
   (a) Inhaled heliox
   (b) Nebulised adrenaline
   (c) Nebulised budesonide
   (d) Nebulised dexamethasone
   (e) Oral dexamethasone
2. A 2-year-old boy is brought to Accident & Emergency with breathing difficulties. A diagnosis of moderate croup is given. Which ONE of the following statements is correct?
   (a) Dexamethasone and adrenaline are always given regardless of severity.
   (b) Inspiratory stridor should be present.
   (c) Stridor does not occur in mild cases.
   (d) The child should be admitted for 48 h monitoring before discharge.
   (e) The child should be monitored for 12–24 h before discharge.
3. In an 18-month-old child suffering from stridor, which ONE of the following condition lists should be considered?
   (a) Asthma, croup, bronchiolitis, trauma
   (b) Croup, epiglottitis, asthma, retropharyngeal abscess
   (c) Croup, epiglottis, bronchiolitis, trauma
   (d) Epiglottitis, foreign body, asthma, retropharyngeal abscess

   (e) Trauma, croup, retropharyngeal abscess, foreign body
4. Bacterial tracheitis and epiglottis are two conditions that need to be differentiated from croup. Which ONE of the following sign or symptoms is associated with tracheitis?
   (a) Onset is sudden.
   (b) Pyrexia is not present.
   (c) Swallowing is normal.
   (d) Cough has a barking sound.
   (e) There is drooling.
5. A patient presents with sudden onset cough and difficulty in swallowing. Which ONE of the following conditions is most likely?
   (a) Abscess
   (b) Croup
   (c) Epiglottitis
   (d) Foreign body
   (e) Tracheitis

Answers
1. e; 2. b; 3. e; 4. d; 5. c

KEY POINTS: CROUP
- Typically caused by parainfluenza virus
- Key symptom is an acute onset barking cough.
- Symptoms usually resolve within 48 h.
- Treatment depends on assessment of severity, but steroids are normally recommended.

WEBSITES

NHS Greater Glasgow and Clyde guidelines – Croup
https://www.clinicalguidelines.scot.nhs.uk/media/2528/
  croup-english.pdf

CASE 39: CHRONIC COUGH

PRESENTATION

A 63-year-old Caucasian man, Mr W, presents to the walk-in clinic asking for advice on his cough. He tells you he has been struggling with it for a few weeks and that he has been troubled with coughs on and off for the past 18 months. He has tried various cough medicines, but they have not helped.

PROBLEM REPRESENTATION

A 63-year-old man presents with a cough of long-standing duration.

HYPOTHESIS GENERATION (LIKELY, POSSIBLE AND CRITICAL DIAGNOSES)

The British Thoracic Society Guidelines (Feb. 2019) state that cough is usually self-limiting and will resolve in 3 or 4 weeks. Coughs of longer duration are classified as chronic and almost always have an identifiable pathological cause. For Mr W, the conditions to consider in the first instance, based on his age and duration, are:

Likely Diagnoses
- Asthma
- Chronic obstructive pulmonary disease (COPD)
- Gastrooesophageal reflux disease (GORD)
- Upper airway cough syndrome (UACS)

Possible Diagnoses
- Bronchiectasis
- Heart failure
- Lung abscess
- Medication
- Nocardiosis
- Sarcoidosis
- Tuberculosis (TB)

Critical Diagnosis
- Malignancy

CONTINUED INFORMATION GATHERING

On further questioning, Mr W tells you that his cough is a bit chesty and he has been getting out of breath. GORD and UACS tend not to cause productive cough and seem less likely than asthma and COPD. To further rule out GORD and UACS questions on any associated symptoms need to be asked. In GORD, heartburn symptoms are usual and UACS shows nasal symptoms and throat clearing. Mr. W has not noticed any cold-like symptoms or dyspepsia but does say that he gets tired easily and has put that down to his cough. These symptoms seem to rule out GORD and UACS. You ask about periodicity (e.g., worse at any time) as you know asthma shows this more compared to COPD. He says his cough is just there and he coughs throughout the day.

His symptoms of productive cough, with no periodicity, causing some breathlessness and associated tiredness more closely align with COPD.

PROBLEM REFINEMENT

COPD is strongly associated with smoking. You ask him if he is a current or previous smoker. He says he smoked for 35 years but gave it up 10 years ago. COPD seems most plausible. Checks on possible causes show these to be unlikely: bronchiectasis and lung abscess would usually show much more sputum production; heart failure and lung abscess are associated with older people; sarcoidosis, nocardiosis and TB exhibit other symptoms such as fever and weight loss.

It would be worth checking Mr W's medical history to make sure he was not taking an angiotensin-converting enzyme (ACE) inhibitor, although a nonproductive cough is usually associated with ACE inhibitor. He tells you he is diabetic and takes metformin. He also takes painkillers for arthritis. It seems medicines are not the cause of his cough.

⚡ RED FLAGS

It appears that Mr W's cough has sinister pathology and chronic obstructive pulmonary disease is likely but lung cancer cannot be totally ruled out, although other symptoms such as loss of appetite and weight loss would be expected.

MANAGEMENT

Self-care Options

Mr W should be advised against trying any further cough medicines.

Prescribing Options

Before any treatment can be considered, your differential diagnosis of COPD needs to be confirmed via spirometry testing. It is also advisable to arrange a chest X-ray to exclude other causes (e.g., lung cancer) and a full blood count to identify anaemia.

Safety Netting

You tell Mr W that his cough is probably due to his smoking history and before any treatment can be given, we need to do some tests. This will involve tests to assess his breathing and an X-ray to look at his lungs. This means a hospital visit will need to be organised.

AIDE MEMOIRE

Likely Diagnoses

Asthma

Asthma is classically characterised by coughing, wheezing, chest tightness and shortness of breath, which tend to be variable and intermittent. Cough can be episodic being worse in the evening or morning. Asthma can also present as 'cough variant asthma', where cough is the predominant symptom, with little or no dyspnoea.

Chronic Obstructive Pulmonary Disease

COPD, beside chronic productive cough, is characterised by breathlessness that progressively worsens over time. Other symptoms include wheeze, reduced exercise tolerance and fatigue. COPD sufferers experience frequent respiratory tract infections. Patients often do not notice early symptoms, or they adjust their lifestyle to make breathing easier. Most people with COPD are current or former smokers, although a small proportion will have occupational exposure to chemicals and dust.

Upper Airway Cough Syndrome

Patients usually present with a runny or blocked nose, nasal dripping and an itchy throat. Purulent discharge and facial pain may suggest concomitant sinusitis. Cough is highly variable, affecting between 10% and 80% of people. Symptoms of an annoying nonproductive cough include abnormal sensations arising from the throat and throat clearing.

Gastrooesophageal Reflux Disease

GORD is associated with classical symptoms of heartburn, but the constant irritation can lead to chronic coughing.

Possible Diagnoses

Bronchiectasis

Besides chronic cough, people with bronchiectasis exhibit dyspnoea, large volumes of purulent sputum (that can be bloody), fever, fatigue and weight loss. It is associated with increased age.

Heart Failure

Often the first symptoms patients experience are fatigue, shortness of breath, orthopnoea and dyspnoea at night. As the condition progresses from mild/moderate to severe heart failure, patients will show ankle swelling and might complain of a productive, frothy cough, which may have pink-tinged sputum and may be worst at night.

Lung Abscess

A typical presentation is initially a nonproductive cough with pleuritic pain and dyspnoea with signs of infection such as malaise and fever. Later, the cough produces large amounts of purulent and often foul-smelling sputum. Fatigue, night sweats and weight loss can also be observed. It is more common in the elderly.

Medication

ACE inhibitors are known to cause chronic cough in up to one-third of patients. Cough may appear immediately or a few months into the therapy. Resolution of the cough usually occurs 2–4 weeks after withdrawal, although it may take a few months to resolve.

Nocardiosis

This is a rare cause of cough. Nocardiosis symptoms are similar to those of pneumonia and TB. Symptoms include chest pain, difficulty in breathing, cough with purulent/blood-tinged sputum, fever, sweats, fatigue and weight loss.

Sarcoidosis

Sarcoidosis is a rare multisystem inflammatory disease usually affecting people under the age of 50 years. Any organ system can be involved but most commonly the lungs. Nonspecific symptoms such as fatigue, weight loss, fever or night sweats can be experienced. Lung-specific symptoms include dyspnoea, dry cough and sometimes wheeze.

Tuberculosis

TB is characterised by its slow onset and initial mild symptoms but should be considered in those at high risk and have symptoms of fever, weight loss, night sweats or malaise. Cough associated with TB is chronic in nature and sputum production can vary from mild to severe with associated haemoptysis, although this feature tends to be late in symptom presentation. In the UK, cases tend to be seen in immigrant populations.

Critical Diagnosis
Malignancy

Lung cancer, especially early in disease expression, has many overlapping signs and symptoms similar to other conditions. However, suspicion should be raised in those people with a new unexplained cough over the age of 40 years, especially if they have a smoking history. They may experience breathlessness, haemoptysis, loss of appetite, fatigue and loss of weight.

MCQs

1. COPD is confirmed via spirometry testing. Which ONE of the following lung function tests is used to confirm the diagnosis?
   (a) FEV_1 before bronchodilator treatment
   (b) FEV_1 after bronchodilator treatment
   (c) Tidal volume before bronchodilator treatment
   (d) Tidal volume after bronchodilator treatment
   (e) Vital capacity
2. A number of risk factors exist in the development of COPD. Which ONE of the following is NOT an associated risk factor?
   (a) Air pollution
   (b) Genetics
   (c) Occupational exposure
   (d) Recurrent chest infection
   (e) Smoking

3. The National Institute for Health and Care Excellence guidance on inhaler choice in COPD advises that choice of inhaled therapy is based on which ONE of the following?
   (a) Minimising the number and types of inhalers used by each person
   (b) Number of hospital admissions
   (c) Side effects
   (d) The medicines' potential to reduce exacerbations
   (e) The person's preferences and ability to use the inhalers
4. Patients with COPD frequently suffer from acute exacerbation of symptoms. Which ONE of the following medicines is used as first-line treatment for such symptoms?
   (a) Long-acting beta-2 agonist
   (b) Long-acting muscarinic antagonist
   (c) Short-acting beta-2 agonist
   (d) Short-acting muscarinic antagonist
   (e) Steroids
5. Long-term oxygen therapy can be given to patients with COPD with severe disease. Which ONE of the following would NOT be an indication for oxygen therapy?
   (a) Cyanosis
   (b) FEV_1 less than 40% predicted
   (c) Oxygen saturation of less than 92%
   (d) Peripheral oedema
   (e) Raised jugular venous pressure

Answers
1. b; 2. d; 3. b; 4. e; 5. b

KEY POINTS: CHRONIC OBSTRUCTIVE PULMONARY DISEASE

- Most cases are associated with a smoking history.
- Key symptoms are persistent cough and breathlessness that worsen over time.
- Treatment options include pulmonary rehabilitation, a combination of inhaled short- and long-acting beta-agonists and steroids.

WEBSITES

Breathing Matters
https://www.breathingmatters.co.uk/

CASE 40: COUGH IN AN ASTHMATIC PATIENT

PRESENTATION

A 27-year-old woman, not known to you, presents with a prescription for salbutamol and beclometasone inhalers. You decide to check her inhaler use and technique as she is a new patient. She tells you she has been an asthmatic for 10 years and these two inhalers have not changed for a number of years. Her inhaler technique seems reasonable. During the conversation she tells you that she has recently developed a cough and would like to buy something for it.

PROBLEM REPRESENTATION

A 27-year-old female asthmatic patient presents with acute onset cough.

HYPOTHESIS GENERATION (LIKELY, POSSIBLE AND CRITICAL DIAGNOSES)

By far, the most common causes of acute cough are infections of the upper respiratory tract and acute bronchitis, although there is symptom overlap between viral cough, the common cold and acute bronchitis. Given our patient is asthmatic, we also need to ensure she is not experiencing an exacerbation of her asthma.

Likely Diagnoses

- Acute bronchitis
- Common cold
- Viral cough
- Worsening asthma

Possible Diagnoses

- COVID-19
- Other infections
  - Pneumonia
  - Whooping cough (not in this case)
- GORD
- Influenza
- UACS
- Vocal cord dysfunction

Critical Diagnoses

- Malignancy
- Pneumothorax
- Pulmonary embolism

CONTINUED INFORMATION GATHERING

We know almost nothing about her symptoms and need to get more information from her. She said the cough is recent in onset, but we need to know how long she has had the cough. Additionally, knowing about the nature of the cough and other associated symptoms is necessary.

The patient tells you that her cough is dry (i.e., non-productive), she has had it for 3 days or so and does not feel 100%.

It appears that cough is the predominant symptom and fits most closely with acute bronchitis. In common cold and viral cough, associated symptoms such as nasal congestion, sore throat and fever tend to be more obvious.

You ask her what she means by 'not 100%'. She reports that she just feels a bit tired and generally not able to function at 100%. You interpret this as mild constitutional symptoms.

The presence of mild constitutional symptoms and lack of other symptoms still suggest acute bronchitis, although she has not reported any dyspnoea or wheeze. The lack of such symptoms also points away from worsening asthma.

PROBLEM REFINEMENT

To rule out worsening asthma checking on how she is using her inhalers now seems appropriate, for example, appropriate use of her steroid inhaler and if she has been using her salbutamol more frequently. In addition, it would be worth seeing if there have been any recent lifestyle changes, for example, new activities/exercise or changes to home or work environments. You find out she has been using the inhalers as prescribed and has not needed to use the salbutamol more than when needed and there is little in the way of changes to lifestyle. Her asthma seems well managed.

Other possible causes seem unlikely: she is not exhibiting any changes to smell/taste (COVID-19) debilitating symptoms (flu), congestion or throat clearing (UACS) pleuritic pain (pneumonia) or stridor (vocal cord dysfunction).

It appears her symptoms fit most closely with acute bronchitis.

⚡ RED FLAGS

Acute onset and lack of other symptoms (cancer) and no shortness of breath or chest pain (pneumothorax) suggest none of the critical diagnoses are responsible for her symptoms.

MANAGEMENT

Self-care Options

First, she should be encouraged to drink more fluid. If the patient is insistent on wanting a cough treatment, then a demulcent would be first-line therapy. Pharmacologically active cough medicines (e.g., dextromethorphan) have poor evidence of efficacy.

Prescribing Options

Beyond self-care measures, there is nothing further to recommend, although as she is asthmatic it would be worth asking her to monitor her peak flow more frequently than normal to assess any deterioration in lung function.

Safety Netting

You tell her viral bronchitis is causing her cough and, beyond simple self-help measures, no medicine is needed. Her cough should clear up in the next 2 weeks. As she is asthmatic, you do warn her that if she notices the symptoms worsening, she should come back.

AIDE MEMOIRE

Likely Diagnoses
Acute Bronchitis

Cough is the predominant symptom, either with or without sputum production. Wheeze is often present, and the person may be breathless. Other symptoms can be present such as mild fever, malaise and sore throat.

Common Cold

The first symptoms noted are usually a sore or irritated throat with associated sneezing, followed closely by profuse nasal discharge and congestion. The sore throat usually resolves quickly, and by the second and third day of illness, nasal symptoms predominate. A cough can develop (approximately 30% of people), typically after nasal symptoms have cleared. Systemic symptoms are uncommon, but people can experience headache, mild to moderate fever and general malaise. If systemic symptoms are present, they are generally not debilitating, and the person can carry on with day-to-day activities.

Viral Cough

The symptoms of viral cough typically present with sudden onset and associated fever; cold symptoms are also often present. Sputum production is minimal, and symptoms are often worse in the evening.

Worsening Asthma

Asthma symptoms are associated with coughing, wheezing, chest tightness and shortness of breath, which tend to be variable and intermittent. Exacerbation of existing asthma can see a worsening of all symptoms.

Possible Diagnoses
COVID-19

COVID-19 presents with a wide range of symptoms, but the most common presentations include a new continuous dry cough, high temperature and a loss or change to sense of smell or taste. Other symptoms that can be experienced include shortness of breath, tiredness, sore throat, headache, nasal congestion, gastrointestinal (GI) disturbances and loss of appetite.

Other Infections – *Pneumonia*

Symptoms are typically sudden in onset, usually over 24–48 h. Cough is the predominant symptom. It can be either productive or nonproductive. Accompanying symptoms include fever, breathlessness, general malaise, sweating, pleuritic pain and tachycardia. The person will be obviously poorly. Other less common symptoms include headache, fatigue and wheeze. In elderly people, confusion is often seen.

Gastrooesophageal Reflux Disease

GORD is associated with classical symptoms of heartburn, but the constant irritation can lead to coughing.

Influenza

The onset of influenza is sudden, within a few hours, and typical symptoms include cold-like symptoms, fever, a nonproductive cough and generalised symptoms such as shivering, chills, malaise, marked aching of limbs, insomnia, fatigue and loss of appetite. Influenza is therefore normally debilitating. Flu is typically seen between December and March.

Upper Airway Cough Syndrome

Patients usually present with a runny or blocked nose, nasal dripping and an itchy or unpleasant sensation in the throat. Purulent discharge and facial pain may suggest concomitant sinusitis. Nonproductive cough is highly variable, affecting between 10% and 80% of people.

Vocal Cord Dysfunction

Vocal cord dysfunction occurs when the vocal cords intermittently malfunction and close when the person inhales, reducing the space available for air to move in and out. It is most common in people aged 20–40 years old, especially women. Symptoms can mimic asthma. Other symptoms include stridor, hoarseness, feeling of choking and frequent clearing of the throat. Symptoms can be triggered, for example, by irritants, temperature changes, odours and exercise.

Critical Diagnoses

Lung Cancer

Common early symptoms include cough and breathlessness. Suspicion should be raised in those people with a new unexplained cough over the age of 40, especially if they have a smoking history. They may experience loss of appetite, fatigue and loss of weight.

Pneumothorax

The main symptoms of a pneumothorax are sudden pleuritic chest pain, shortness of breath and cough. The severity of symptoms depends on the extent of lung collapse. The patient is likely to show signs of distress.

Pulmonary Embolism

Predominant symptoms are dyspnoea, pleuritic chest pain, fever and leg pain/swelling. Cough can also be present with haemoptysis.

▮ M C Q s

1. Several risk factors are known to contribute to people developing asthma. Which ONE of the following is not a risk factor?
   (a) Low body mass index
   (b) Personal or family history of atopic disease
   (c) Respiratory infections in infancy
   (d) Social deprivation
   (e) Workplace exposures

2. Asthma is a common chronic condition affecting over 8 million people in the UK. Which ONE of the following patient groups is asthma most prevalent in?
   (a) Adult men
   (b) Adult women
   (c) Children
   (d) Elderly men
   (e) Elderly women

3. Asthma is characterised by respiratory symptoms. Which ONE of the symptom clusters best describe asthma?
   (a) Cough and wheeze
   (b) Cough and chest tightness
   (c) Cough, wheeze and chest tightness
   (d) Cough, wheeze, chest tightness and shortness of breath
   (e) Cough, wheeze, chest tightness and orthopnoea

4. British Thoracic Society/Scottish Intercollegiate Guideline Network guidance in 2019 defined what complete asthma control looked like. Which ONE of the following is not classed as complete asthma control?
   (a) Exercise is not limited by asthma.
   (b) No daytime symptoms
   (c) No need for rescue medication
   (d) No night-time awakening due to asthma
   (e) Only very occasional asthma attacks

5. Beta-2 agonists are a mainstay of asthma management. In which ONE of the following patient groups should they be used with caution?
   (a) Diabetes insipidus
   (b) Hypothyroidism
   (c) Hyperthyroidism
   (d) Osteoporosis
   (e) Parkinson's disease

Answers

1. a; 2. c; 3. d; 4. e; 5. c

KEY POINTS: ACUTE BRONCHITIS

- Commonly caused by influenza A and B, adenovirus, respiratory syncytial virus and rhinovirus
- Key symptom is an acute onset nonproductive cough.
- Symptoms should resolve within 14–21 days.
- No treatment is necessary.

WEBSITES

Asthma and Lung UK
https://www.asthmaandlung.org.uk/
Roy Castle Lung Cancer Foundation
https://roycastle.org/

CASE 41: UPPER RESPIRATORY TRACT SYMPTOMS

PRESENTATION

Mr T, a man in his early 40s, presents to you on a Friday afternoon in late September complaining of a sore throat, nasal discharge and cough. He has had the symptoms for about 4 days now and also says he feels 'a bit rough'.

PROBLEM REPRESENTATION

A middle-aged man presents with a 4-day history of generalised upper respiratory symptoms.

HYPOTHESIS GENERATION (LIKELY, POSSIBLE AND CRITICAL DIAGNOSES)

The prevalence of the common cold makes this the most likely diagnosis as adults tend to contract two to three incidents of cold per year, although influenza and COVID-19 are also common and need to be considered.

Likely Diagnoses

- Common cold
- COVID-19
- Influenza

Possible Diagnoses

- Allergic rhinitis
- Glandular fever (unlikely in this case)
- Pharyngitis

Complications

- Otitis media (unlikely in this case)
- Rhinosinusitis

Critical Diagnosis

- Meningitis (unlikely in this case)

CONTINUED INFORMATION GATHERING

Cold, flu and COVID-19 present with similar overlapping symptom profiles (see comparison table). In Mr T's case, we need to establish how debilitating his symptoms are. We know he feels 'a bit rough', and he has presented himself which implies his symptoms are not too debilitating. This seems to strengthen a common cold diagnosis over influenza or COVID-19. Additionally, the time of year (September) also points more toward his symptoms being a cold.

It would be helpful to understand how his symptoms developed and to explore if any other symptoms are present. You find out that Mr T's symptoms started with a sore throat, which is now less sore, but he has developed a lot of nasal congestion and over the last 24 h has started coughing. He says he has recently developed a headache and feels hot.

The way in which his symptoms presented best fits with a common cold.

PROBLEM REFINEMENT

To help rule out COVID-19 it would be worth asking about loss of taste/smell. He reports his taste and smell are fine and he has not been in contact with anyone with COVID-19 as far as he is aware.

He seems to be exhibiting some classic symptoms of allergic rhinitis but has not reported any nasal itching or eye symptoms and, in addition, seems to be experiencing some systemic symptoms. As his sore throat is now less troublesome, it seems to suggest pharyngitis is not the cause. Age seems to rule out glandular fever and meningitis.

At this point, it appears Mr T is suffering from a common cold.

⚡ RED FLAGS

He seems to be exhibiting no warning signs or symptoms of meningitis.

MANAGEMENT

Self-care Options

Mr T should be advised to take measures to reduce the opportunity for viral spreading such as using disposable tissues rather than handkerchiefs, wash his hands frequently, not to share towels and avoid trying to touch his nose and eyes.

You advise him to increase his fluid intake and take adequate rest. Symptoms can be managed with analgesia and decongestants.

Prescribing Options

No specific prescribing of medication is required.

Safety Netting

You tell Mr T you think he has a cold and symptoms should disappear in the next 4–7 days but if symptoms persist or he starts getting facial pain, then he needs to return to get his symptoms reassessed.

AIDE MEMOIRE

Likely Diagnoses
Common Cold

The first symptoms noted are usually a sore or irritated throat with associated sneezing, followed closely by profuse nasal discharge and congestion. The sore throat usually resolves quickly, and by the second and third day of illness, nasal symptoms predominate. A cough can develop (approximately 30% of people), typically after nasal symptoms have cleared. Systemic symptoms are uncommon, but people can experience headache, mild to moderate fever and general malaise. If systemic symptoms are present, they generally not debilitating, and the person can carry on with day-to-day activities.

COVID-19

COVID-19 presents with a wide range of symptoms, but the most common presentations include a new continuous dry cough, high temperature and a loss or change to sense of smell or taste. Other symptoms that can be experienced include shortness of breath, tiredness, sore throat, headache, nasal congestion, GI disturbances and loss of appetite.

Influenza

The onset of influenza is sudden – within a few hours – and typical symptoms include cold-like symptoms, fever, a nonproductive cough and generalised symptoms such as shivering, chills, malaise, marked aching of limbs, insomnia, fatigue and loss of appetite. Influenza is therefore normally debilitating. Flu is typically seen between December and March.

Possible Diagnoses
Allergic Rhinitis

This can present with a similar symptom complex to the common cold, exhibiting rhinorrhoea and nasal congestion, sneezing and cough. However, it is usual to experience nasal or conjunctival itching/redness. A family history of atopy is often present, and symptoms also tend to be more long-standing.

Glandular Fever

Seen most commonly in adolescents/young adults, symptoms of fatigue/general malaise are usually experienced before signs of sore throat, fever and lymph node enlargement. A maculopapular rash on the trunk is seen in about 10% of patients. Fatigue can persist for a number of weeks after the acute symptoms disappear.

Pharyngitis

Sore throat can be an isolated symptom or as part of a cluster of symptoms that include rhinorrhoea (rare), cough, malaise, fever, headache and hoarseness. Differentiation between viral and bacterial causes is difficult but cough tends to absent in bacterial causes.

Complications
Otitis Media

Acute otitis media is most common in children up to the age of 4 years old. Symptoms develop rapidly. Young children often hold or rub their ear or have nonspecific symptoms such as fever, crying, poor feeding and restlessness. In older children, ear pain/earache is the predominant feature and tends to be throbbing. An examination of the ear should reveal a red/yellow and bulging tympanic membrane with a loss of normal landmarks.

Rhinosinusitis

It can affect any age group although it is more common in adults. Symptoms that are highly suggestive of sinusitis are nasal obstruction and discharge, and facial pain. Other symptoms include frontal headache, fever, loss of smell and tenderness over the cheekbones. The pain can also increase on lying down or bending over.

Critical Diagnosis
Meningitis

Meningitis can present with upper respiratory tract-like symptoms such as sore throat, cold and nasal congestion although these are less prominent than symptoms of lethargy, fever, irritability, headache, joint pain, stiff neck, photophobia and nonblanching rash. Table 7.2 summarises these diagnosis.

TABLE 7.2   Condition Summary of the Common Cold, Flu and COVID-19

Symptoms	COVID-19	Flu	Cold
Sore throat	Sometimes	Sometimes	Common
Cough	Common	Common	Approximately 30% of patients
Rhinorrhoea/nasal congestion	Rare	Sometimes	Common
Fatigue	Sometimes	Common	Rare
Fever	Common	Common	Rare
Headaches	Sometimes	Common	Rare
Loss of taste or smell	Common	Rare	Rare
Sneezing	No	No	Common
Gastrointestinal symptoms	Sometimes	Sometimes	No

MCQs

1. Approximately what proportion of general practice consultations are taken up by upper respiratory tract infections?
   (a) 2%
   (b) 5%
   (c) 8%
   (d) 10%
   (e) 15%

2. The mother of a 16-year-old boy is worried about her son as he is complaining of a cough, headache, fever and feeling generally poorly. Which ONE of the following conditions is the most likely cause?
   (a) Common cold
   (b) Influenza
   (c) Meningitis
   (d) Sinusitis
   (e) Tension-type headache

3. Mr F presents complaining of a blocked nose, facial pain and a reduced sense of smell. Upon further questioning he adds that he suffers from hay fever and was playing football in a field with his friends yesterday. Which ONE of the following is the most likely diagnosis?
   (a) Allergic rhinitis
   (b) Common cold
   (c) Influenza
   (d) Sinusitis
   (e) UACS

4. Which ONE of the following symptoms is not a common symptom of flu?
   (a) Cough
   (b) Fatigue
   (c) Fever
   (d) Gastrointestinal disturbance
   (e) Headache

5. Which ONE of the following persons is most likely to contract flu?
   (a) A 41-year-old man with high blood pressure
   (b) A 74-year-old man with angina
   (c) A healthy 6-year-old girl
   (d) A pregnant woman
   (e) An 18-year-old man with asthma

Answers

1. d; 2. b; 3. d; 4. d; 5. b

KEY POINTS: THE COMMON COLD

- Rhinovirus is the most common cause.
- Key symptoms are sore throat, nasal symptoms and cough.
- Symptoms should resolve within 7 days but can last longer.
- Treatment is symptomatic, including analgesia and decongestants.

WEBSITES

Meningitis now
https://www.meningitisnow.org/

8

Women's Health Issues

CASE 42: ABNORMAL UTERINE BLEEDING

PRESENTATION

Miss T, a Caucasian 33-year-old woman, presents with heavy menstrual bleeding. She tells you it has been going on for a number of months now and seems to be getting progressively worse. She describes the symptoms as interfering with her daily routine, as the bleeding means that she has to change sanitary towels almost hourly. Her periods are regular and last about a week.

PROBLEM REPRESENTATION

A 33-year-old woman presents with a chronic history of heavy menstrual bleeding that is progressively worsening.

HYPOTHESIS GENERATION (LIKELY, POSSIBLE AND CRITICAL DIAGNOSES)

Abnormal uterine bleeding can be defined as bleeding from the uterus that is longer than usual or that occurs at an irregular time. Abnormal bleeding can be considered structural (e.g., polyps, malignancy) or nonstructural (e.g., coagulopathy, ovulatory dysfunction). The age of the patient will have a bearing on your hypothesis generation; for example, in older women (perimenopausal or postmenopausal) malignancy should always be considered. For Miss T, we need to consider the following as the likely causes of her symptoms.

Likely Diagnoses

- Adenomyosis
- Fibroid
- Polyp
  - Endometrial
  - Cervical

Possible Diagnoses

- Complications of pregnancy
- Endometriosis
- Medicines
- Ovarian cyst (benign)
- Pelvic inflammatory disease (PID)
- Polycystic ovary syndrome
- Salpingitis
- Systemic
  - Hypothyroidism
  - Coagulation disorders
- Uterine myoma

Critical Diagnosis

- Malignancy

CONTINUED INFORMATION GATHERING

Further exploration of her menstrual cycle history, as well as determining if she has any associated symptoms is needed.

She says her periods are pretty regular, usually occurring every 28–32 days; they last between 5 and 7 days and are generally painful but not debilitating. Her last period was a week ago, and she again experienced very heavy bleeding. This has now been happening for the last 6 months or so. She says that the last couple of months she has experienced lower back pain and hip pain and struggled with going to the toilet while experiencing constipation-like symptoms.

This description seems to best fit a differential diagnosis of fibroids. Polyps seem less likely due to the presence of gastrointestinal (GI) symptoms and pain other than dysmenorrhoea. Adenomyosis is more likely than polyps but tends not to exhibit GI/urinary symptoms.

PROBLEM REFINEMENT

When considering fibroids as the diagnosis, we could check if Miss T has any risk factors for their development. Risk factors include age, onset of menarche, pregnancy, ethnicity and obesity. Miss T tells you that she started her periods when she was about 11 or 12 years old and has no children. You observe that she seems overweight. This seems to suggest she does have risk factors – early age of menarche, nulliparity and being overweight, which strengthens your differential diagnosis of fibroids.

We still have not specifically ruled out other causes of her bleeding (possible diagnosis list) although we know she is not pregnant, and she does not describe any intermenstrual bleeding (seen with cysts, PID, salpingitis). Other conditions seem unlikely. Poly cystic ovarary syndrome is noted for infrequent periods; endometriosis (and salpingitis) has pain rather than bleeding as the main symptom; coagulation disorders will present earlier in life, and hypothyroidism is seen generally in older age groups.

Medicines can be ruled out/in by taking a medication history. She tells you that she is not taking hormonal contraception but uses barrier methods. She takes no medication bought or prescribed on a regular basis.

> ## ⚡ RED FLAGS
> Malignancy always needs to be considered, although this tends to be seen in older patients. She tells you she is up to date with her cervical screening, the results of which were normal.

MANAGEMENT

Treatment options for fibroids are mainly governed by the woman's fertility wishes. In Miss T's case, you confirm that she wants to continue with contraceptive measures and has no desire currently to become pregnant.

Self-care Options

Not applicable.

Prescribing Options

Short-term use of tranexamic acid (500 mg three or four times a day) could be tried to control bleeding. Beyond controlling bleeding, a range of tests need to be considered. Anaemia is often associated with heavy bleeding, and therefore, a full blood count should be performed. Although hypothyroidism is unlikely, it would seem sensible to check thyroid function if checking for anaemia.

Safety Netting

You tell Miss T that you think the bleeding might be due to fibroids, and you want to send her for a pelvic ultrasound scan. You would also like to take a blood sample and run tests for anaemia and thyroid function.

AIDE MEMOIRE

Likely Diagnoses

Adenomyosis

Adenomyosis occurs when endometrial tissue grows into the myometrium and can cause dysmenorrhoea and heavy periods, lower abdominal discomfort/pressure and bloating.

Fibroids

Fibroids are common and thought to occur in 20%–50% of women older than 30 years of age, with the incidence increasing during the reproductive years and declining after menopause. They are frequently asymptomatic. If symptoms are experienced, menstrual irregularity is prominent and accompanied with dysmenorrhoea, pelvic discomfort/pain or back pain, abdominal bloating and urinary tract (frequency, urgency and incontinence) and GI (constipation) symptoms. A number of risk factors have been identified and include family history; early menarche; nulliparity; and Causcasian, Black and Asian ethnicity.

Polyps

Uterine polyps are growths attached to the inner wall of the uterus that extend into the uterine cavity. They are usually benign and asymptomatic, and affect women of all ages.

Abnormal menstrual bleeding is the most common symptom and appears to increase with age. This is often irregular and unpredictable, for example, having frequent, variable length and excessively heavy periods. Intermenstrual and postcoital bleeding can also be seen. Dysmenorrhoea is uncommon. Table 8.1 summarises how these likely diagnoses present.

TABLE 8.1	Condition Summary of Signs/Symptoms for Polyps, Adenomyosis and Fibroids				
	Dysmenorrhoea	Pain Other Than Dysmenorrhoea	Painful Sex	Abdominal Discomfort	Urinary and gastrointestinal tract Symptoms
Polyp	Uncommon	No	No	Uncommon	No
Adenomyosis	Common	Pelvic pain	Possible	Common	Unusual
Fibroid	Common	Pelvic and back pain	Possible	Common	Sometimes

Possible Diagnoses

Complications of Pregnancy

Vaginal bleeding in a pregnant woman may indicate miscarriage or ectopic pregnancy.

Endometriosis

Endometriosis is a relatively unusual cause of bleeding and represents less than 5% of all cases. Pain is experienced in the lower abdomen and pelvis, and starts prior to menstruation but symptoms worsen during menses. Patients may experience period-related GI and urinary symptoms.

Medicines

Medicines are often implicated with menstrual bleeding. These include sex hormones (e.g., contraceptive hormones, hormone replacement therapy), monoamine oxidase inhibitors, tamoxifen and anticoagulants, as well as intrauterine contraceptive devices.

Ovarian Cyst (Benign)

An ovarian cyst is a fluid-filled sac that forms on or in the ovary. These cysts are often asymptomatic, but can sometimes cause heavy periods or bleeding between periods. Other symptoms that can be experienced are low back pain, intermittent pelvic pain, abdominal bloating, pain during intercourse, increased urinary frequency and constipation.

Pelvic Inflammatory Disease

Patients are often asymptomatic or exhibit mild symptoms. Vaginal bleeding between periods and after sex can be experienced, and periods themselves can be painful and heavy. Other symptoms include lower abdominal and pelvic pain, vaginal discharge, painful sex, fever and dysuria. PID is almost always caused through a sexually transmitted disease (STD) and is therefore most commonly seen in younger women, especially those with multiple sexual partners.

Polycystic Ovary Syndrome

Women with polycystic ovary syndrome have infrequent periods or no periods; this can lead to difficulties in getting pregnant. Skin problems occur such as hirsutism (usually on the face, chest and back), acne and rough dry skin. Patients are often overweight and have a positive family history.

Salpingitis

Bilateral lower abdominal pain, fever and vaginal discharge are the predominant symptoms. Irregular menstrual bleeding (e.g., spotting between periods), nausea and vomiting, and urinary tract infection (UTI) symptoms can also be experienced.

Systemic Causes

Hypothyroidism. This can cause frequent and heavy periods. However, other symptoms should be obvious such as fatigue, weight gain, cold intolerance, dry and coarse hair and forgetfulness.

Coagulation disorders. A history of heavy menstrual bleeding since menarche accompanied with other indicators of haemorrhage should be present such as dental-related bleeding, bleeding gums, epistaxis and bruising easily.

Uterine Myoma

This is usually asymptomatic but can present with heavy and/or irregular menstrual bleeding. Pelvic examination may show an enlarged, nodular pelvic mass that can vary in size and shape.

Critical Diagnoses

Malignancy

Endometrial cancer. Almost all (90%) are diagnosed in postmenopausal women. Bleeding is the main symptom. Bleeding is initially slight and intermittent but may become constant and heavy. Other symptoms can be pelvic discomfort and pain (late symptom), pain during sex and difficult/painful urination.

Ovarian cancer. Typically seen in older people, especially from 50 years upwards. Symptoms include abdominal bloating, feeling full, loss of appetite (leading to weight loss), pelvic/abdominal pain, urinary symptoms such as frequency and urgency, and irritable bowel syndrome-like symptoms. Other symptoms can include abnormal bleeding, dyspepsia and nausea.

Cervical cancer. The most common symptoms of cervical cancer include unusual vaginal bleeding, pain during sex and low back and hip pain. Cervical cancer is most common in women in their 30s and 40s.

Vulval and vaginal cancer. These are relatively rare cancers. Both can be associated with bleeding between periods. However other symptoms will be present. Persistent itch is common to both cancers as well as palpable lump/growth. In vaginal cancer, discharge that smells or is blood stained is often seen.

MCQs

1. Fibroids are a common cause of uterine bleeding. Which ONE of the following is NOT a risk factor associated with developing fibroids?
   (a) Black or Asian ethnicity
   (b) Increasing age
   (c) Late menarche
   (d) Obesity
   (e) Older age at first pregnancy
2. A 39-year-old woman presents with period pain. On questioning, you ascertain that the pain, which can be quite severe, seems to be worse about a week before her period and is also worse during intercourse. Which ONE of the following conditions is she most likely to be suffering from?
   (a) Cervical carcinoma
   (b) Endometrial carcinoma
   (c) Endometriosis
   (d) PID
   (e) Primary dysmenorrhoea
3. A patient presents with menstrual bleeding accompanied with dysmenorrhoea, pelvic pain and dysuria. Which ONE of the following conditions is most likely?
   (a) Adenomyosis
   (b) Fibroid
   (c) Polyp

   (d) Salpingitis
   (e) Vulval cancer
4. Medicines are frequently implicated in causing bleeding. Which ONE of the following medicines is most likely to be associated with this side effect?
   (a) Apixaban
   (b) Evorel patches
   (c) Microgynon
   (d) Phenelzine
   (e) Tamoxifen
5. Symptoms of bleeding, pelvic pain, bloating and nausea are most suggestive of which ONE of the following types of cancer?
   (a) Cervical cancer
   (b) Endometrial cancer
   (c) Ovarian cancer
   (d) Vaginal
   (e) Vulval cancer

Answers
1. c; 2. c; 3. b; 4; e; 5. b

KEY POINTS: FIBROIDS

- The exact cause is unknown but is linked to hormonal changes.
- Key symptoms are heavy bleeding and pain.
- Can spontaneously resolve and often shrink after the menopause

WEBSITES

British Fibroid Trust
http://www.britishfibroidtrust.org.uk/

CASE 43: SUSPECTED URINARY TRACT INFECTION

PRESENTATION

It is a Monday morning and a 27-year-old-Asian woman, Miss J, asks you for advice on getting some treatment for cystitis. She says she has been experiencing a burning sensation when going to the toilet for the last 3 days.

PROBLEM REPRESENTATION

A 27-year-old woman presents with a 3-day history of acute dysuria symptoms.

HYPOTHESIS GENERATION (LIKELY, POSSIBLE AND CRITICAL DIAGNOSES)

In Miss J's case, based on her presenting symptoms and age, the likely conditions to consider in the first instance would be:

Likely Diagnoses

- Acute uncomplicated cystitis
- Pyelonephritis
- STDs

Possible Diagnoses

- Current pregnancy
- Foreign body
- Interstitial cystitis (painful bladder syndrome)
- Medicine-induced cystitis
- Vaginitis

Critical Diagnosis

- Malignancy

CONTINUED INFORMATION GATHERING

A 3-day history of burning when passing urine does point to cystitis, but it is important to know more about Miss J's symptoms as one would expect other symptoms to be present such as urgency and frequency. In addition, the major complication of cystitis, pyelonephritis needs to be eliminated from your thinking.

Miss J tells you she is going to the toilet more frequently and gets pain on passing urine, but denies any flank pain, systemic symptoms or vaginal discharge. This seems to rule out pyelonephritis or retained foreign body.

A social and medical history should be taken to exclude other causes of her symptoms such as pregnancy, adverse drug reactions and STDs. You find out she is in a stable relationship, is unlikely to be pregnant and has no medical history but does take occasional nonsteroidal antiinflammatory drugs for back pain.

At this point, her symptoms strongly point to a differential diagnosis of acute uncomplicated cystitis.

PROBLEM REFINEMENT

You ask about previous episodes of similar symptoms. Miss J says she has had cystitis before, but only once and that was about 3 years ago. This cleared up after a course of antibiotics from the doctor. This seems to rule out any long-term chronic problem such as interstitial cystitis.

You make a differential diagnosis of acute uncomplicated UTI.

> ### ⚡ RED FLAGS
>
> Prior to any actions being taken, even though she is young and did not report signs of haematuria, a final check should be made, as blood in the urine can suggest malignancy.
>
> Miss J confirms she has not seen any blood in her urine.

MANAGEMENT

Self-care Options

Over-the-counter treatments are available, for example, a 2-day course of sachets of sodium or potassium citrate, although evidence of effectiveness is poor and using them should be discouraged. Tell her to keep hydrated and, if needed, use simple analgesia for the pain.

Prescribing Options

If symptoms persist, then antibiotics could be instigated, but in about a third of women with an uncomplicated UTI, the infection will resolve after approximately 1 week without the need for antibiotics.

Safety Netting

You tell Miss J you believe she has cystitis and symptoms should clear up in a further 5 days. Antibiotics are not needed at this time as her symptoms appear relatively mild; however, you can give her a delayed antibiotic prescription. This means she can get the prescription from the pharmacy and start taking the antibiotics if her symptoms worsen or fail to improve after 48 h.

AIDE MEMOIRE

Likely Diagnoses
Acute Uncomplicated Cystitis

Acute uncomplicated cystitis is very common, especially in those aged 15–34 years. Typically, a patient will present with discomfort, pain, burning, tingling or stinging when passing urine. Acute uncomplicated cystitis is also associated with frequency, urgency, nocturia and changes to urine appearance (e.g., cloudy or change in colour).

Pyelonephritis

Pyelonephritis tends to be a complication of cystitis due to bacteria ascending the urinary tract. The classic triad of flank pain, fever and nausea are typical. Onset is usually sudden.

Sexually Transmitted Diseases

STDs most commonly affect young women – mostly those aged 15–34 years – and can present with dysuria, increased or altered (usually purulent) vaginal discharge, lower abdominal pain and pain during sex. A sexual history often reveals a history of unprotected sex, multiple sexual partners or a new sexual partner.

Possible Diagnoses
Current Pregnancy

During pregnancy, urinary tract changes predispose women to infection. Cystitis presents with the same symptoms seen in nonpregnant individuals.

Foreign Body

Ongoing use of a catheter can increase the risk of bacterial infection. Additionally, retention of a foreign body (e.g., tampon) in the vagina may result in a foul-smelling discharge. Contact dermatitis may occur leading to inflammation and irritation.

Interstitial Cystitis

Interstitial cystitis is a chronic condition that causes lower abdominal pain, persistent urgency and frequency. The pain ranges from mild discomfort to severe pain. Pain is often worse whilst the bladder fills and relieved on urination. The condition is a part of a spectrum of diseases known as painful bladder syndrome and is often a diagnosis of exclusion.

Medicine-induced cystitis. Nonsteroidal antiinflammatory agents, especially tiaprofenic acid, opioids, nifedipine (dysuria – uncommon), cyclophosphamide (cystitis – very common) and ketamine (rare), have been shown to cause symptoms of cystitis.

Vaginitis

Vaginitis is usually associated with vaginal discharge and pain during sex. It can cause cystitis-like symptoms, although typically it is not associated with urgency or frequency. Postmenopausal women (atrophic vaginitis) experience thinning of the endometrial lining because of a reduction in the levels of circulating oestrogen in the blood. This can also lead to symptoms of vaginal dryness and itching.

Critical Diagnoses
Malignancy

Kidney cancer. If symptoms are present, haematuria is the most common symptom. Other symptoms may be present, but are vague and include weight loss, fever, flank pain, tiredness and loss of appetite. It is most common in people over the age of 60 years.

Bladder cancer. Painless haematuria is the predominant symptom. Less commonly UTI-like symptoms are experienced, for example, frequency, urgency and burning. It is most common in people over the age of 70 years and rarely seen in people under the age of 40 years.

Ovarian cancer. Typically seen in older people, especially from 50 years upwards. Symptoms can include persistent or frequent increased urinary urgency and/or frequency. However, other symptoms such as abdominal bloating, feeling full, loss of appetite (leading to weight loss), pelvic/abdominal pain, abnormal uterine bleeding and irritable bowel syndrome-like symptoms can also be present.

▌MCQs

1. Recurrent UTIs are relatively common and associated with certain risk factors. Which ONE of the following is least associated with being a risk factor?
   (a) Atrophic vaginitis
   (b) Catheterisation
   (c) Diabetes
   (d) History of UTIs
   (e) Urinary incontinence

2. A 23-year-old woman presents with urgency on urination. Further questioning reveals she also has lower back pain and type 1 diabetes. Which ONE of the following conditions is the most likely cause?
   (a) Cystitis
   (b) Kidney stones
   (c) Malignancy
   (d) Pyelonephritis
   (e) STD

3. As a practitioner without an independent prescribing qualification, which ONE of the following signs/symptoms would not alert you to consider onward referral?
   (a) Flank pain
   (b) Frequent passing of urine
   (c) Nausea and/or vomiting
   (d) Not passing urine all day
   (e) Shivering or chills
4. Which ONE of the following symptoms should alert you to an ascending UTI?
   (a) Micturition is frequent.
   (b) Their urine is cloudy.
   (c) They are suffering from a high temperature.
   (d) They are suffering from dysuria.
   (e) The onset of the attack is sudden.
5. Which ONE of the following patient groups is NOT considered at risk of developing an upper UTI?
   (a) Diabetic patients
   (b) Immunocompromised patients
   (c) Patients with an indwelling catheter
   (d) Patient history of kidney stones
   (e) Patients with gout

Answers

1. c; 2. d; 3. b; 4. c; 5. e

KEY POINTS: UNCOMPLICATED URINARY TRACT INFECTION

- *Escherichia coli* from the gastrointestinal tract is the most common pathogen implicated.
- Frequency, dysuria and urgency are the most common symptoms.
- Most resolve within 7 days.

CASE 44: VAGINAL DISCHARGE

PRESENTATION

A female Caucasian patient, Mrs D, approximately 38 years of age, presents to the pharmacy saying she has thrush. She says she has a white discharge and her symptoms have been present for the last 2 days. She is otherwise healthy and has no medical problems.

PROBLEM REPRESENTATION

A 38-year-old woman presents with a 2-day history of white vaginal discharge.

HYPOTHESIS GENERATION (LIKELY, POSSIBLE AND CRITICAL DIAGNOSES)

Abnormal discharge is most commonly caused by infection. Given Mrs D's age, the two likely conditions we need to initially consider would be:

Likely Diagnoses

- Bacterial vaginosis (BV)
- Thrush

Possible Diagnoses

- Herpes simplex virus infection
- PID
- Retained foreign body (e.g., tampon)
- STDs (Chlamydia, gonorrhoea, trichomoniasis)
- Vaginitis

Critical Diagnosis

- Malignancy

CONTINUED INFORMATION GATHERING

Patient self-labelling has been reported as unreliable, and it will be necessary to establish if thrush is correct. Questions centred on the nature of discharge and any other associated symptoms should be asked. Both thrush and BV are associated with a white discharge, although thrush is described as curd or cottage cheese-like and BV as thin. Discharge of thrush has little or no odour whereas BV is malodorous. Mrs D describes the discharge as white and thin, and she denies any unpleasant odour. Itch is a prominent feature of thrush, but Mrs D says that she is not really affected by itching.

As her symptoms do not fit a classical presentation of thrush, it seems appropriate to ask more questions with respect to a diagnosis of BV.

PROBLEM REFINEMENT

Certain risk factors increase the chances of developing BV and therefore these could be explored with the patient. These include being sexually active or recent changes in sexual partner, use of vaginal products, having an intrauterine device fitted or being a smoker.

She tells you she is in a stable relationship and takes the pill and never uses vaginal products and is a nonsmoker.

She therefore appears to have no risk factors to support a differential diagnosis of BV. It therefore appears thrush is probable even though she says itch is not prominent. At this point, it would be worth exploring any previous episodes of discharge she has experienced and comparing those symptoms to this presentation. She tells you she had exactly the same symptoms about 18 months ago and these cleared up quickly after taking a single dose capsule from the doctor (the capsule in all likelihood being fluconazole). This history supports a diagnosis of thrush.

At this point it is worth making sure that other possible causes are considered. STDs seem very unlikely – due to nature of discharge and being in a stable relationship. She has also not reported any UTI-like symptoms (PID, foreign body, vaginitis) or fever (foreign body, herpes simplex, PID).

> ## ⚡ RED FLAGS
> No unusual vaginal bleeding has been reported, which seems to rule out malignancy.

MANAGEMENT

Self-care Options

The patient could buy fluconazole or an imidazole product, especially if they pay for prescriptions as they are cheaper than the current National Health Service prescription charge.

Prescribing Options

Fluconazole is a single-dose treatment. Imidazoles, depending on formulation, can range from a single-dose pessary to a short course of pessaries or cream. Treatment choice will be driven by patient preference.

Safety Netting

You agree with Mrs D that she probably has thrush. With treatment, her symptoms should resolve in 72 h. Mrs D should return if her symptoms persist beyond a week.

AIDE MEMOIRE

Likely Diagnoses
Bacterial Vaginosis

If patients exhibit symptoms, then it is characterised by a thin grey/white discharge with a strong fishy odour. Odour is worse after sexual intercourse and may worsen during menses and after intercourse. Itching and soreness

are not usually present. Sexual activity, smoking, intrauterine devices and Black ethnicity are known risk factors.

Thrush

The cardinal symptoms of vaginal candidiasis are vulval pruritus and vaginal soreness/burning. Discharge (in approximately 20% cases) has little or no odour and is described as cottage cheese- or curd-like.

Possible Diagnoses
Herpes Simplex Virus Infection

Multiple painful blisters/ulcers on the external genitalia are the main clinical feature. Other symptoms that can be experienced, although rare, include headache, fever, dysuria and vaginal discharge.

Pelvic Inflammatory Disease

PID is often asymptomatic, but if signs and symptoms are experienced, they range from lower abdominal pain, pain during sex and associated bleeding after sex, intermenstrual bleeding, frequent and painful urination, fever and large amounts of unusual vaginal discharge.

Retained Foreign Body (e.g., Tampon)

Signs of a retained object include malodorous coloured discharge, vaginal itching, fever and dysuria.

Sexually Transmitted Infections

Risk factors in contracting an STI are increased level of sexual activity and multiple sexual partners.

Chlamydia. A majority (75%) of women with chlamydia are asymptomatic. When symptoms are experienced, these can range from vaginal discharge, which may be purulent, pelvic pain, intermenstrual bleeding, pain during sex and dysuria.

Gonorrhoea. The most common symptoms include an increased vaginal thick green/yellow discharge, lower abdominal pain and dysuria.

Trichomoniasis. Up to 50% of patients are asymptomatic. When present, common symptoms include a profuse, frothy, greenish-yellow and fishy-smelling discharge. Other symptoms include vulvar itching and soreness, vaginal spotting, dysuria and lower abdominal pain.

Vaginitis

Vaginitis is usually associated with vaginal discharge and pain during sex. It can also cause cystitis-like symptoms, although typically it is not associated with urgency or frequency. Postmenopausal women (atrophic vaginitis) experience thinning of the endometrial lining as a result of a reduction in the levels of circulating oestrogen in the blood. This can also lead to symptoms of vaginal dryness. Vaginitis caused by a streptococcal infection (rare) tends to cause more severe signs and symptoms than other causes of vaginitis.

Critical Diagnosis

Malignancy (Cervical, Vulval and Vaginal Cancers)

Unusual vaginal bleeding is most associated with malignancy. Other symptoms can include back and hip pain, vaginal itching and rarely blood-tinged vaginal discharge. Cervical cancer is most common in women in their early 30 and 40s, but vulval and vaginal cancers are most common in women over 75 years.

▮ M C Q s

1. A 26-year-old woman asks for your advice. She has been experiencing a colourless cream-white curd-like vaginal discharge. She explains that there is no smell, however, she is experiencing a lot of itching. Which ONE of the following is the most likely diagnosis?
   (a) BV
   (b) Chlamydia
   (c) Gonorrhoea
   (d) Trichomoniasis
   (e) Vaginal candidiasis

2. A 32-year-old woman tells you she has been experiencing vaginal discharge which has an unpleasant fishy smell. She describes the discharge as thin and green-yellow in colour. Which ONE of the following is the most likely diagnosis?
   (a) BV
   (b) Cystitis
   (c) Gonorrhoea
   (d) Trichomoniasis
   (e) Vaginal candidiasis

3. A 25-year-old woman presents to the pharmacy complaining of intense vaginal itching accompanied by a nonsmelling colourless discharge. You take a social history and find that the patient has had three sexual partners in the last 2 months and used a barrier protection method with two of them. She also mentions she recently completed a course of antibiotics for a UTI. Which ONE of the conditions is the most likely diagnosis?
   (a) BV

   (b) Chlamydia
   (c) Gonorrhoea
   (d) Trichomoniasis
   (e) Vaginal candidiasis

4. Recurrent *Candida* infection is defined as four or more episodes in 12 months. A number of possible risk factors have been identified. Which ONE of the following is not known to be a risk factor?
   (a) Diabetes mellitus
   (b) HIV infection
   (c) Recent antibiotic use
   (d) Rheumatoid arthritis
   (e) Use of local irritants

5. A 23-year-old woman presents with a history of lower abdominal pain, abnormal vaginal discharge, dyspareunia, fever, nausea and vomiting for 5 days. From the following conditions, which ONE is the most likely diagnosis?
   (a) Acute appendicitis
   (b) Acute pyelonephritis
   (c) Atrophic vaginitis
   (d) Herpes simplex
   (e) PID

Answers
1. e; 2. a; 3. e; 4. d; 5. e

KEY POINTS: THRUSH

- *Candida albicans* (90%) and *Candida glabrata* (5%) are responsible for thrush.
- Recent antibiotic use and local irritants can precipitate thrush.
- Key symptom is itch.
- The incidence of recurrent infections (four or more attacks in a year) is low (5%).

▮ CASE 45: VAGINAL ITCHING

PRESENTATION

Mrs P, a 47-year-old Asian mother of two and well known to you, asks for some advice. She tells you she has been suffering from vaginal itching and some vulval soreness over the last few days. She bought some cream (clotrimazole) from the pharmacy a couple of days ago as she thought it was thrush, but her symptoms have not improved. She wants to know if there is anything else she could try.

PROBLEM REPRESENTATION

A 47-year-old woman presents with acute onset vaginal symptoms possibly unresponsive to clotrimazole.

HYPOTHESIS GENERATION (LIKELY, POSSIBLE AND CRITICAL DIAGNOSES)

The most common causes of vaginal itching/soreness affecting a woman of our patient's age is thrush (see Table 8.2).

Likely Diagnosis

- Thrush

Possible Diagnoses

- BV
- Trichomoniasis
- Vaginitis (older women)

Critical Diagnosis

- Malignancy

CONTINUED INFORMATION GATHERING

Mrs P's symptoms do fit with a diagnosis of thrush, although failure of clotrimazole to resolve her symptoms would be unusual given its effectiveness. Further questions about other symptoms, a medical history and use of clotrimazole need to be asked. Mrs P says she has not noticed any discharge, takes no regular medicines from the doctor and her description of using the clotrimazole seems appropriate.

It would seem reasonable at this point to believe the patient is suffering from vaginal thrush and is receiving appropriate treatment (although she might not have been using it for long enough). Conditions causing similar symptoms, for example, BV and trichomoniasis, have discharge as a prominent symptom (see summary information below). Mrs P is also in a stable relationship, which supports thrush as the diagnosis rather than BV or trichomoniasis.

PROBLEM REFINEMENT

It would be useful to establish from Mrs P a history of previous bouts of thrush, as some women will develop recurrent thrush, which can be attributed to undiagnosed type 2 diabetes. This is especially true in Asian people, who are known to be two to four times more likely to develop type 2 diabetes. It would also be advisable to establish if Mrs P is currently suffering from excessive thirst, urination or fatigue – all hallmark symptoms of diabetes, although these are insidious in onset and may go unnoticed.

Mrs P reports having thrush symptoms a couple of times over the last 18 months or so, but denies any other symptoms.

⚡ RED FLAGS

Mrs P has no alarm symptoms such as abnormal bleeding.

MANAGEMENT

Self-care Options

Not applicable.

Prescribing Options

Mrs P should be told to continue using clotrimazole for a further 5 days to help clear the current episode of thrush. However, her previous symptoms of thrush,

TABLE 8.2	Condition Summary for Thrush, Bacterial Vaginosis and Trichomoniasis			
	Timing	**Discharge**	**Odour**	**Itch**
Thrush	Acute and onset quick	White curd- or cottage cheese-like (one in five patients)	Little or none	Prominent
Bacterial vaginosis	Acute but onset slow	White and thin (one in two patients)	Strong and fishy, which might be worse during menses and after sex	Slight
Trichomoniasis	Acute but onset slow	Green-yellow and can be frothy	Malodorous	Slight

coupled with potential treatment failure, require further investigation.

Safety Netting

You tell Mrs P that because she has had more than one episode of thrush recently, it would be a good idea to check if there is anything causing these episodes. You tell her that multiple bouts of thrush are sometimes a symptom of diabetes, and you would like to do some tests to make sure this is not causing her symptoms.

AIDE MEMOIRE

Likely Diagnosis
Thrush

The cardinal symptoms of vaginal candidiasis are vulval pruritus and vaginal soreness/burning. Discharge (in approximately 20% cases) has little or no odour and is described as cottage cheese- or curd-like.

Possible Diagnoses
Bacterial Vaginosis

If patients exhibit symptoms, then it is characterised by a thin grey/white discharge with a strong fishy odour. Odour is worse after sexual intercourse and may worsen during menses and after intercourse. Itching and soreness are not usually present. Sexual activity, smoking, intrauterine devices and being Black are known risk factors.

Trichomoniasis

Up to 50% of patients are asymptomatic. When present, common symptoms include a profuse, frothy, greenish-yellow and fishy-smelling discharge. Other symptoms include vulvar itching and soreness, vaginal spotting, dysuria and lower abdominal pain.

Vaginitis

Vaginitis is usually associated with vaginal discharge and pain during sex. It can also cause cystitis-like symptoms, although typically it is not associated with urgency or frequency. Postmenopausal women (atrophic vaginitis) experience thinning of the endometrial lining as a result of a reduction in the levels of circulating oestrogen in the blood. This can also lead to symptoms of vaginal dryness and itching. Vaginitis caused by a streptococcal infection (rare) tends to cause more severe signs and symptoms to other causes of vaginitis.

Critical Diagnosis
Malignancy (Vulval and Vaginal Cancers)

These are relatively rare cancers. Both can be associated with bleeding between periods. However other symptoms will be present. Persistent itch is common to both cancers as well as palpable lump/growth. In vaginal cancer, discharge that smells or is blood stained is often seen. Vulval and vaginal cancers are most common in women over the age of 75 years.

▌ M C Q s

1. Which ONE of the following set of symptoms most closely matches that of vaginal thrush?
   (a) Itch and discharge described as having an offensive odour
   (b) Itch and burning sensation and curd-like discharge
   (c) Little itching but frothy yellow discharge
   (d) Little or no itch but increased urgency and pain on passing urine
   (e) Little itching but associated with blood-stained discharge
2. Which ONE of the following symptoms is commonly associated with trichomoniasis?
   (a) Clear, watery vaginal discharge
   (b) Cottage cheese-like vaginal discharge
   (c) Frothy, green-yellow vaginal discharge
   (d) Small ulcers on the external genitalia
   (e) White, fishy-smelling vaginal discharge
3. A 21-year-old student asks for advice about some 'women's symptoms'. Which ONE of the following set of symptoms is least indicative of referral to the doctor?
   (a) Itch and discharge described as having an offensive odour
   (b) Itch and burning sensation and curd-like discharge
   (c) Little itching but frothy yellow discharge
   (d) Little itching but associated with blood-stained discharge
   (e) No itching but increased urgency and pain on passing urine with flank pain
4. Diabetes can manifest with a wide range of signs and symptoms. Which ONE of the following is not a symptom associated with diabetes?
   (a) Fatigue
   (b) Frequent urination
   (c) Itchy skin

(d) Muscle pain

(e) Thirst

5. Which ONE of the following is not a risk factor for type 2 diabetes?

(a) Family history

(b) Hypertension

(c) Obesity

(d) Polycystic ovarian syndrome

(e) Poor dietary habits

Answers

1. b; 2. c; 3. b; 4. d; 5. b

KEY POINTS: UNDIAGNOSED TYPE 2 DIABETES

* Estimated that there are 1 million people with undiagnosed type 2 diabetes
* Risk factors include obesity (especially abdominal circumference), over 40 years of age, ethnicity and recurrent infection.
* Key symptoms include polyuria and polydipsia, fatigue and unexplained weight loss.

WEBSITES

Diabetes UK
https://www.diabetes.org.uk/
Desmond Educational programmes
https://www.desmond.nhs.uk/about-us

9

General Physical Problems

CASE 46: INSOMNIA

PRESENTATION

Mr L, a 48-year-old man, presents with difficulty in falling asleep. He says it takes him at least an hour to fall asleep after going to bed. He has been experiencing this for the last 4–6 weeks.

PROBLEM REPRESENTATION

A 48-year-old man presents with a 6-week history of sleep disturbance.

HYPOTHESIS GENERATION (LIKELY, POSSIBLE AND CRITICAL DIAGNOSES)

Insomnia can occur at any age, but the incidence increases with age. It is more common in women than men.

Insomnia is defined as difficulty in getting to sleep, struggling to maintain sleep, waking up frequently in the night or a tendency to wake up early and be unable to go back to sleep, or having sleep of poor quality that results in impaired daytime functioning. Short-term insomnia is typically described as lasting a few days to a few weeks (it is classified as chronic insomnia if present for more than 3 months). In short-term cases (sometimes referred to as adjustment insomnia), there is usually an identifiable precipitating cause or risk factor. Conditions to consider are:

Likely Diagnoses

- Acute episodes of stress
- Circadian rhythm disorders
  - Shift work
  - Jet lag

- Environment – noise, temperature, etc.
- Medicines
- Preexisting medical conditions

Possible Diagnoses

- Parasomnia
- Periodic limb movement disorder
- Restless legs syndrome
- Sleep apnoea

Critical Diagnosis

- Narcolepsy

CONTINUED INFORMATION GATHERING

A thorough understanding of Mr L's sleeping patterns and taking a medical and social history are needed to try and identify the cause of his symptoms.

Mr L tells you that he is normally not affected by poor sleep; in fact, this is the first time he has experienced such symptoms. He says that he has a lot on his mind, and when he goes to bed, he finds it hard to stop thinking about stuff. His poor sleeping has been keeping his wife awake at night too, as he has been quite restless and kicking his legs a lot. He lost his sister about 3 months ago – she died of breast cancer. He is generally in good health and has no medical problems.

The death of his sister appears to be the precipitating event as to the cause of his insomnia.

PROBLEM REFINEMENT

At this point, it would be useful to see if there are any other factors that could be contributing to his poor sleeping and determine what he has been doing to cope with the death of his sister.

He tells you he has thrown himself into his work (as a sales director for a coffee company) to keep himself busy, but it is when he is at home in the evenings that he is not coping too well. He admits to drinking more alcohol than usual in the evenings. His bedtimes are variable, and he has noticed that he has been getting tired at work; hence, he has been drinking more coffee during the day to perk himself up. He has not been going to the gym as often, as he has lost motivation.

Increased alcohol and caffeine intake coupled with erratic times of going to bed will all contribute to his sleeping difficulty. This additional information confirms your thinking that the death of his sister is the cause of his insomnia, and his coping strategies are contributing to his insomnia.

> ⚡ **RED FLAGS**
>
> He has no symptoms suggestive of narcolepsy, for example, excessive drowsiness or sudden attacks of sleep.

MANAGEMENT

Self-care Options

You talk to Mr L about how he can improve his sleep. The options include:

- Maintain a regular bedtime and awakening time.
- Reduce the amount of coffee he is drinking, especially in the evening.
- Try to limit or avoid alcohol in the evening, especially just before going to bed.
- Try to go back to the gym, but do not exercise too late in the evening.
- Make sure the bedroom is comfortable – avoid it being too warm.
- Do not watch TV, use the computer or read in bed (e.g., avoid mental activity).
- If unable to get to sleep, get up and do something, and return to bed when sleepy.

Prescribing Options

Besides managing the acute presentation of insomnia, there is a need to explore how he can better cope with managing his grief and assessing if he is depressed.

A referral to a grief counsellor should be considered along with potential instigation of a sleep aid (nonbenzodiazepine) for up to a week. If depression is diagnosed, the use of a selective serotonin inhibitor (SSRI) may be warranted. However, some SSRIs can aggravate insomnia. Therefore, if instigated, daytime dosing of SSRIs is advisable. Mr L agrees to try zopiclone for a few nights and improve his sleep patterns.

Safety Netting

You discuss with Mr L that you believe his insomnia has been triggered by the death of his sister. The short-term measures put in place will hopefully help, but you would like to see him again in 1–2 weeks to check up on how he is.

AIDE MEMOIRE

Likely Diagnoses

A number of risk factors associated with short-term insomnia can be identified and include shift or night work, noise or light during the night, uncomfortably high or low temperatures and travelling to different time zones that can disturb the sleep–wake cycle.

Medical Conditions

A large number of conditions can disturb sleep due to symptoms ranging from pruritus, pain, breathing difficulties and excessive sweating. Table 9.1 lists those frequently implicated with disturbing sleep.

Medicines

Medicines and using nonpharmacological drugs (e.g., caffeine, nicotine, alcohol, illicit drugs) can have central nervous system-related adverse effects that can affect sleep patterns, as shown in Table 9.2 (this list is not exhaustive).

TABLE 9.1 Conditions that can Cause Insomnia	
Cardiovascular	Heart failure, arrhythmia, coronary artery disease
Pulmonary	Chronic obstructive pulmonary disease, asthma
Neurologic	Stroke, Parkinson's disease, depression, dementia
Gastrointestinal	Gastroesophageal reflux
Renal	Chronic renal failure
Endocrine	Diabetes, hyperthyroidism
Rheumatologic	Rheumatoid arthritis, osteoarthritis, fibromyalgia
Gynaecological	Pregnancy, menopause

TABLE 9.2 **Medicines Known to Cause Insomnia**	
Stimulants	Caffeine, theophylline, sympathomimetics amines (e.g., pseudoephedrine), monoamine oxidase inhibitors – especially in early treatment
Antiepileptics	Carbamazepine, phenytoin
Alcohol	Low to moderate amounts can promote sleep, but when taken in excess or over a long period, it can disturb sleep.
Beta-blockers	Can cause nightmares, especially propranolol
Calcium channel blockers	Can cause somnolence
Selective serotonin inhibitor (SSRIs)	Especially fluoxetine
Diuretics	Ensure these are not taken after midday to stop the need to urinate at night.
Cholinesterase inhibitors	Donepezil (abnormal dreams and nightmares), galantamine
Metoclopramide	
Alpha-blockers	

Possible Diagnoses

Parasomnia

Parasomnia relates to unusual behaviours that people experience prior to falling asleep, while asleep or during the arousal period between sleep and wakefulness. It is associated with unnatural movements, behaviours, emotions, perceptions and dreams. In some cases, it is severe or persistent enough to cause significant sleep disruption and distress or injury to the patient or bed partner. Examples are sleep walking, night terrors and sleep-related hallucinations.

Periodic Limb Movement Disorder

This is characterised by involuntary movements of the legs, occurring every 20–40 s, consisting of dorsiflexion of the ankle and flaring of the toes. The leg movements are often accompanied by repetitive, brief arousals from sleep that the patient is often not aware of. The disruption to sleep may result in nonrefreshing sleep and daytime fatigue.

Restless Legs Syndrome

Restless legs syndrome is often confused with periodic limb movement disorder; however, the symptoms of restless legs syndrome occur while the person is still awake, although symptoms are typically worse in the evenings. The person experiences uncomfortable tingling or crawling sensations in the legs, accompanied by an uncontrollable urge to move the legs to feel relief.

Sleep Apnoea

Sleep apnoea is associated with a variety of symptoms related to poor sleeping. It should be suspected in individuals who suffer from unrefreshing sleep, excessive day time fatigue and sleepiness. It is also associated with being male or obese.

Critical Diagnosis

Narcolepsy

Narcolepsy is characterised by overwhelming daytime drowsiness and sudden attacks of sleep. People with narcolepsy often find it difficult to stay awake for long periods of time. Symptoms also include disrupted sleep and cataplexy (sudden loss of muscle tone that results in conscious collapse), often in response to intense emotions such as laughter, surprise or anger. Narcolepsy typically presents from the midteens onwards.

▌ M C Q s

1. A 20-year-old student has had trouble sleeping for 2 weeks accompanied by general daytime lethargy. Which ONE of the following is the most likely cause?
   (a) Hypersomnia
   (b) Long-term insomnia
   (c) Narcolepsy
   (d) Short-term insomnia
   (e) Transient insomnia

2. Which ONE of the following statements about insomnia is FALSE?
   (a) Affects one-third of the population
   (b) Chronic insomnia rarely remits spontaneously.
   (c) Common in the elderly
   (d) Insomnia of >1 year is a risk factor for depression.
   (e) More common in men
3. If pharmacological intervention is deemed appropriate, which ONE of the following agents is considered first line?
   (a) Benzodiazepines
   (b) Melatonin
   (c) Sedating antihistamines
   (d) Z drugs
   (e) None of the above
4. From the list of medicines, which ONE is not associated with sleep disturbances?
   (a) Beta-blockers
   (b) Calcium channel blocking agents
   (c) Statins
   (d) Sympathomimetic agents
   (e) Theophylline
5. Chronic insomnia is associated with:
   (a) Acute stressful situations
   (b) Change to shift patterns
   (c) Excessive caffeine intake
   (d) Foreign travel
   (e) None of the above

Answers

1. d; 2. e; 3. d; 4. c; 5. e

KEY POINTS: INSOMNIA

- Short-term insomnia is associated with triggers and chronic insomnia, and often associated with an underlying medical condition.
- Key symptoms are difficulty falling asleep or maintaining sleep and lacking refreshment from sleep.
- Avoid benzodiazepines and use z drugs short-term.

WEBSITES

International Sleep Charity
https://www.internationalsleepcharity.org/
The Sleep Charity
https://thesleepcharity.org.uk/
Sleep Foundation
http://www.sleepfoundation.org/

British Snoring & Sleep Apnoea Association
https://britishsnoring.co.uk/
Mental Health Foundation – How to sleep better
https://www.mentalhealth.org.uk/explore-mental-health/
   publications/how-sleep-better

CASE 47: LEG SWELLING

PRESENTATION

A 23-year-old woman presents to you complaining of a swollen and tender right calf. She says she first noticed her calf aching a couple of days ago and it has slowly gotten worse. She is otherwise fit and healthy but does take the combined oral contraceptive pill for birth control.

PROBLEM REPRESENTATION

A 23-year-old healthy woman presents with a 2-day history of worsening calf pain and associated swelling.

HYPOTHESIS GENERATION (LIKELY, POSSIBLE AND CRITICAL DIAGNOSES)

Lower limb oedema is a common and challenging diagnostic problem, often with a significant impact. It is defined as swelling caused by an increase in interstitial fluid that exceeds the capacity of physiologic lymphatic drainage. Fluid collection can be a result of many aetiologies, including a range of local or systemic disorders. Symptoms can be debilitating and subsequently impact quality of life.

Likely Diagnoses

- Cellulitis
- Deep vein thrombosis (DVT)
- Medicines
- Musculoskeletal injuries
- Systemic disease: heart failure

Possible Diagnoses

- Compartment syndrome
- Complex regional pain syndrome
- Lipoedema
- Lymphoedema – primary and secondary
- Systemic disease
  - Hepatic (cirrhosis)
  - Hypothroidism
  - Renal (nephrotic syndrome)

- Thrombophlebitis
- Venous insufficiency

Critical Diagnosis

- Compartment syndrome (acute)
- Malignancy

CONTINUED INFORMATION GATHERING

As we are dealing with an acute presentation in a young woman, the conditions from the 'likely diagnoses list' that need to be considered are cellulitis, DVT, medicines and musculoskeletal injuries. Heart failure can be excluded as this is a condition of the elderly.

Initially, questioning should establish the exact site of swelling and if it is affected by the time of day or the person's position, and to ensure it is only unilateral. The level of pain should also be explored.

She confirms it is just her right calf, and you confirm this on examination. There is obvious localised calf swelling on her right leg compared with her left leg, and the patient complains that it hurts when you apply pressure. Her calf does not feel hot, there is no visible signs of rash or pitting oedema. She tells you the pain is more aching discomfort than debilitating pain.

At this point, cellulitis seems unlikely as the patient appears well (e.g., afebrile), the skin is normal temperature and there is no rash present. Additionally, as the pain and swelling have come on relatively slowly, a musculoskeletal injury is also unlikely. We know she takes the combined pill, and this can cause leg swelling as a side effect, although this tends to be bilateral. Establishing any causality is needed to see if the pill might be a cause of her symptoms. You find out she has taken the same pill for the last 2 years, there have been no dose changes and she takes it as prescribed. An adverse drug reaction does not seem to be the cause of her symptoms, although taking the pill is a known risk factor for developing a DVT.

As DVT is now suspected, you explore if she has any other risk factors for DVT, such as smoking, recent prolonged travel or a history of a DVT. She tells you she does smoke, but it is more a social thing rather than every day.

DVT does seem to be the most plausible diagnosis.

PROBLEM REFINEMENT

Other acute unilateral presentations of leg swelling should be ruled out from your thinking. These include compartment syndrome and complex regional pain syndrome. However, compartment syndrome is associated with trauma and, in both conditions, pain will be severe. Therefore, both these problems can be discounted from our thinking.

The Wells' criteria for DVT should be used to shape your thinking and decision making. You decide that she scores '2' due to calf tenderness and the size of the swelling. A score of 2 or more suggests that DVT is likely. As she takes the pill, this will be classed as a provoked DVT as per guidance from the National Institute for Health and Care Excellence.

> ⚡ **RED FLAGS**
>
> Our patient has not reported any signs of breathlessness or chest pain, which seems to rule out pulmonary embolism.

MANAGEMENT

Self-care Options

Not applicable.

Prescribing Options

The patient needs to have a leg ultrasound, with the results available within 4 h. If a DVT is confirmed, oral anticoagulants will be initiated, and an alternative contraceptive/contraceptive method will need to be instigated.

Safety Netting

Anticoagulant therapy is usually for a minimum of 3 months. Therefore, a follow-up consultation will be required after a month or so to make sure there are no problems.

AIDE MEMOIRE

Likely Diagnoses
Cellulitis

Typically, a break in the skin allows *Streptococcus* or *Staphylococcus* bacteria to invade, causing acute onset swollen and tender skin that is red and painful to the touch. It is almost always unilateral affecting the lower limb. Systemic symptoms can also be present, including fever and malaise. It can spread rapidly, and recurrence is common.

Deep Vein Thrombosis

DVT results in obstruction to venous flow. Findings that suggest DVT include acute, unilateral pitting oedema, usually in the calf, associated with throbbing pain, redness, warmth and tenderness. Patients who develop DVT commonly have risk factors, such as increasing age, obesity, active cancer, recent surgery or trauma, hospitalisation, immobilisation, pregnancy, a preceding long flight or oral contraceptive use. Using Wells' scoring helps to assess the probability of a DVT, but diagnosis requires confirmation of a blood clot by venous ultrasound imaging.

Medicines

Medicine-induced leg swelling is relatively common. Presentation is usually acute and bilateral. Medicines implicated include hormone therapy, gabapentinoids and antihypertensives (especially calcium channel blockers) and anticancer drugs such as docetaxel.

Musculoskeletal Injuries

Sprains, strains and fractures affecting the lower limb can cause localised swelling and pain. A recent history of trauma should be present. A ruptured Baker's cyst (rare) can present with similar symptoms of a DVT or acute thrombophlebitis. Symptoms of popliteal swelling with associated vague pain precede rupture symptoms.

Systemic Causes: Heart Failure

Onset of symptoms tends to be slow, insidious and non-specific, making an early diagnosis challenging. Typically, shortness of breath, night-time cough, fatigue, decreased exercise tolerance and painless bilateral ankle and lower limb swelling are seen. It is a condition of the elderly with increasing prevalence with increasing age.

Possible Diagnoses

Compartment Syndrome

Compartment syndrome develops when swelling or bleeding occurs within a compartment, causing increased pressure on the capillaries, nerves and muscles. Acute presentations usually develop after a severe injury and cause intense pain with associated paraesthesia and constitute a medical emergency. Chronic presentations most often occur in the calf. Onset is gradual (months) and causes swelling, pain and sometimes paraesthesia. Tenderness and tightness of the muscle are common. It is often seen in runners as it is associated with strenuous activity. Rest will alleviate symptoms.

Complex Regional Pain Syndrome

This must be considered with a significantly painful chronically swollen limb. Onset usually follows after an injury to the leg. Pain can be intense, even from slight contact, and can persist for prolonged periods. Skin texture changes and discolouration are seen over time.

Systemic Disease Other Than Heart Failure

Systemic disease will cause bilateral leg swelling. New onset or exacerbations of renal, hepatic and endocrine issues may be a cause.

Renal (nephrotic syndrome). Nephrotic syndrome causes hypoalbuminaemia or hypoproteinaemia and manifests with a wide range of signs and symptoms. Diffuse oedema is the predominant symptom, including lower leg oedema. Other symptoms include breathlessness, signs of infection, dizziness and fatigue. It is frequently accompanied by dyslipidaemia, abnormalities in coagulation, reduced renal function and immunological disorders.

Hepatic (cirrhosis). Leg swelling is a recognised symptom of cirrhosis as a result of increased pressure in the portal vein. Accompanying symptoms include fatigue, loss of appetite, bruising easily, weight loss, itching or yellow discolouration of the skin.

Hypothyroidism. One of the symptoms of hypothyroidism is swollen feet/lower limbs. However, more obvious symptoms of tiredness, dry skin, hair loss, weight gain, constipation, cold intolerance and difficulty concentrating are seen.

Venous Insufficiency

Chronic venous insufficiency typically causes chronic leg or ankle oedema accompanied with discomfort/heaviness in the legs, aching, itching and skin discolouration/eczema or sometimes skin breakdown. People often have a history of hypertension, smoking, obesity or inactivity or there is a family history.

Lymphoedema – Primary and Secondary

Lymphoedema is a chronic, progressive swelling of tissue that occurs as a result of excess accumulation of lymph due to inadequate drainage. It is caused by a congenital abnormality or dysfunction in the lymphatic system (primary) or acquired (secondary), such as from trauma, infection and malignancy. Typically, it initially presents with painless unilateral limb swelling, including the foot, with pitting oedema present in early disease. The patient may also complain of a feeling of heaviness in the limb, especially at the end of the day and in hot weather. Over time, the skin becomes thicker and rougher and skin turgor is increased. In severe cases, the skin can break down.

Lipoedema

Lipoedema is almost always bilateral nonpitting oedema of the legs with sparing of the feet. Swelling tends to worsen as the day progresses or in hot weather. Legs might take on a lumpy texture and people may find walking difficult. Disproportionate pain, tenderness and an unusual tendency to bruise easily for no obvious cause is also experienced. It is more common in women and only very rarely affects men.

Thrombophlebitis (Superficial Vein Thrombosis)

Occurs in the lower legs and usually results from having varicose veins. Pain and swelling typically develop over hours to days and tend to resolve over days/weeks. The skin over the vein becomes red, and the area feels warm and tender. The vein feels like a hard cord under the skin, not soft like a varicose vein.

Critical Diagnoses

Compartment Syndrome – Acute

See earlier.

Malignancy

Occult (site of primary tumour cannot be found) cancers may be present with apparently idiopathic DVT. A history of unexplained weight loss or adenopathy might suggest malignancy.

MCQs

1. A middle-aged male patient presents with acute, pitting oedema and pain in his right lower extremity that started yesterday. Physical examination detects redness, warmth and tenderness in the limb. Based on these findings, which ONE of the following is the most likely diagnosis?
   (a) Chronic venous insufficiency
   (b) DVT
   (c) Heart failure
   (d) Lipoedema
   (e) Nephrotic syndrome
2. Which ONE of the following scenarios is most appropriate for antibiotics to be initiated in primary care for cellulitis?
   (a) Mild systemic upset with no comorbidities
   (b) Mild systemic upset with multiple comorbidities
   (c) No systemic symptoms but has poorly controlled diabetes

   (d) No systemic symptoms but has controlled diabetes
   (e) No systemic upset and has no comorbidities
3. A 78-year-old man presents with a 5-month history of nonpainful bilateral leg oedema. Which ONE of the following is the most likely diagnosis?
   (a) Cellulitis
   (b) DVT
   (c) Heart failure
   (d) Lipodema
   (e) Lymphoedema
4. A number of risk factors are known in the development of DVT. Which ONE of the following is least associated as a risk factor?
   (a) Diabetes
   (b) Inactivity
   (c) Obesity
   (d) Older age
   (e) Smoking
5. Leg swelling can be acute or chronic and affect one or both legs. Which ONE of the following tends to be an acute presentation affecting one leg?
   (a) Cellulitis
   (b) Heart failure
   (c) Lipoedema
   (d) Lymphoedema
   (e) Venous insufficiency

Answers

1. b; 2. e; 3. c; 4. a; 5. a

KEY POINTS: DEEP VEIN THROMBOSIS

- A thrombus that partially or completely blocks blood flow and can be classified as provoked (associated with a risk factor) or unprovoked (absence of risk factors)
- Unilateral localised pain and tenderness and calf swelling are normal presenting symptoms.
- Referral is needed, but if not possible, anticoagulation should be started.

WEBSITES

Wells' scoring for DVT
https://www.mdcalc.com/calc/362/wells-criteria-dvt
Venous thromboembolic diseases: diagnosis, management and thrombophilia testing
https://www.nice.org.uk/guidance/ng158

CASE 48: TIRED ALL THE TIME

PRESENTATION

A 53-year-old Caucasian woman presents stating she always feels tired and exhausted and has not been sleeping well. She says the symptoms have been going on for months but has just been getting on with things and has put it down to the menopause, for which she takes Evorel (oestradiol) patches and Utrogestran (progestogen) capsules. She also complains of generalised muscle aching.

PROBLEM REPRESENTATION

Postmenopausal Caucasian woman with chronic tiredness, sleeping difficulties and associated musculoskeletal symptoms.

HYPOTHESIS GENERATION (LIKELY, POSSIBLE AND CRITICAL DIAGNOSES)

Tiredness is a normal part of life, but it is also a vague and nonspecific symptom of many conditions, including serious illnesses. It is also associated with being overweight and early pregnancy. A diagnosis is made in less than half of patients with fatigue.

Likely Diagnoses

- Anxiety/stress
- Chronic fatigue syndrome (myalgic encephalomyelitis)
- Depression
- Diabetes
- Fibromyalgia
- Work/life balance

Possible Diagnoses

- Addison's disease
- Anaemia
- Cushing's disease
- Gastrointestinal (GI) conditions
- Heart failure
- Infection
- Medicines
- Neurological conditions
- Obstructive sleep apnoea
- Thyroid disease

Critical Diagnosis

- Cancer

CONTINUED INFORMATION GATHERING

To help determine the cause it is important to clarify what the patient actually means by tiredness. Is it a lack of energy, do they experience daytime sleepiness or are they feeling low? The patient repeats that she just feels tired all the time and exhausted. Often she has to stop during the day for a rest or a sleep. This additional information does not really help with establishing a diagnosis, and at this time any one of the likely diagnoses is still a possibility.

She has reported musculoskeletal symptoms. Further clarification of where these symptoms are experienced is needed. She tells you she tends to have general aching, but especially in her hips, shoulders and hands. She also says that sometimes her fingers are swollen but this seems to happen randomly.

The history of tiredness and widespread aches and pains seems to be more consistent with fibromyalgia. You ask if she has any other symptoms. She tells you she gets some irritable bowel syndrome symptoms and has had these on and off for quite a time. This predates her current symptoms. She says she has not noticed any excessive thirst or going to the bathroom more, nor is she overly anxious. She does say that the continual tiredness is making day-to-day functioning difficult, and it is getting her down.

This further information seems to point away from anxiety, depression and diabetes.

PROBLEM REFINEMENT

You ask her about her job. She tells you she currently works part-time and mainly from home, which works well, although at times it can be stressful near deadline dates. She does not feel that work is the cause of her symptoms but does acknowledge that it might make symptoms worse when she is stressed.

Again, this seems to further support fibromyalgia as symptoms are known to worsen in times of stress. Chronic fatigue syndrome also seems less likely now as this is characterised by day-to-day activities being severely impaired. Her age and sex tend to suggest that heart failure and sleep apnoea can be discounted.

An examination of her joints reveals them to be normal. You arrange for blood tests to be performed, including oestrogen levels regarding her hormone replacement therapy (HRT). The results come back all in the normal range, indicating problems such as anaemia, thyroid dysfunction, diabetes, Cushing's syndrome and rheumatoid arthritis can be discounted.

Again this seems to further support fibromyalgia as symptoms are known to worsen in times of stress but based on current findings you are not certain.

> ## ⚡ RED FLAGS
>
> Tiredness is often present with various forms of cancer. Given her nonspecific symptoms and uncertainty of the diagnosis, cancer cannot be discounted. The patient will require monitoring and follow-up. No focal deficits are reported or observed, which seems to rule out neurological conditions at this time.

MANAGEMENT

Self-care Options

On the basis of a tentative diagnosis of fibromyalgia, the patient should be encouraged to exercise. You find out she has a gym membership but has not been going as regularly as she would like because of her symptoms. You encourage her that this is something she should aim to keep doing as exercise has been shown to help with symptoms. In addition, you can recommend a general healthy lifestyle and diet and discuss sleep hygiene measures.

Prescribing Options

Antidepressants can be tried (e.g., amitriptyline), but at this point you feel these are not warranted.

Safety Netting

You share your thoughts about it possibly being fibromyalgia, but you tell her you are not sure. You ask her to come back in a month's time to see how her symptoms are and to review if the self-care measures are helping. You also tell her that if she gets any new symptoms, she should get in touch straight away.

Depending on the review, a rethink on the diagnosis maybe needed. If you still suspect fibromyalgia, talking therapies could be an option as well as sign posting to charities that can provide additional support.

AIDE MEMOIRE

Likely Diagnoses
Anxiety/Stress

Anxiety and stress, besides manifesting with psychological symptoms such as irritability, difficulty concentrating and restlessness, can exhibit physical symptoms, including headaches, palpitations, shaking, shortness of breath, poor sleep and tiredness.

Chronic Fatigue Syndrome (Myalgic Encephalomyelitis)

Chronic fatigue syndrome may be suspected if the person reports having longstanding, debilitating fatigue that is worsened by activity and not significantly relieved by rest, having unrefreshing sleep or sleep disturbance (or both) and experiencing cognitive difficulties (sometimes described as 'brain fog').

Depression

Besides psychological symptoms, commonly depression can manifest with physical symptoms of poor sleep, changes in appetite, poor concentration and fatigue.

Diabetes (Type 2)

Tiredness is a common symptom of diabetes. Other common symptoms include polydipsia, polyuria, blurred vision, unexplained weight loss and recurrent infections.

Fibromyalgia

Fibromyalgia is a very common disorder, particularly in middle-aged women, characterised by diffuse chronic musculoskeletal pain, fatigue, low mood, nonrestorative sleep and normal blood results. The American College of Rheumatology has established diagnostic criteria for the disease, which include a history of widespread pain in association with 11 of 18 specific tender point sites (see website link for further details). Patients with fibromyalgia often report dropping things due to pain and weakness. It has been associated with irritable bladder, irritable bowel syndrome, headaches and temporomandibular joint pain.

Work/Life Balance

Long working hours, shift or night work can affect the pattern of waking and sleeping, leading to fatigue and tiredness. Life events can also contribute to general tiredness, such as caring responsibilities and parental duties to young children.

Possible Diagnoses
Addison's Disease

A diagnosis can be difficult due to the nonspecific nature of a range of common symptoms experienced.

Fatigue is a very early common symptom seen in most patients. Other early symptoms include low mood, muscle weakness, weight loss and loss of appetite, increased urination and increased thirst. Over time, these symptoms worsen and other symptoms such as diarrhoea, abdominal pain, nausea/vomiting, dizziness, cramps and darkening of the skin can occur.

Anaemia

Anaemia is commonly caused through dietary restriction, medicines or blood loss (e.g., menstruation). Typically, fatigue is prominent along with headache, dyspnoea, pallor and dry skin and hair changes.

Cushing's Disease

Tiredness can be experienced but is not a prominent symptom. The main signs/symptoms of Cushing's disease are round red face, hump on the back of the neck, skin changes such as stretch marks or acne and unusual rapid weight gain, especially around the belly.

Gastrointestinal Conditions

A number of GI conditions can exhibit tiredness as a general symptom, for example, inflammatory bowel disease (IBD), irritable bowel syndrome, coeliac disease and hepatitis. For IBD, bloody diarrhoea would be prominent; for irritable bowel syndrome, lower abdominal pain; for coeliac disease, diarrhoea; for hepatitis fever, nausea.

Heart Failure

Tiredness and lethargy are the most prevalent symptoms in heart failure patients and are accompanied with breathlessness, leg swelling, loss of appetite, poor exercise tolerance and productive cough.

Infection

Some infections will have tiredness as a prominent symptom such as glandular fever. Other infections can also have tiredness as a symptom, including influenza, COVID-19, pneumonia, tuberculosis and HIV. However, more prominent symptoms associated with each infection will be present.

Medicines

Many medicines can cause weakness and fatigue, and include antidepressants, high blood pressure medicines (angiotensin-converting enzyme inhibitors, beta-blockers, calcium channel blockers), statins and antianxiety medicines.

Neurological

Fatigue is commonly reported in many neurologic illnesses, including multiple sclerosis, Parkinson's disease, myasthenia gravis and stroke. Fatigue contributes substantially to quality of life and disability in these illnesses.

Obstructive Sleep Apnoea

This is more common in obese men of increasing age. It should be suspected in those who are fatigued, are excessively sleepy through the day and are known to snore when asleep. People often complain of unrefreshing sleep and difficulty in concentrating.

Thyroid Disease

Tiredness is associated with both hypo and hyperthyroidism. In hyperthyroidism, symptoms such as breathlessness, dysphagia, nervousness and hyperactivity are often present; in hypothyroidism, symptoms include cold intolerance, weight gain, constipation and dry skin.

Critical Diagnosis
Cancer

Most forms of cancer exhibit general signs and symptoms, including fatigue. Cancer-related fatigue tends to be chronic and not relieved by rest or sleep.

MCQs

1. A 60-year-old woman, who has recently been diagnosed with hypertension and takes atenolol, presents saying she is tired all the time, struggling to concentrate and feels nauseous, which has led to her not feeling like she wants to eat. You ask if she has any aches and pains. She tells you she has been experiencing some knee joint pain but puts this down to age. She also says she been finding concentrating difficult. Which ONE of the following is the most likely diagnosis?
   (a) Chronic renal failure
   (b) Hepatitis
   (c) Hyperparathyroidism
   (d) Medication side effects
   (e) Osteoarthritis

2. A 52-year-old woman presents with pain in multiple joints, especially her hands and back. She says her hands intermittently are swollen and her grip is weak. She tells you she is always tired. However, on examination, there is no discernible swelling of the hands although there appears to be widespread tenderness. Blood tests are performed but all are normal. Which ONE of the following is the most likely diagnosis?
   (a) Fibromyalgia
   (b) Hypothyroidism
   (c) Myalgic encephalomyelitis
   (d) Osteoarthritis
   (e) Rheumatoid arthritis
3. A 35-year-old woman stopped taking the combined oral contraceptive pill 6 months ago as her blood pressure was continually raised. Since stopping her combined oral contraceptive pill, she reports feeling 'rubbish'. She says she is constantly tired, her face is a red mess and she has put on weight. Which ONE of the following is the most likely diagnosis?
   (a) Alcohol use disorder
   (b) Coeliac disease
   (c) Cushing's disease
   (d) Polycystic ovary syndrome
   (e) Stress
4. A 47-year-old woman complains of a 6- to 12-month history of aching all over. She is sleeping poorly and is tired all the time. The pain is pretty much constant but flares up without any real reason. After tests, which rule out causes such as arthritis, a diagnosis of fibromyalgia is reached. Which ONE of the following therapeutic options would be most appropriate?
   (a) Aerobic exercise
   (b) Acupuncture
   (c) A nonsteroidal antiinflammatory drug
   (d) An SSRI
   (e) Methotrexate
5. Medicines can cause tiredness. Which ONE of the following is reported to cause tiredness most frequently?
   (a) Aspirin
   (b) Atenolol
   (c) Atorvastatin
   (d) Ramipril
   (e) Sertraline

Answers

1. c; 2. a; 3. c; 4. a; 5. e

KEY POINTS: FIBROMYALGIA

- Disease of abnormal central nervous pain processing associated with amplification of nociceptive stimuli
- Characterised by diffuse musculoskeletal pain, fatigue and nonrestorative sleep
- Exercise, talking therapies and antidepressants (to manage the pain) form the main treatment modalities.

WEBSITES

Diagnostic Criteria for Fibromyalgia: Critical Review and Future Perspectives
https://www.ncbi.nlm.nih.gov/pmc/articles/PMC7230253/
Fibromyalgia Action UK
http://www.fmauk.org
UK Fibromyalgia
https://ukfibromyalgia.com

CASE 49: UNEXPLAINED (UNINTENTIONAL) WEIGHT LOSS

PRESENTATION

You have an appointment with a mother and her 14-year-old daughter, Miss D. Both are known to you as you have seen them over the years for various minor illnesses. Miss D is generally shy and not very forthcoming with information. Her mother has brought her today as she is concerned about her daughter's weight. She reports that her daughter is thin and recent clothes purchases now appear large on her and suspects she has lost weight. Miss D does not really say too much, other than she likes to have her clothes baggy and that is why her mum thinks she has lost weight.

PROBLEM REPRESENTATION

A mother presents with her adolescent daughter who is usually healthy but may be suffering from acute weight loss.

HYPOTHESIS GENERATION (LIKELY, POSSIBLE AND CRITICAL DIAGNOSES)

Unintentional weight loss has been defined as weight loss of at least 5% that occurs over the last 6–12 months and is not the expected consequence of treatment of a known illness. An assessment for the presence of cancer is always a high priority, although a wide range of causes of unintentional weight loss need to be considered. Dementia and depression should be considered in elderly patients and eating disorders in younger adults. However, in up to 25% of cases, no identifiable cause can be found.

Likely Diagnoses

- Any advanced malignancy – especially GI
- Gastrointestinal conditions
  - Coeliac disease
  - IBD
  - Peptic ulcer
- Psychiatric causes
  - Anxiety
  - Depression
  - Eating disorders

Possible Diagnoses

- Addison's disease
- Alcoholism
- Chronic obstructive pulmonary disease (COPD)
- Dementia
- Diabetes
- Heart failure
- Infection (serious)
  - HIV
  - Tuberculosis
- Medicines
- Parkinson's disease
- Thyrotoxicosis

Critical Diagnoses

- Endocarditis
- Malignancy

CONTINUED INFORMATION GATHERING

Given we are dealing with an adolescent girl, we can initially rule out a number of likely and possible causes of weight loss, such as peptic ulcer disease, Addison's disease, alcoholism, COPD, infections, heart failure, medicines, Parkinson's disease and thyrotoxicosis. The most likely conditions we need to first consider are mental health and GI disorders and diabetes.

We need to better understand if Miss D is indeed losing weight or underweight. You calculate her body mass index is 19.0, so although in the healthy range (<18.5 is classed as underweight), this is on the low side. When you ask specifically about losing weight,

Miss D says she has not weighed herself recently and does not volunteer that she feels she has lost weight.

Given weight loss can be associated with mental health disorders and you noticed she seemed somewhat withdrawn, asking about triggers for stress and asking screening questions for depression seems appropriate. She tells you she is fine and there is nothing like exams happening that might make her feel upset. You ask if she has started her periods and, if she has, what are they like. She says she has had them for about a year now and they seem fairly regular, but she does get some cramping pain with them, for which takes occasional paracetamol. Normal periods tend to point away from an eating disorder.

It seems your initial questions centred on establishing if a mental health disorder is responsible for her symptoms may not be the cause of her symptoms, although denial of symptoms in such cases is common.

PROBLEM REFINEMENT

A GI cause or diabetes will present with a range of symptoms other than weight loss. You ask if she has experienced any sort of symptoms over the last few weeks.

She tells you that she has been going to the toilet a lot recently and despite her mother thinking she has lost weight, she is always hungry and eats a lot. She denies any GI symptoms such as abdominal pain and diarrhoea.

Although your first thinking was that she was suffering from a suspected eating disorder, her symptoms seem to be pointing toward a diagnosis of type 1 diabetes.

⚡ RED FLAGS

Cancer and endocarditis would be very unlikely in a 14-year-old girl as both are rare in this age group. Cancer also tends to decrease appetite, not increase it, and in endocarditis other symptoms such as fever are present.

MANAGEMENT

Self-care Options

Not applicable.

Prescribing Options

Onward referral to a paediatric specialist is needed.

Safety Netting

You share your thoughts about your suspicion that it could be diabetes, but tests are needed to see if this is the case. You make arrangements for the girl to be seen at the local hospital. Two days later you receive confirmation from the paediatric diabetes team that she does indeed have diabetes and that she has been discharged on a biphasic insulin regimen, offered educational support and signposted to diabetes UK. The girl is due to go back to the hospital for reassessment in 2 weeks. You arrange an appointment for after this hospital visit to provide ongoing support.

AIDE MEMOIRE

Likely Diagnoses
Any Advanced Malignancy – Especially Gastrointestinal

The probability of malignancy is suggested by progressive onset of symptoms over weeks or months, which include change of bowel habit, rectal bleeding, neurological deficit, haemoptysis, appetite loss and unintended weight loss.

Gastrointestinal Conditions

Coeliac disease. Symptoms are often nonspecific but adult patients will have persistent GI symptoms that include steatorrhoea, bloating and abdominal pain, accompanied with unintentional weight loss. Prolonged fatigue (often due to anaemia) and persistent mouth ulcers can also be present. It can occur at any age put has two peaks of onset; shortly after weaning and people in their 20s and 30s.

Inflammatory bowel disease. Crohn's disease and ulcerative colitis are characterised by GI disturbance – either as persistent diarrhoea or bloody diarrhoea associated with urgency and tenesmus. Both exhibit lower abdominal pain. In Crohn's disease, the most common place for it to start is at the end of the small intestine (ileum), causing right lower quadrant pain. In ulcerative colitis, the pain is more common in the left lower quadrant. Over time, weight loss can be observed.

Both are also associated with extraintestinal symptoms, affecting between 25% and 40% of patients, and include arthritis, mouth ulcers, red eye and fatigue (due to anaemia). Other nonspecific symptoms such as malaise and fever can be present. Young adults (20–40 years old) are most affected.

Peptic ulcer. Typically, the patient will have well-localised, midepigastric pain described as 'constant', 'annoying' or 'gnawing/boring'. In gastric ulcers, the pain is usually triggered by food (and not relieved by antacids)

and experienced shortly after eating. In duodenal ulcers, the pain occurs 2–5 h after meals, which is relieved by food and often awakens a person at night. Gastric ulcers are also more commonly associated with weight loss and GI bleeds than duodenal ulcers. Peak incidence of duodenal ulcers is between 45 and 64 years of age, whereas incidence of gastric ulcers increases with age.

Psychiatric Causes

Anxiety. Anxiety may often present with only physical symptoms. These can be variable but include headache, insomnia, back pain and GI symptoms. Symptoms included in international diagnostic criteria (e.g., DSM-5 or ICD-11) when establishing a diagnosis of generalised anxiety disorder are restlessness, poor concentration, irritability and sleep disturbance. Excessive anxiety and worry can lead to weight loss.

It is worth noting that normal life events (e.g., marriage/divorce, bereavement) can precipitate anxiety symptoms and would not necessitate a formal diagnosis such as generalised anxiety disorder.

Depression. Depressive episodes are associated with sleep issues, poor concentration, social withdrawal and lack of interest in usual activities. Like anxiety, depression can present with physical symptoms only, including loss of weight (which is one of the DSM-5 symptoms). To help with a diagnosis, it is recommended that two screening questions are asked: 1. During the last month, have you often been bothered by feeling down, depressed or hopeless? 2. During the last month, have you often been bothered by having little interest or pleasure in doing things? If either question is answered 'yes', further evaluation of symptoms is needed.

Eating disorders. These include anorexia, bulimia, binge eating disorder and atypical eating disorder, the latter being the most common. It is seen almost exclusively in women (90%), especially those who are adolescents or young adults. In addition to weight loss (which can be rapid), other physical symptoms include GI problems and hormonal disturbances (e.g., amenorrhoea). Typically, mental health problems are observed such as depression, anxiety, stress and low self-esteem. Overconcern with body weight and shape is very common.

Possible Diagnoses
Addison's Disease

This a rare condition affecting those aged 30–50 years. Symptoms can be nonspecific and common to other conditions. Early symptoms include low mood, fatigue, muscle weakness, weight loss and loss of appetite, increased urination and increased thirst. Over time, these symptoms worsen and other symptoms such as diarrhoea, abdominal pain, nausea/vomiting, dizziness, cramps and darkening of the skin can occur.

Alcohol Use Disorder

Weight loss can be seen in those who are drinking at unsafe levels. This tends to be part of a wider pattern of self-neglect, although alcohol's effect on organ function, for example, the liver's inability to process fatty acids, leads to symptoms such as steatorrhoea that contributes to weight loss.

Chronic Obstructive Pulmonary Disease

COPD, beside chronic productive cough, is characterised by breathlessness that progressively worsens over time. Other symptoms include wheeze, reduced exercise tolerance and fatigue. COPD sufferers experience frequent respiratory tract infections. Patients often do not notice early symptoms, or they adjust their lifestyle to make breathing easier. Most people with COPD are current or former smokers, although a small proportion will have occupational exposure to chemicals and dust. Unintended weight loss is seen in severe cases or the later stages of the disease.

Dementia

Weight loss is often seen in the later stages of the disease. This may be because of a loss of appetite, pain or difficulties with swallowing and chewing.

Diabetes

Clinical features of type 1 diabetes show ketosis and rapid weight loss in children and young adults. Sometimes people refer to type 1 diabetes symptoms as the '4t's': toilet (polyuria); thirsty; tired; and thinner. For type 2 diabetes, polydipsia, polyuria, blurred vision, recurrent infection, tiredness and unexplained weight loss can be experienced.

Heart Failure

Often the first symptoms patients experience is fatigue and breathlessness on exertion, at rest or on lying flat. As the condition progresses from mild/moderate to severe heart failure, patients will show ankle swelling and might complain of a productive, frothy cough which may have pink-tinged sputum and may be worst at night. Occasionally, people develop cardiac cachexia leading to weight loss.

Infection (Serious)

HIV. After initial contraction of the HIV infection, most people experience flu-like symptoms for a few weeks. Other nonflu like symptoms include rash, diarrhoea, cough and weight loss.

Tuberculosis. Symptoms of active TB disease usually begin gradually and worsen over a few weeks. Besides respiratory symptoms, the person may develop fever, chills, night sweats, tiredness and weight loss.

Medicines

A number of medicines are known to cause weight loss as an adverse drug reaction. These include metformin, acarbose, exenatide, zonisamide, topiramate, bupropion and fluoxetine.

Parkinson's Disease

Weight loss can be a problem with those diagnosed with Parkinson's disease. This is probably multifactorial and includes difficulty in self-feeding, dysphagia and having a decreased appetite.

Thyrotoxicosis

Signs and symptoms of an overactive thyroid are numerous and can therefore be hard to diagnose. Symptoms include insomnia, fatigue, hyperactivity, mood swings, heat sensitivity, altered periods and weight loss despite having an increased appetite. Signs include shaking, palpitations, hair loss and goitre. In most cases, people aged between 20 and 40 years are most affected.

Critical Diagnoses
Endocarditis

Endocarditis (subacute). This usually develops insidiously and progresses slowly. Early symptoms are vague, and include fever, malaise, night sweats and weight loss.

Malignancy

Most forms of cancer can exhibit general signs and symptoms. Unexplained weight loss is associated with many forms of cancer.

MCQs

1. In people with unexplained weight loss and an increased appetite, which ONE of the following may be the cause?
   (a) An adverse drug reaction
   (b) Cancer
   (c) Depression
   (d) Hyperthyroidism
   (e) None of the above
2. People with fever, fatigue and night sweats may have which ONE of the following disorders?
   (a) Addison's disease
   (b) Cancer
   (c) Diabetes
   (d) Heart failure
   (e) Hyperthyroidism
3. Adverse drug reactions are known to cause weight loss. Which ONE of the following is most likely to cause weight loss?
   (a) Bupropion
   (b) Digoxin
   (c) Exenatide
   (d) Levodopa
   (e) Zonisamide
4. Type 1 diabetes can present with a range of signs and symptoms. Which ONE of the following is least likely?
   (a) Blurred vision
   (b) Excessive thirst
   (c) Fatigue
   (d) Polyuria
   (e) Weight loss
5. When trying to establish the cause of weight loss, understanding about the person is useful. For which ONE of the following would appetite be increased?
   (a) Adverse drug reactions
   (b) Anxiety
   (c) Cancer
   (d) Depression
   (e) Hyperthyroidism

Answers
1. d; 2. b; 3. e; 4. a; 5. e

KEY POINTS: TYPE 1 DIABETES
- Caused by an absolute deficiency of insulin
- Typically presents in young adults who exhibit low body mass index with fatigue, rapid weight loss and hyperglycaemia

- Insulin therapy needs to be tailored to the individual.
- HbA1C should be <6.5% to minimise long-term complications.

WEBSITES

Diabetes UK
https://www.diabetes.org.uk/
Beat eating disorders
https://www.beateatingdisorders.org.uk/
Drinkaware
https://www.drinkaware.co.uk/
Body Mass Index Calculator
https://www.nhs.uk/live-well/healthy-weight/bmi-calculator/

CASE 50: VOIDING PROBLEMS

PRESENTATION

An elderly man of 79 years of age is having trouble going to the toilet. He has a history of increasing difficulty going to the toilet. He says that it is hard for him to actually urinate. Sometimes he can be in the toilet for ages before he urinates and then he tends not to pass much urine. He also says that sometimes, despite his best efforts, he cannot go at all. Despite this, sometimes he finds that after going to the bathroom, he ends up having little accidents and his wife has now got some pads for him. He is not happy about this but seems resigned to this fact. He would really like to get the problem sorted as it is getting him down. He has a complicated medical history, having had a coronary artery bypass graft at the age of 53 years and more recent transient ischaemic attacks, age-related macular generation and vascular dementia. In addition, he has bilateral leg oedema and is being investigated for heart failure. He also has had one or two minor falls in the last 6 months. He is obviously frail and requires a stick to walk about the house and now needs to use a wheelchair to get out of the house.

PROBLEM REPRESENTATION

An elderly man with multimorbidity presents with progressively worsening urinary symptoms.

HYPOTHESIS GENERATION (LIKELY, POSSIBLE AND CRITICAL DIAGNOSES)

Lower urinary tract symptoms (LUTS) are a common problem in older men, with up to 30% of men over 65 years of age reporting troublesome symptoms.

Various 'umbrella terms' such as overactive bladder syndrome are used to categorise symptoms, but LUTS can be broadly grouped into problems of:

Voiding: weak or intermittent urinary stream, hesitancy, dribbling and incomplete emptying

Storage: increased frequency, urgency, nocturia and incontinence

In older men, as in our case, the commonest cause of LUTS is benign prostatic hyperplasia (BPH).

Likely Diagnoses

- BPH

Possible Diagnoses

- Bladder stones
- Infection
- Medication
- Neurological disease
- Prostatitis
- Urethral stricture

Critical Diagnosis

- Bladder and prostate cancer

CONTINUED INFORMATION GATHERING

This patient seems to be experiencing classical voiding symptoms, such as decreased urinary stream, hesitancy and postmicturition dribble, which are all associated with BPH. Bladder stones, prostatitis and infection seem unlikely as he has not reported nocturia or any abdominal pain. Confusion can be seen with infection, but this may be difficult to assess given he has vascular dementia, although dementia may be contributing to his symptoms. At this stage, urethral stricture cannot be discounted, although this is often associated with trauma through insertion of catheters or endoscopes.

PROBLEM REFINEMENT

Medicines are known to cause LUTS. As our patient has multimorbidity, it is important to take a drug history. Investigation of his records reveals:

Clopidogrel 75 mg 1 od
Isosorbide mononitrate MR 60 mg 1 od
Furosemide 40 mg mane and 40 mg at midday
Cetirizine 10 mg od
Amlodipine 10 mg od
Ramipril 10 mg 1 od
Ranolazine 500 mg bd

Fybogel sachets 1 bd prn
Paracetamol 2 qds prn
Ranibizumab 0.5 mg as intravitreal injection each month

Review of his medicines does implicate ramipril as a potential causative agent of LUTS. However, ramipril tends to increase urine output (uncommon), which is not consistent with his symptoms. It seems medicines are not the cause of his symptoms.

> ### ⚡ RED FLAGS
> Renal and urinary cancers are associated with haematuria. This has not been reported by the patient. A dipstick urine test shows no indication of leucocytes, proteins or blood. Cancer seems unlikely and further prostate-specific antigen testing should be performed to assess prostate cancer risk.

MANAGEMENT

Self-care Options

He has reported that he has begun to use pads for the occasional dribbling episodes, and this should be encouraged. He should be advised that he should maintain fluid intake but reduce caffeine intake from drinks such as tea and coffee. He has a history of constipation. This can worsen symptoms of LUTS and so a healthy diet with plenty of fibre should be reinforced to reduce the episodes of constipation he has.

Prescribing Options

Initially, it seems appropriate to arrange for prostate-specific antigen testing and gain a baseline International Prostate Symptom Score (0–35, where <7 = mild symptoms, 8–19 = moderate and >20 = severe) and consider urodynamic testing. Depending on the results, it is likely he will be offered a 5-alpha-reductase inhibitor (e.g., finasteride) as an alpha-blocker would be unsuitable due to his fall history and current medication.

Safety Netting

It is important to make the gentleman aware of the symptoms of acute urinary retention, for example, abrupt (over a period of hours) development of the inability to pass urine with associated increasing pain and swollen bladder. He should be told if he experiences these symptoms he must go straight to Accident and Emergency.

AIDE MEMOIRE

Likely Diagnoses

Benign Prostatic Hyperplasia

BPH is a progressive enlargement of the prostate gland caused by long-term exposure of the prostate to testosterone. Enlargement puts pressure on the urethra obstructing the flow of urine. Additionally, the bladder wall muscle may thicken, and a loss of elasticity may reduce the volume of urine it may hold. Symptoms tend to be both voiding and storage related. Storage symptoms include increased frequency, urgency, nocturia and incontinence, with patients describing frequent trips to the toilet, getting up in the night or anxiety that they might not reach the toilet in time. Voiding symptoms refer to decreased flow of urine, hesitancy, incomplete emptying, intermittency and dribbling. Patients may use terms such as stopping and starting or dribbling.

Possible Diagnoses

Bladder Stones

Bladder stones can present with LUTS, such as increased frequency associated with difficulty passing urine and nocturia. However, it also presents with lower abdominal pain, cloudy or bloody urine.

Infection

Lower urinary tract infections present with typical LUTS – urgency, frequency, nocturia. There may also be dysuria, suprapubic pain and cloudy/bloody urine. In more elderly men, confusion may also be present.

Medication

Medicines are frequently implicated in causing or contributing to voiding issues. These include angiotension-converting enzyme inhibitors, antipsychotics, tricyclic antidepressants, sedative antihistamines, opioid analgesics, benzodiazepines and diuretics.

Neurological Disease

A number of neurological conditions can show LUTS, for example, multiple sclerosis, Parkinson's disease, dementia and diabetic neuropathy, but these will be incidental symptoms when compared with the major presenting symptoms of each condition.

Prostatitis

Acute prostatitis presents with a combination of urinary tract infection and LUT symptoms. Additionally, low back, rectal or penile pain can be experienced. Prostatitis can become chronic (defined as symptoms for at least 3 months).

Urethral Stricture

Narrowing of the urethra occurs generally due to the formation of scar tissue caused by trauma, for example, catheter use or medical procedures. Typical voiding LUTS are experienced.

Critical Diagnosis

Bladder and Prostate Cancer

Bladder cancer. Haematuria is the most common symptom. Dysuria and urinary frequency are also seen. If the cancer is locally advanced or has metastasised, then unexplained weight loss, low back pain and fatigue may be present.

Prostate cancer. Symptoms closely mimic BPH but can also show haematuria, lethargy and weight loss. Risk of developing prostate cancer increases with age, a family history of the disease and being of Black ethnicity. A raised prostate-specific antigen level, relative to age, will help determine if cancer is a cause of symptoms.

▮ MCQs

1. Which ONE of the following is not recognised to exacerbate LUTS?
   (a) Fizzy drinks
   (b) High alcohol intake
   (c) High caffeine intake
   (d) High fibre diet
   (e) High fluid intake in the evening
2. Which ONE of the following would classically be a voiding symptom?
   (a) Frequency
   (b) Hesitancy in micturition
   (c) Incontinence
   (d) Nocturia
   (e) Urgency
3. Which ONE of the following medications is often considered first line in patients with voiding symptoms with a history of postural hypotension?
   (a) Desmopressin
   (b) Finasteride
   (c) Oxybutynin
   (d) Tamsulosin
   (e) Tolterodine

4. A 74-year-old man who was started on antihypertensive medication 5 days ago presents with his first episode of urinary retention. Which ONE of the following medicines is most likely to have caused urinary retention?
   (a) Angiotensin-converting enzyme inhibitors
   (b) Angiotensin II receptor blocker
   (c) Beta-blocker
   (d) Calcium channel blocker
   (e) Thiazide diuretic

5. A 61-year-old man who was diagnosed with BPH 6 weeks ago and takes tamsulosin presents back to the general practitioner complaining of dizziness. He is a heavy goods vehicle driver, and he is concerned about his ability to keep on driving. Which ONE of the following is the most likely problem?
   (a) Benign positional paroxysmal vertigo
   (b) Labyrinthitis
   (c) Postural (orthostatic) hypotension
   (d) Prostate cancer
   (e) Side effect of tamsulosin

Answers

1. d; 2. b; 3. b; 4. d; 5. e

KEY POINTS: BENIGN PROSTATIC HYPERPLASIA

- BPH is extremely common with ageing but only sometimes causes symptoms.
- Patients should be provided with information on signs of acute urinary retention and what they need to do.
- Consider relieving troublesome obstructive symptoms with alpha-adrenergic blockers or 5-alpha-reductase inhibitors.

WEBSITES AND FURTHER READING

National Institute for Health and Care Excellence (NICE) Guidance: Lower urinary tract symptoms in men: management
https://www.nice.org.uk/guidance/cg97
Prostate Cancer UK
https://prostatecanceruk.org/
International prostate symptom score
https://www.ruh.nhs.uk/patients/urology/documents/patient_leaflets/form_ipss.pdf
Bladder & Bowel Community
https://www.bladderandbowel.org/
Rees, J., Bultitude, M., & Challacombe, B. (2014). The management of lower urinary tract symptoms in men. *BMJ, 348*, g3861. https://doi.org/10.1136/bmj.g3861.
Simpson, R. J., Lee, R. J., Garraway, W. M., King, D., & McIntosh, I. (1994). Consultation patterns in a community survey of men with benign prostatic hyperplasia. *The British Journal of General Practice : the journal of the Royal College of General Practitioners, 44*(388), 499–502.

INDEX